D1087213

Antique Medical Instruments

Elisabeth Bennion

Sotheby Parke Bernet
University of California Press

First published in 1979 for
Sotheby Parke Bernet Publications by
Philip Wilson Publishers Ltd,
Russell Chambers,
Covent Garden, London WC2

Published in the United States and Canada by
University of California Press,
Berkeley and Los Angeles

ISBN: 0 85667 052 9 (UK edition)
ISBN: 0 520 03832 0 (US edition)
Library of Congress catalog card no: 78-55189

Designed by Peter Ling and George Evans
Printed in Great Britain by BAS Printers Ltd, Over Wallop, Hampshire
and bound by Mansell (Bookbinders) Limited, Witham, Essex

Foreword

In the course of a surgical career most surgeons acquire some interest in the history of certain instruments but few of them have any profound knowledge of the subject. Some surgeons, and especially young ones, are keen to develop new instruments though experience often teaches them that there is much to be said for keeping the range of tools as simple as possible. When a surgeon does develop the itch to design a new instrument, he will often be well advised to browse around the showroom or workshop of a first class instrument firm: such a visit will often reveal virtually the precise tool which he was wanting but which was designed many years before for an entirely different purpose.

Many schoolchildren become familiar with trepanning instruments. As medical students we generally learnt a little about René Laennec and his monaural stethoscope. Occasionally, as surgical dressers, and especially when working in some of our more ancient hospitals, our curiosity would be fired by some antique device lying on the instrument shelves, but few of us were keen to learn much about surgical instruments. Only that rare person with the collector's instinct showed any obsessive regard for antique instruments.

Although one may marvel that men should have been boring holes in each other's skulls five or six thousand years ago, most of us are less likely to marvel at the ingenuity of their toolmakers. It requires the medical Arthur Negus amongst us to appreciate the skill of the craftsmen who manufactured those instruments, sometimes of exquisite elegance, which were used by our predecessors. And even the few medical men and women who have antiquarian interests are only likely to publish papers concerning the tools and appliances related to their own specialist work.

When I was invited to write a foreword to this book I found myself wondering what could be original about it. However, a little research with the librarian at one of the finest surgical libraries in the world quickly convinced me of the singular absence of any comprehensive work in this field. There are therefore many reasons why we should be grateful to Mrs Elisabeth Bennion for having produced this truly impressive volume. A study of her wide range of sources, and of her detailed directory of surgical instrument makers known to be at work before 1870, should quickly convince anyone that here we have a truly remarkable and highly industrious researcher.

Though the greater part of this book is concerned with surgical instruments, the author has included additional interesting commentary on medicine receptacles, infant and invalid feeding utensils, and other articles of medical association. Mrs Bennion has visited many places in Britain and overseas during the course of her researches, and she has assembled an impressive series of photographs of instruments in private and public collections. She has also managed to insert some delightful snippets of information. Thus, as President of a Surgical College which is always in need of funds for surgical research, I could not suppress a feeling of envy when I read the author's reference to that decree of 1505, north of the border, which determined that the Barber-Surgeons of Scotland had a monopoly on the manufacture and sale of whisky!

I am confident that this work will attract a keen, though specialised, readership and that it will rapidly become accepted as the most important reference source. I warmly congratulate Elisabeth Bennion on her industry and scholarship and I am delighted to have had the opportunity of reading the typescript of this book.

REGINALD MURLEY
President

Royal College of Surgeons of England

Contents

List of colour plates

Acknowledgements

One of the pleasantest aspects of writing this book has been the help and kindness shown me by those whom I have approached, and the feeling that perhaps the book might, in some way, unite my fellow enthusiasts.

Principally, my most grateful thanks are due to Mr Maurice Freeman and the Directors of Simon Kaye Ltd for their encouragement and indulgent co-operation; to those whose perseverance in the chase brought me the pieces that engendered the interest in the first place; to the staff of I. Freeman & Son Inc. of New York for their research on the other side of the Atlantic; and to Mr Wynne Weston-Davies for his help with the Directory.

Finally, I must thank Mr R. Lindsay Doig for his professional advice and meticulous care in reading my manuscript, which has been invaluable.

Those by whose courtesy the illustrations have been published are:

H.M. The Queen, Royal Libraries, Windsor Castle

Armouries, H.M. Tower of London
Ashmolean Museum, Oxford

Bedford Museum, Bedford
Birmingham Assay Office
British Museum (Sir Ambrose Heal Collection)
British Optical Association, Library and Museum

Castle Museum, York
College of Physicians of Philadelphia
Commanding Officer, *H.M.S. Victory*, Portsmouth

Department of Obstetrics, University of Edinburgh
Dollond and Aitchison Museum, Yardley

Anthony Finch, London

Germanisches Nationalmuseum, Nuremberg

Institute of Medical History, Vienna

Simon Kaye Ltd, London (whose photographs were taken by Raymond Fortt Studios Ltd)
Nicole Kramer, Village Suisse, Paris
Kunstgewerbemuseum, West Berlin

Manchester City Art Gallery (Thomas Greg Collection)
Musée Crozatier, Puy, France
Musée de l'Histoire de la Médecine de Paris (Cliché Assistance
    Publique)
Musée d'Histoire des Sciences, Geneva
Musée le Secq des Tournelles, Rouen
Museum Boerhaave, Leiden
Museo del Prado, Madrid
Museum of English Rural Life, Reading
Museum of Historical Medicine, Copenhagen

National Army Museum, London
Norfolk Museums Service (Castle Museum, Norwich)
Norfolk Museums Service (Strangers' Hall Museum, Norwich)

Pharmaceutical Society of Great Britain Museum
Pitt Rivers Museum, Oxford

W. Radcliffe (from *Milestones in Midwifery*, John Wright, Bristol)
Radio Times Hulton Picture Library, London
Ramstein Collection, Basle
Royal Army Medical Corps Museum, Aldershot
Royal College of Physicians of England
Royal College of Physicians of Ireland
President and Council of Royal College of Surgeons of England
Royal College of Surgeons of Edinburgh
Royal College of Veterinary Surgeons Library, London

St John's College, Oxford
St Thomas' Hospital, London
Sheffield City Museum
Smithsonian Institute, Washington D.C., Division of Medical Sciences,
    National Museum of History and Technology
S. J. Shrubsole Ltd, London
Society of Antiquarians, Newcastle upon Tyne
Sotheby Parke Bernet & Co. Ltd, London
Stedelijk Museum, Amsterdam

The General Infirmary, Leeds
The Parker Gallery Ltd, London

University College Hospital Medical School, London

John Weiss & Sons Ltd, London
Wellcome Institute Trustees, London
Woolstaplers' Hall Museum, Chipping Camden
Worshipful Company of Barbers, London
Wye College, Kent

ELISABETH BENNION

'It is no small presumption to dismember the image of God.'

JOHN WOODALL (1556–1643)

CHAPTER ONE

Introductory account of the history of the profession

Note: The dimensions given throughout are approximate

The history of medical and surgical instruments is an almost uncharted field. There is little bibliography, and research into the subject has been slow and difficult, but the rewards of discovering early instruments of intricate and beautiful workmanship have engendered quite unexpected enthusiasm and goodwill among those who have co-operated in it. One problem has been knowing where to stop. For many, the book will have stopped too soon and omitted too much, and yet there may be others who feel it tells them more about medical instruments than they care to know. It represents the history of man's humanity to man, fought against intolerable odds imperfectly understood.

Another new window has been opened on the past and one of a poignancy seldom equalled. Almost every instrument can be seen as a piece of social comment on its day, The Curator of one of the Museums in Nuremburg, said to the writer when discussing some pieces, 'How can one presume to understand the work of Dürer without accepting that this was a surgical instrument of his day?' Indeed, the piece in question might be said to have been the drawings of Dürer embodied in a saw. This must be the answer to the squeamish who might well find the subject gruesome. With respect, this would seem to be a limited and unimaginative approach and, as the poet–philosopher George Santayana has said, 'He who is inclined to ignore the past must be prepared to repeat it.' When Queen Victoria visited her soldiers, returned from the Crimean War to hospital in London, some were rebuked for describing to the Queen the details of their wounds and operations, to which she replied that if her soldiers were brave enough to undergo these sufferings, then she must be brave enough to hear of it. We, too, owe an enormous debt to all those who in earlier days endured unspeakable agony under operation, and to those who have attempted to alleviate it.

Many of the pieces described in this book owe their origin to similar pieces used in the early Middle Ages and beyond, and many virtually identical ones occur in the catalogues of today, if made of different materials. The human body has not changed and it is

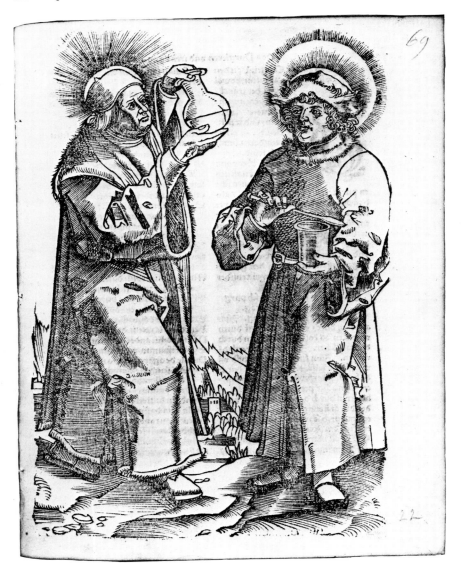

1. *St Cosmas and St Damian, twin Arab brothers and surgeons who were converted to Christianity and martyred c. A.D. 303. They became the Patron Saints of the Barber–Surgeons. Woodcut from Hans von Gersdorff, c. 1520.*
(Germanisches Nationalmuseum Nuremberg)

interesting to note how early the right instrument for each operation was devised. The two events that revolutionised technique and the chances of recovery were the introductions of anaesthesia and antisepsis, not advances in instrument design. Nevertheless, the speed required to operate without anaesthetic restricted the scope of surgery and precluded so many of the operations possible today.

It must be remembered that many of the conditions experienced by our forebears made treatment necessary that would not occur so often today. Not many women, for example, wish to have their right breast amputated to save it from the bowstring as the Amazons did.

2

Aneurysms and urethral stricture were common, chiefly resulting from untreated syphilis; and the nobility and gentry who spent long hours in the saddle, often in heavy rain, suffered considerably from fistula-in-ano. We are often inclined, indeed encouraged, to think that we are weaklings compared with the physical strength of our ancestors who hewed and hauled and pushed and heaved weights that leave us breathless. The truth is abundantly obvious to the student of medical history—they were called upon to perform physical feats far beyond their strength with the result that herniae or ruptures were the occupational hazard of the working man.

This account is principally concerned with English pieces though it is fully conceded that the medical profession in Italy and France before the eighteenth century was more advanced than ours. The School of Medicine at Salerno was founded in the ninth century, and the Faculties of Medicine at both Montpellier and Bologna were also very early foundations. The first Lecturer in Medicine at Oxford, Nicholas Tingewick, a fellow of Balliol, was appointed in the time of Edward I.

The year of 1870 has been chosen as the latter end of the survey as, with the introduction of antisepsis in 1867 by Joseph Lister (1827–1911) and the eventual acceptance of sterilisation for all instruments, they necessarily became plainer and less interesting; wood, ivory, tortoise-shell, and other decorative materials were proscribed from use. Even so, a catalogue of 1897 said, 'We do not think that the day when metal-handled instruments will replace ebony and ivory is near at hand.'

The earliest instrument makers were the Armourers, joined and later superseded by the Cutlers. Working parallel with them for the finer, more sophisticated, pieces were the Silversmiths. Specialist instrument makers did not appear until the eighteenth century (see Directory of surgical instrument makers). Although no great innovations were made by the English makers themselves, their superior workmanship made their pieces better than those from the Continent and English-made pieces were in great demand there.

Throughout the history of medicine it has to be noted that advance was perpetually opposed by that apparently healing body, the Church. Time and again one reads of new discoveries meeting with the disapproval of Holy Church, which ordained that suffering was a visitation of God and its alleviation the action of presumptuous, impious man. Even winnowing-machines, when their time came, were said to be ungodly; only God had the right to raise the wind. Natural remedies, such as herbs, were approved as being God-given, but each advance in surgery had obstacles to overcome—thus starting the distinction in approval between physicians and surgeons almost before their professions had started.

The most primitive tribes have held their medical practitioners in veneration, even when it was not merited. Many sets of rules were laid down for professional conduct, among the earliest those by Archimathaeus in 1100 B.C. Lanfranc of Milan (d. 1315), who was banished for political reasons and took Italian surgery to Paris, wrote, 'A Surgian must have handes wel shaped. Long smale fyngres and his body not quaking and all must be of subtle wit.' John of Arderne (*fl.* 1370) had very high ethical principles; in *de Arte Medicinae* he recommended courtesy, sobriety, piety, and compassion—and the acquisition of a public image. Until the early Middle Ages medicine and surgery had been almost entirely the provenance of the monastery; the earliest hospitals in this country, St Bartholomew's and St Thomas's were both monastic foundations started in the twelfth century. Manuscript illustrations bear this out abundantly. But in 1215, a papal edict of Pope Innocent III decreed that no priest who had touched blood might consecrate the Host. However, the small repository of surgical skill and knowledge resided in the monasteries, and it was there that the sick came to be cured, so use was made of the itinerant barbers who regularly called to shave the tonsures and trim the beards. At first they operated under the supervision of the monks but gradually grew independent. It was difficult for them to gain public confidence: barbers at bath-houses might undertake shaving, bleeding, and minor surgery or a lucky break was sometimes provided at a joust, when ghastly accidents were opportunities for cures with maximum audience and publicity.

The Hundred Years' War (1337–1453) and the Wars of the Roses (1453–97) created a great demand for military surgeons. Wars were expensive, soldiers were well paid, and therefore a large financial investment—their health and lives had money value—so surgeons became important in the army. They were not united in any army corps but served individual commanders or noblemen, then, as early as 1369, forming themselves into a society, the Military Guild. Apprentices were bound for six years, then examined by Masters of the Guild and, if passed, were admitted to membership. Civil Barber–Surgeons formed a Guild before 1300; they took on apprentices, taught them with lectures, dissections, and practical demonstrations, examined them and then licensed them to practise in the city of the guild. In 1462 the guild was incorporated and henceforth known as a company. Curious privileges and hindrances were accorded them. In Scotland, a decree of 1505 granted the Barber–Surgeons a monopoly of the making and selling of whisky. In 1540 an Act of Parliament was passed forming the United Company of Barbers and Surgeons, but declaring that surgeons should not barber, nor barbers act as surgeons, although they were united in the same legal corporation. Later, this rule appears to have been stretched and it was 1745 before Surgeons set up on their own. The surviving relic of the Barber–Surgeons is the barber's pole, the filet representing a bandage.

Physicians, however, did not have to be licensed until the Royal College of Physicians was set up in 1518, though it needed only a slight acquaintance with ancient Greek ideas on medicine to acquire the licence, especially for those intending to practise in the provinces. London doctors were required to have a little more learning—'no man shall us mysterie of Physick unless he has studied it in some universitie.' Galen (A.D. 130–200), Greek adviser to Marcus Aurelius, said to his student physicians, 'If you do not wish to learn Greek, then you are a barbarian.' Leche was the term applied to the early surgeons, but the physician was called medicine, implying some scholarship and greater social standing. In the fifteenth century it was noticed that the medical profession was a link between the middle and upper classes; but whereas the physicians mingled with the nobility, surgeons considered it a high honour to be received into the ranks of the physicians. It was probably the required knowledge of Greek that set the physician apart from the surgeon on the social scale, a division which still survives in terms of address today.

In fact, although the physicians claimed to have a remedy for every ill, they had virtually no idea, at this date, of the causes of disease, and the surgeons had few opportunities to improve their skill and knowledge. Their charter gave the Company the right to dissect the bodies of only four criminals a year. These dissections were frequently a matter of general entertainment for the layman. In 1662, Samuel Pepys visited the Hall of the Barber–Surgeons and heard a lecture. 'We had a fine dinner and good learned company.' Afterwards he attended a dissection. 'Methought it was a very unpleasant sight.' Many therefore, felt compelled to study abroad where unrestrained dissection was legal, resulting in much more advanced surgery than in this country. Leonardo da Vinci presumably suffered no lack of corpses for his anatomical studies. He, and other artists such as Donatello and Michelangelo, were the first real students of anatomy (pl. 2). It was in Padua that William Harvey (1578–1657) first discovered the circulation of the blood,

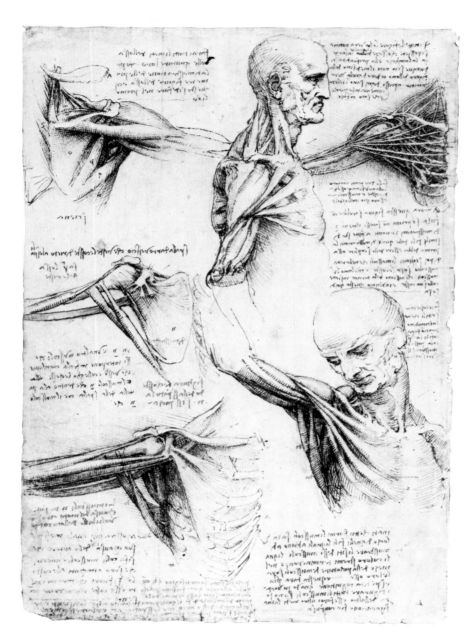

2.   *Anatomical drawing by Leonardo da Vinci (1452–1519).*
(Copyright reserved, Royal Libraries, Windsor Castle)

but when his book on the subject was published here, he was dismissed as a crank. When one considers that the official list of Drugs in 1618 included Bone-Marrow, Sweat, Blood, and Shavings from the skull of an executed criminal, one can understand the setting into which Harvey's discovery fell. In the City of London, apothecaries had formed themselves into a distinct section of the

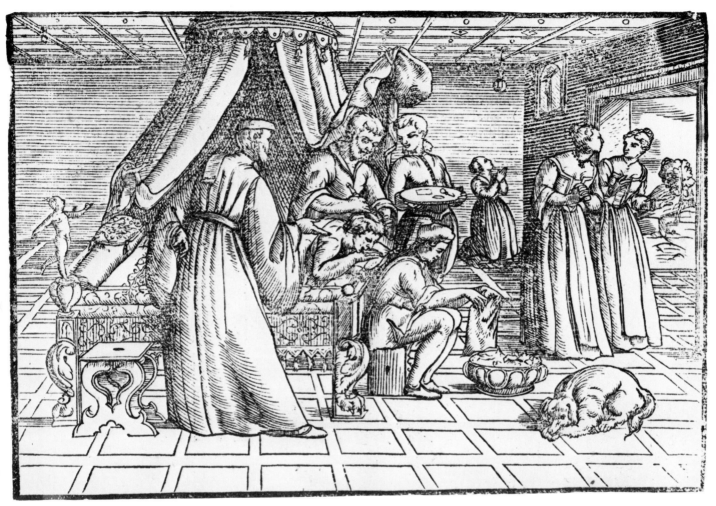

3. *Surgeon operating for skull fracture.*
Woodcut from Andreas della Croce's
Chirurgiae, *1573.*
(Wellcome Collection Library)

Grocers' Company but were separated from them in 1617 under a charter of James I. The Society of the Apothecaries of London was then set up.

The difficulties that beset doctors in this country were manifold apart from the restriction of corpses. The necessity for an arts degree before studying medicine meant that there were 13 years from entering university to achieving a doctorate. Occasionally, it was possible to obtain a licence to practise after a cursory study of medicine and, in fact, there was little actual teaching. At both Oxford and Cambridge the Regius Chairs were political appointments, and at neither place was there a hospital until the second half of the eighteenth century; in addition, only members of the established Church were eligible. Herman Boerhaave (1668–1738) at Leyden, not

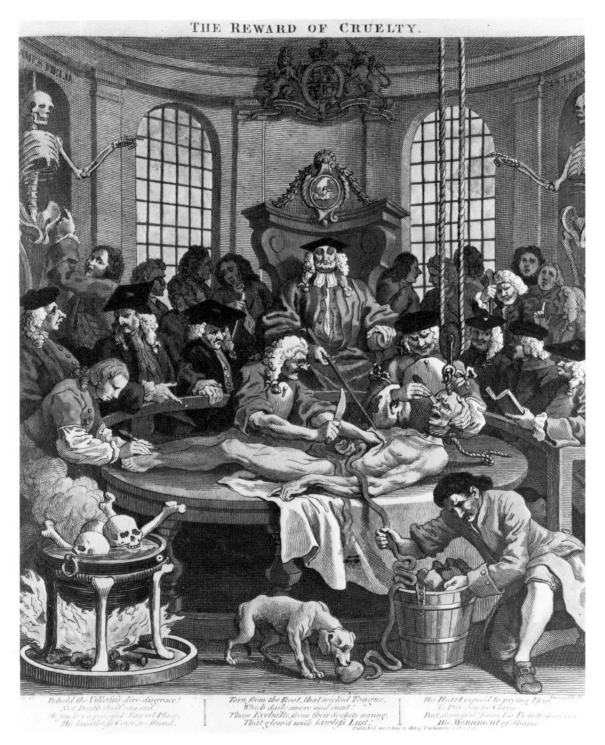

only one of the greatest physicians of his time, but a great teacher, attracted the largest number of pupils from England and Scotland. The influence of this select band on British medicine is untold, so many of them were afterwards elected to offices of high honour and distinction.

The surgeons were, nevertheless, at a greater disadvantage; they either had to learn from their patients—which was often too late—or else break the law by buying bodies offered to them by the 'resurrection-men'. Matters improved a little in 1745 when the new Surgeons' Company with Headquarters at Surgeons' Hall was allowed a regular supply of felon corpses, though in some places (notably Edinburgh, where the first medical school for the training of doctors was set up) the demand for bodies was far greater than the supply of criminals. The London resurrectionist, Crouch, set a record by abstracting the body of a hydrocephalic boy in thirty minutes in daylight, evading a whole corps of grave watchers. Undoubtedly, murders committed by the infamous Burke and Hare in Edinburgh, and by Williams in London, were for surgical purposes. Relations had to fit a 'mortsafe' over the grave of the newly dead, a heavy iron grid that was bolted down. The well-known engraving by Hogarth entitled 'The Reward of Cruelty' shows a felon, the noose still round his neck, being dissected by hack-surgeons while the lecturer directs proceedings with a staff, to the assorted horror, distaste, and interest of his students; a dog meanwhile gobbles up the entrails on the floor (pl. 4). Sir Astley Cooper (1768–1841), Surgeon to George IV, in giving evidence to a committee of the House of Commons said, 'There is no person, let his situation in life be what it may, whom if I were disposed to dissect, I might not obtain. The law only enhances the price, and does not prevent the exhumation.' The Anatomy Act, which ended this situation, was not passed until much later, in 1832.

But similarly, medicine, despite the greater respect it exacted, weltered in a sea of confusion. Riches and importance were of little avail—they merely multiplied the doctors and cures at one's disposal. It is thought that the untimely death of Charles II in 1685 might well have been the result of the doctors who worked on him, night and day, seldom fewer than four at a time, for three days. During that time they let blood, then let more blood, and then had pans of hot coal placed on his body to bring him round again. They gave him laxatives and emetics; they let blood yet again at regular intervals; they put burning plasters on him to raise blisters; gave him sneezing powders and made lots of little cuts on various parts of his body, no doubt with dirty lancets. As he grew weaker, they

4. *William Hogarth,* The Reward of Cruelty, *c. 1750.*
(The Parker Gallery Ltd, London)

9

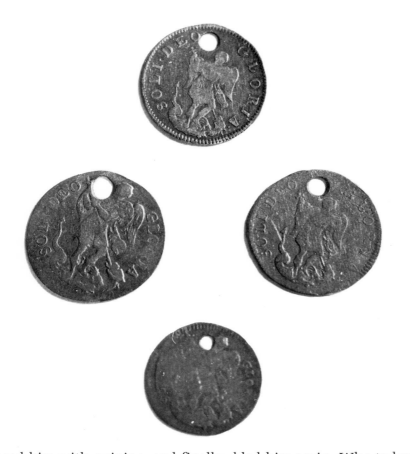

5.   *Superstition relating to 'The King's Evil'*
was firmly entrenched for many centuries.
Four scrofula touch-pieces, c. 1700.
(Strangers' Hall Museum, Norwich)

dosed him with quinine, and finally, bled him again. Who today, starting in the very best of health, could withstand all that?

Even those of more moderate standing than the King had to endure terrible ordeals in their illnesses. Dr Rowland Davies, afterwards Bishop of Cork, writing in September 1689, says 'I ordered a clyster for Mrs Patty and a plaster to her poll, which caused a great blister but her distemper altered not by it.' Next day—'and it was ordered that blisters should be raised behind the ears; leeches having applied to the temples and a cephalic hysterical emulsion, with peony seeds only, should be made for her.' On ensuing days, she is reported with 'convulsive motions, many fits and convulsions—whereon I had her cupped on both shoulders, which brought her a little to her senses'! Pigeons were applied to her head . . . 'But she came not to herself today.'—Despairing of death, the doctor mercifully resorts to prayer rather than more remedies and a few days later the pigeons (presumably putrefying by now) can be removed and all is well.

Faith in one's doctor meant much. Alexander Pope wrote:

> 'I'll do what Mead and Cheselden advise
> To keep these limbs and preserve these eyes.'

Nevertheless, doctors were very expensive, particularly in London, with the result that only the rich could afford a physician. This meant that the apothecary, with a wide range of cures, flourished.

The eighteenth century saw the flowering of quack patent medicine—newspapers carrying patent advertisements such as the following in 1774:

> 'Grant's incomparable and never failing
> drops (price one shilling the bottle) a speedy
> cure for Coughs, Colds, Asthmas, Phisic,
> Wheezings, difficult breath, shortness of
> breath and all sorts of Consumptions, even
> when so far advanced as not to be cured by
> any other Medicine in the World.'

However, the apothecary was still beyond the range of the really poor who had to rely on superstitions (pl. 5), and the traditional herbal cures of the past. One is inclined to believe they may have been the best off in the end.

John Hunter (1728–93), a very original thinker and stimulator of the profession, found surgery little better than a trade when he entered it, but succeeded for the first time in giving it stature, resulting in the establishment of the Royal College of Surgeons in 1800. However, Smollett, a surgeon himself who trained with William Smellie (see Chapter 6), described in *Roderick Random*, written in 1748, his hero's final examination in surgery like this:

> 'I was conducted into a large hall, where I saw about a dozen of grim faces sitting at a long table one of whom bade me come forward in such an imperious tone that I was actually for a minute or two bereft of my senses. He then proceeded to interrogate me about my age, the town where I had served my time, with the terms of my apprenticeship; and when I informed him that I had served three years only, he fell into a violent passion: (and) swore it was a shame and a scandal to send such raw boys into the world as surgeons. This reduced me to such a situation that I was scarce able to stand. A plump gentleman who sat opposite to me with a skull before him, examined me touching the operation of the trepan, and was very well satisfied with my answers. The next person who questioned me was a wag who began by asking if I

11

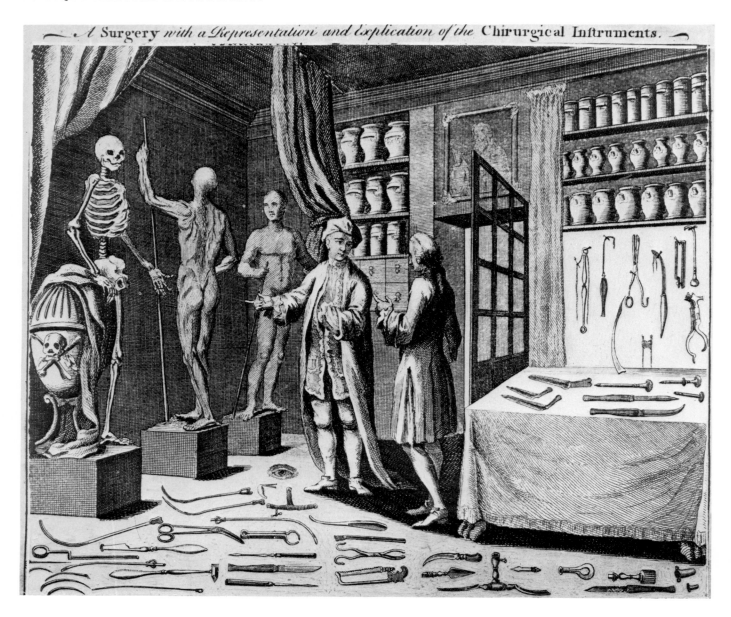

A Surgery with a Representation and Explication of the Chirurgical Instruments.

had ever seen an amputation performed; and I replying in the affirmative, he shook his head, and said, "What! upon a dead subject I suppose? Suppose you was called to a patient of plethoric habit, who had been bruised by a fall, what would you do?" I answered I would bleed him immediately. "What", said he, "before you had tied up his arm?" But this stroke of wit not answering his expectation, he desired me to advance to the gentleman who sat next to him, who with a pert air, asked what method of cure I would follow in wounds of the intestines. I repeated the method of cure as it prescribed by the best chirurgical writers; which he heard to an end and then said, with a supercilious smile, "So you think by such treatment the patient might recover? Did you ever know of a case of this kind succeed?" I answered that I did not, and was about to tell him I had never seen a wounded intestine; but he stopped me by saying, with some precipitation "Nor never will. I affirm that all wounds of the intestines, whether great or small, are mortal." "Pardon me, brother," says the fat gentleman, "there is very good authority . . ." Here he was interrupted by the other (and) all the examiners espoused the opinion of one or other of the disputants, and raised their voices all together, when the chairman commanded silence, and ordered me to withdraw. In less than a quarter of an hour I was called in again, received my qualification sealed up, and was ordered to pay five shillings.'

6. *An eighteenth-century surgery.*
(Radio Times Hulton Picture Library)

Surgical operations were virtually only those to set or amputate limbs, let blood, or cut for stone. They were so hazardous and necessitated a state of excruciating pain before anyone could bring themselves to the point of contemplating an operation; the courage of those that did defies belief. The diarist, John Evelyn, describes an amputation on board ship during the Third Dutch War (1672–4): 'the stout and gallant man enduring it with incredible patience and that without being bound to his chair, as is usual in such painful operations, or hardly making a face or crying Oh!; I had hardly courage to be present.' Operations were mainly carried out in the patient's own home and illustrations of the time show the patient sitting in his drawing-room, often in a velvet covered chair with merely a friend, and sometimes not even that, to hold his hand. Hospitals were the resort of the really poor, and almost until the end of the nineteenth century spelled death for those who were admitted to them. One hospital only admitted patients who brought with them the price of their burial, and Sir James Simpson (1811–70) said 'A soldier has more chance of survival on the field of Waterloo than a man who goes into hospital.' The filth and stench of hospitals made them a byword, and conditions did not improve until firstly Florence Nightingale and then Lister brought in their reforms, though the one could never accept the other. 'Germs,' said the redoubtable Miss Nightingale, '*I've* never seen one'! Nevertheless, St Thomas' Hospital, before it was rebuilt on its present site, had a notice admitting, 'Clean patients 5s. Foul ones 10s.'

13

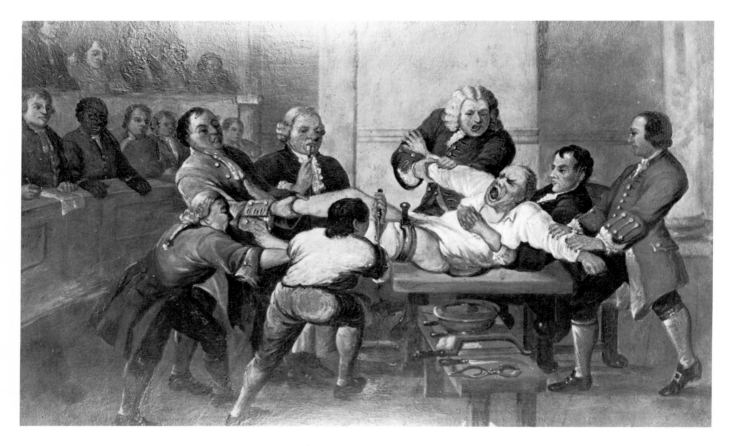

The conditions of nineteenth-century operations were hardly edifying. The best picture can be drawn by visiting the old operating theatre of St Thomas's in the loft of the Wren Church which now forms the Chapter House of Southwark Cathedral (pls. 7 and 8). It was in use between 1821 and 1862 and is the only surviving example of its kind. The table stands in the centre of a horseshoe of raised galleries from which the students looked down; close friends of the surgeon being accommodated on horsehair chairs near the table. A cabinet on the wall held the unwashed instruments, and some pegs the filthy stained coats that the surgeon and his assistants wore to save their own good ones. Beneath the table was a box of sawdust to be kicked into place wherever the blood was dripping most freely. It takes little imagination to feel the galvanising terror of the patient who, primed only with a modicum of laudanum and a piece of leather to bite on, entered the theatre to be strapped to the table. The young Charles Darwin, a medical student at Edinburgh, wrote: 'I attended on two occasions the operating theatre and saw

7. *An oil painting by an unknown artist showing an operation in progress in the operating theatre of St Thomas' Hospital, c. 1780. The surgeon is performing the 'tour de force' (see Chapter 3). (Royal College of Surgeons of England)*

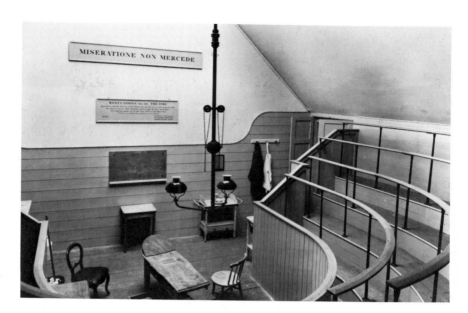

8. *Operating theatre of St Thomas' Hospital, in the loft of St Thomas' Church as it was in 1820. (St Thomas' Hospital)*

two very bad operations, one on a child, but I rushed out before they were completed. Nor did I ever attend again, for hardly any inducement would have been strong enough to make me do so. The two cases fairly haunted me for many a long year.'

With the introduction of anaesthesia for operations in 1846, there was less need for the appalling speed that had hitherto characterised surgery, and more care could be taken. The discovery of the anaesthetic properties of ether came slowly and painfully, and was clouded by William Morton's attempt to keep it a secret and patent it, both actions ethically unacceptable. An account of the first operation under anaesthesia in this country is related in Chapter 3. In 1847, James Simpson (see Chapter 6) introduced chloroform for operations, though principally for use in childbirth, thus setting up a long controversy as to who first discovered anaesthesia. On his death-bed, however, Simpson conceded the point to Morton. There was much heated opposition to the use of anaesthetics in childbirth, a large faction feeling that God willed women to suffer in labour. When Queen Victoria proposed to have it administered by Dr John Snow for the birth of Prince Leopold in 1853, a deputation of Bishops pleaded with her not to do so. However, '*We* are having the baby,' she told them firmly, striking a blow for all women, 'and *we* shall have the chloroform.'

In the nineteenth century, generally, came an improvement in the examination of patients and the keeping of records. The year of 1841 saw the formation of the Pharmaceutical Society of Great

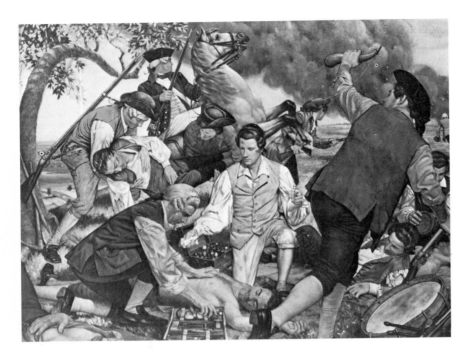

9.   *America's first Apothecary-General, Andrew Craigie (1725–83). He served American forces at the Battle of Bunker Hill and through the War of Independence. (The Parker Gallery Ltd, London)*

Britain, and advances escalated through the nineteenth century culminating in Lister's momentous introduction of antisepsis, following which the mortality rate after operations fell from 43 per cent to 15 per cent. With these advances came an improvement in social standing for the profession. George Eliot's Lady Chettam in *Middlemarch*, speaking of a new doctor who is said to belong to a good family, said 'For my part, I prefer a medical man to be more on a footing with the servants.' But Lady Chettam adds in dismay, 'he is often the cleverer'! In addition, Trollope's Doctor Thorne was never fully accepted by the Ladies of the House however much they required his ministrations. Nevertheless, by the last quarter of the century an undeniable code of ethics had evolved which brought the profession to an unequalled position of respect, before the advent of National Health revolutionised its organisation.

In the fourteenth century, John of Mirfield (*fl.* 1393) in *Breviarium Bartomolomaei* said 'When Physick's dearly bought, it doth much healing bring. But when 'tis freely given, 'tis ne'er a useful thing.'

16

CHAPTER TWO

Saws, trephines and phlebotomy instruments

Trepanning is the oldest known operation, and during the later Neolithic or New Stone Age, it was practised presumably to allow the escape of a demon causing headaches, melancholia, or epilepsy. A flint knife was employed for the purpose and a number of skulls found where the reinserted piece of skull has fused bear testimony to the sometime success of the operation. The second oldest operation is amputation, and in some ancient societies fingers were amputated as a sign of mourning or of caste. Amputation became a lost art when Lister dispelled the ghost of gangrene. We know of illustrations of saws used by the Egyptians, and flint saws from prehistoric communities in Europe, but it was probably the Romans who invented the metal-bladed saw as we know it today. Pliny believed that intrepid inventor Daedalus was responsible and that he conceived the idea from using the jaw of a serpent to cut a piece of wood.

Saws

By the twelfth and thirteenth centuries we know that both the bow and tenon saw were used in England, and one manuscript illustration shows the blades held rigid by plates connected with the back. John Wryghtson's saw of *c.* 1350 was on the bow principle with an angular prow. The earliest illustration of an amputation in this country, one of 1517, shows a leg being taken off below the knee over a barrel of sand. The saw would appear to be at least 30 cm long with a narrow blade inserted into a frame; the stump would then have been covered with a beef or pig bladder. Fabricius (1560–1634), about the year 1590, experimented with a red-hot saw for amputations which, he said cauterised at the same time, was less painful, and lost less blood. From the sixteenth century, Continental influence induced craftsmen to enrich the design of their saws with ornate mounts and elaborate handles of wood, bone, and ivory (pl. 1). Gradually, surgeons evolved different types of saw suited to the type of amputation. These they would have had made to their own specification, though their pupils, who would have become

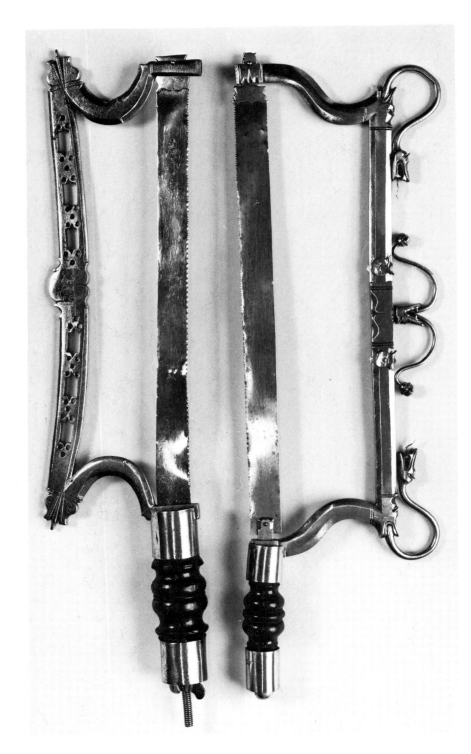

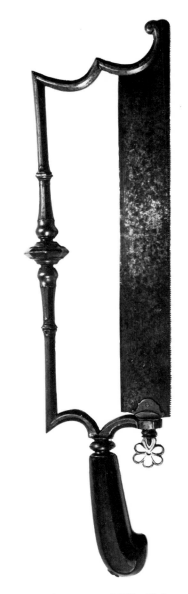

1. *Two exceptionally large amputating saws, showing screw through handle. Left c. 1640, right c. 1550. 50 cm. (Germanisches Nationalmuseum, Nuremberg)*

2. *Amputating saw, c. 1740. 45·5 cm. (Musée le Secq des Tournelles, Rouen)*

3. *An amputation of 1750.*
(Radio Times Hulton Picture Library)

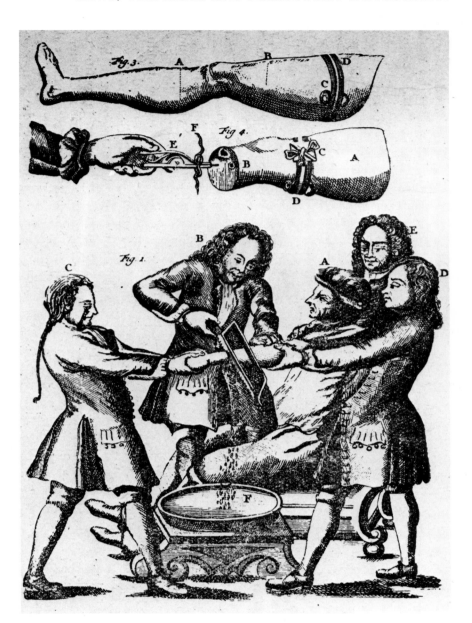

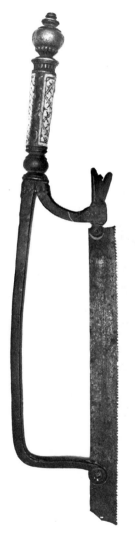

4. *Bone saw, probably German, with carved bone handle, c. 1750. 35·5 cm.*
(Sheffield Museum)

accustomed to a particular design of instrument, had them copied and the saws would then become known by the name of the Master-Surgeon. By the comparatively sophisticated time of the late eighteenth century, when specialist instrument makers were starting in business, this practice had become common, and the ingenuity of one surgeon became accessible to all. Indeed, adaptations of some of the early designs are still used today.

19

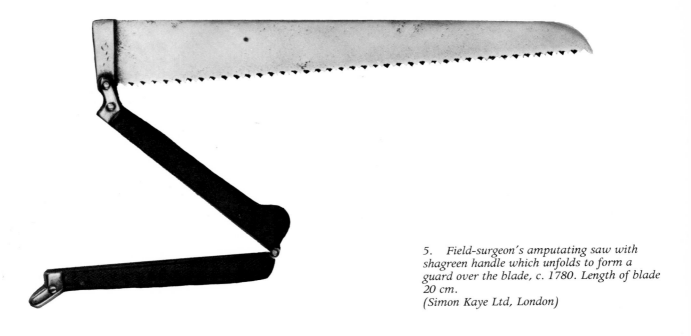

5.   Field-surgeon's amputating saw with shagreen handle which unfolds to form a guard over the blade, c. 1780. Length of blade 20 cm.
(Simon Kaye Ltd, London)

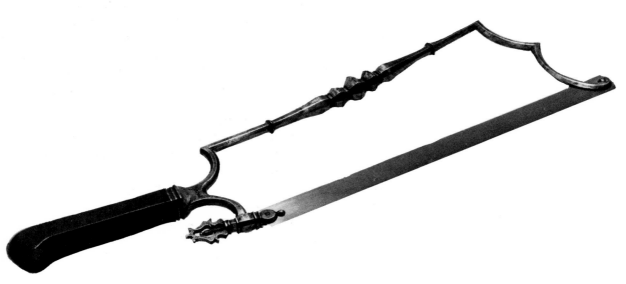

6.   Amputating saw, c. 1750. 35·5 cm.
(Museum Boerhaave, Leiden)

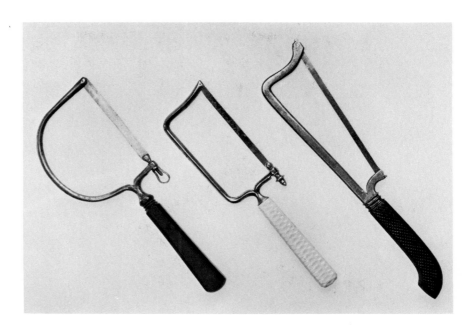

7. *Benjamin Bell's bow saw, c. 1780; fine-toothed bone saw, ivory handle, c. 1820; Evans', bone saw, curved handle, c. 1790. 20 cm, 17 cm, 20 cm. (Simon Kaye Ltd, London)*

The earlier saws were very fine-toothed, undoubtedly to obviate splintering, although this had its own problem, as will be seen. As with all instruments, the earlier ones were of considerable weight and were of much heavier, coarser design with none of the refinements that, with hindsight, now seem obvious. Indeed, saws of the fifteenth, sixteenth, and seventeenth centuries are so large and heavy it is difficult to see how they could have been manipulated with any accuracy or finesse—the very handles were often carved in grotesque shapes that defied an easy grasp. It is sometimes difficult to distinguish them from the saws of a hunting trousse (see Chapter 10). A saw with a screwed-in, removable blade was introduced from Germany *c.* 1520 (pl. 1), and another, *c.* 1550, had a device for tightening the blade while in use. By the mid-seventeenth century, John Scultetus of Ulm (1595–1645), whose book *The Chirurgeon's Store-House* was published in English in 1674, could describe a saw with a screw passing through the handle, which was afterwards modified by Perret at the end of the eighteenth century into a saw that combined this advantage with the general shape of Wryghtson's saw. The eighteenth century saw the introduction of a wealth of new ideas both in the general principle and in the detail of decoration. Only by about 1770 did handles that had been turned and were circular in section become hexagonal for an easier grasp. Around 1790 saw the start of the criss-cross serrations (pls. 7,8) in the ebony handles that were to be

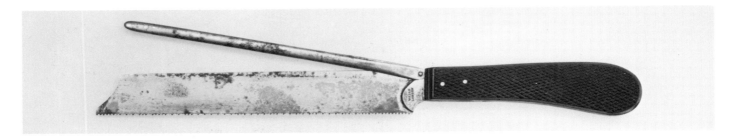

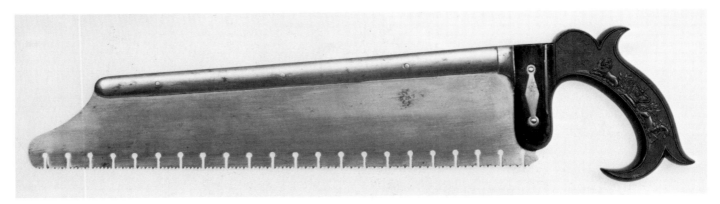

practically standard until the introduction of sterilisation made them obsolete.

Among the new ideas was a complicated invention for cutting the bone while protecting the softer parts. This guarded, amputation saw consisted of a blade enclosed at either end by metal guards, a clip between the two preventing complete closure. Other ingenuities were circular saws, some operated by a coiled spring wound by a complicated system of wheels within wheels. Needless to say, there is little evidence of their having been much used. Judging from the not infrequent examples found on the market, a saw that did see use was Benjamin Bell's metacarpal saw which he introduced in 1780 (pl.7). Bell (1749–1806) published his *A System of Surgery* in 1782. About the same time came a gradual preference for the straight tenon blade for amputation, like that used in carpentry. It eventually took the name of Percivall Pott who recommended it highly. Pott (1715–88), of St Bartholomew's Hospital wrote many learned and forward-looking treatises that revolutionised treatment. He was the first to set bones after compound fracture, having himself been thrown from a horse in Kent Street, Southwark and suffered accordingly. He stressed that the least number of instruments should be used at any operation, and those to be of the simplest design. He himself simplified many

8. *Bone saw, hinged spine, c. 1820, Weiss. 25·5 cm.*
(Simon Kaye Ltd, London)

9. *Bone saw with serrations to prevent clogging of teeth (as introduced in catalogue of 1831) with pressed horn handle, Royal Arms and inscription 'Razor Makers to His Majesty', c. 1835, Weiss. 30·5 cm.*
(Simon Kaye Ltd, London)

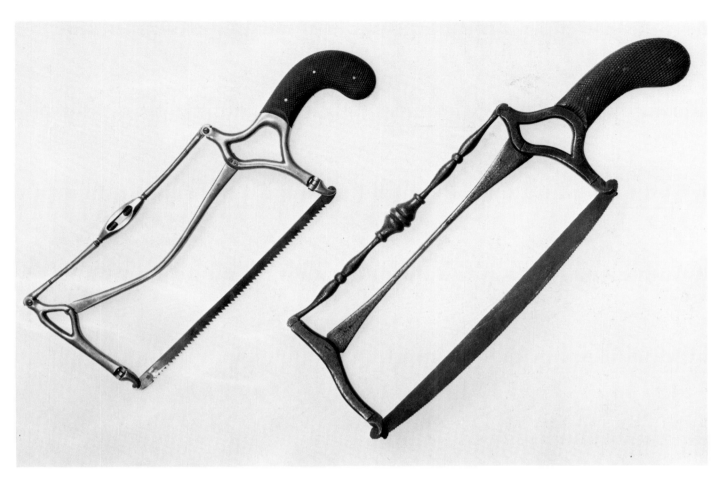

10.   Left, Dr Butcher's saw c. 1860, Aitken, York; right an early forerunner, c. 1790. 25·5 cm, 30·5 cm. (Simon Kaye Ltd, London)

existing designs; he particularly condemned 'artistic bandaging' such as is still shown in First Aid books today. His view of the tenon blade was afterwards shared by William Ferguson (1808–77) and Lister. Ferguson specified that a saw should have a blade 23 cm long and 6·5 cm deep, with an ebony handle similar to that of a cabinet maker (pl. 9). Some of this type had a heavy spine for rigidity. By about 1820 Weiss and others were making these with a hinge on the spine to swing back when the blade was completely submerged in in the bone (pl. 8).

When John Weiss published his first catalogue in 1831 he introduced his improved amputation saw which, he explained, was particularly designed to prevent clogging as he had noticed that as many as three saws were sometimes needed for one amputation. The new saw combined a fine tooth with deep slits at intervals. A rare find is the one illustrated in pl. 8, on the pressed-horn handle of

23

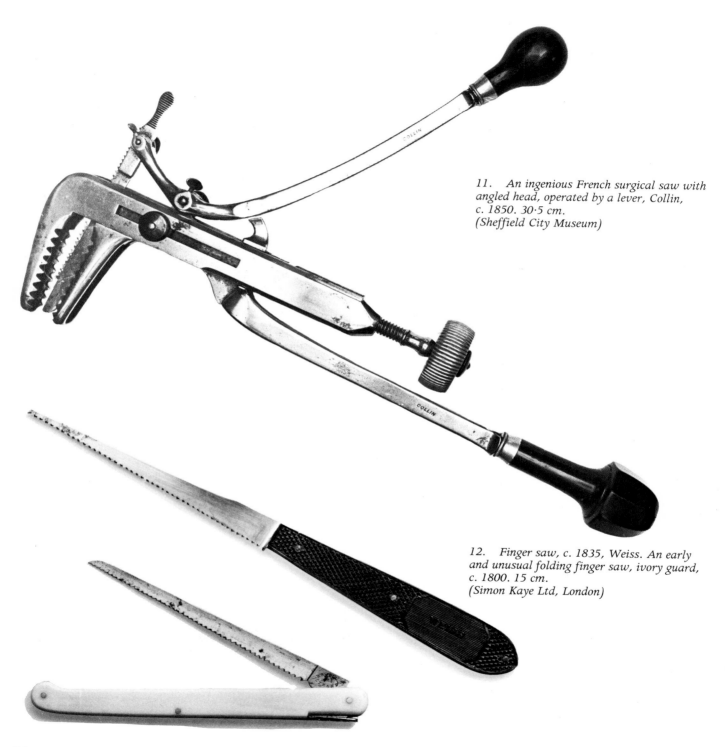

11. *An ingenious French surgical saw with angled head, operated by a lever, Collin, c. 1850. 30·5 cm. (Sheffield City Museum)*

12. *Finger saw, c. 1835, Weiss. An early and unusual folding finger saw, ivory guard, c. 1800. 15 cm. (Simon Kaye Ltd, London)*

which is written 'Razor Makers to His Majesty' which nicely dates it between 1831 and 1837. In 1851 the felicitously named Dr Richard Butcher (1819–95) evolved a type of saw that bore his name for half a century. Finding that the wretched patient, if inexpertly held down, might move during the operation, resulting in breakage of the blade and other ensuing complications, he designed a saw that held the blade on a hinge with a screw tension spring behind the frame on the carpentry principle. In comparing the two illustrated in pl. 10, it is interesting to note how the forerunner, the coarse heavy saw of *c.* 1790, has become the delicate and refined instrument of 60 years later. Butcher felt his saw had two advantages; it could cut in a curve with ease and could be fitted between the flaps without bruising. Chain saws, with ebony, ivory, or steel handles, rarely appeared before 1800. More frequent finds are narrow-bladed finger saws, sometimes folding into an ivory or tortoise-shell guard (pl. 12). These often form part of small cases of minor operating instruments, the handle then being detachable on a spring-socket as a space-saving measure.

13.   An early skull saw as described by Scultetus, c. 1720; Hey's saw, c. 1820, Weiss. 15·5 cm, 15·5 cm. (Simon Kaye Ltd, London)

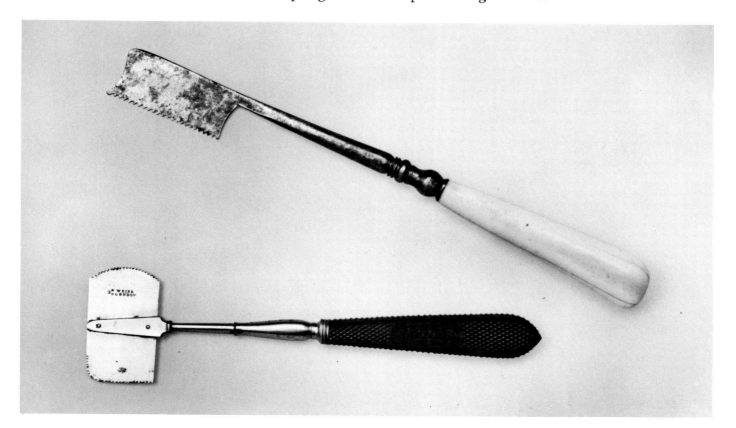

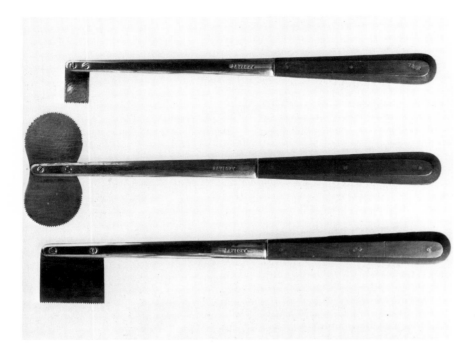

14. *The original Hey's saws made for the personal use of Sir William Hey. Savigny, 1803. 15·5 cm.*
(General Infirmary, Leeds)

SKULL SAWS

It is certain, from manuscripts at St John's College, Oxford, that the earliest skull saws used in this country took the form of those used by John Wrightson (*fl.* 1350) in the fourteenth century; a crescent-shaped blade with the serrations on the outer curve, indispensable for cutting into a convex surface. It is probable that this type continued in use until several other types were introduced from the Continent during the sixteenth century. These were mostly variations on a halberd shape with a saw on either side of the central shaft. An early skull saw of *c.* 1720 in pl. 13 is exactly as described by Scultetus in 1674, and is the forerunner of the Hey's saw. In 1783, Dr Cockell of Pontefract reintroduced the use of the skull saw with a semi-circular edge in preference to the trephine. Sir William Hey, F.R.S. (1736–1819), designed his skull saw in 1803 while working at the Leeds General Infirmary. He used a whole range of double and singled bladed saws with every degree of curve in the blade, so useful, he said 'when the thickness of the cranium which is to be sawed through is very unequal' (pl. 14).

No set of trepanning instruments was afterwards complete without its complement of Hey's saws, and one was included in all large cases of general surgical instruments (col. pl. I).

Trephines and other trepanning instruments

It is difficult now to imagine anyone willingly undergoing a trepanning operation without anaesthetic in the prevailing conditions of medieval surgery (pl. 3, p. 7). A manuscript at Trinity College, Cambridge, shows one being performed with a knife, the blade of which is at least 25·5 cm long, and the forceps of similar size, the poor unfortunate patient being held down by two men. Undoubtedly, many such operations were perpetrated on the insane who had no say in the matter, but it seems unbelievable that some were carried out for wholly valid reasons and were successful. James Yonge (1646–1721) recorded in 1670 at least two successful operations for fracture of the skull with laceration of the brain, and

15.   Jan Sanders van Hemessen (c. 1500–1575), The Surgeon *(showing trepanning operation). (Museo del Prado, Madrid)*

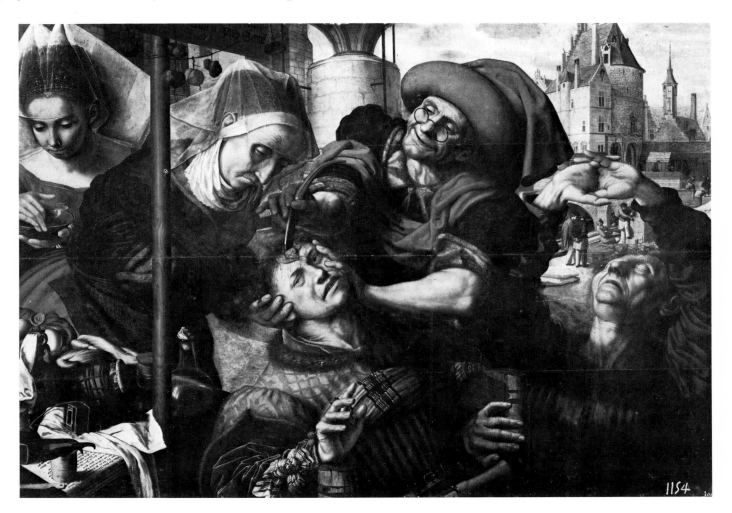

27

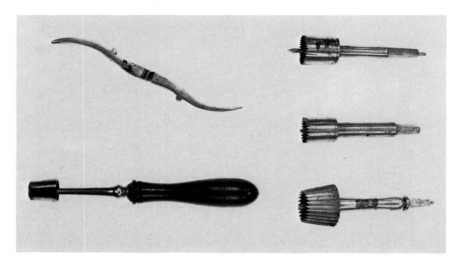

16.   *Trephines and an elevator, c. 1653, Prujean Collection.*
(Royal College of Physicians of England)

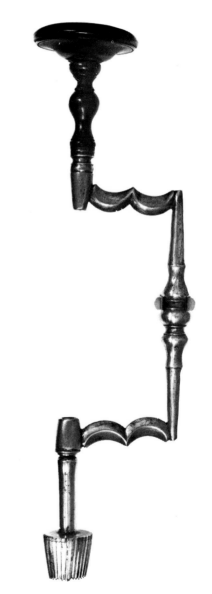

Percivall Pott did much valuable work on external injuries to the head nearly a century later. 'Potts's Puffy Tumour' was an early condition he described, associated with osteomyelitis of the skull.

This description from *Practical Cases and Observations in Surgery*, 1751, is worth quoting:

'A lad received a Blow or Kick from one of the horses in a cart, which fractured the Frontal bone on the left side in several pieces and bent the Forehead inwards, like to a large Bruise in a tin, copper or pewter Vessel; the Depressure reached near down to the Minor Canthus; a Neighbouring Quack-Surgeon, spiritually authorised to lop, dismember, etc. was fetched in to the boy's assistance, who immediately promised a perfect Cure and in a short time—but after having him under his care for five or six days, dressing the wounds (I doubt not) but with his Samaritan Balsam, never failing Plaisters, and suchlike Nostrums, the patient became raving and was afflicted wth convulsive Spasms. On which the Boaster much affrighted took his leave and pronounced him irrecoverable. Early in the Morning I was called out of my Bed to the Patient when I found him delirious, with an Inflammation on his Head and Face of the Erysipalous kind and swoln to so great a degree that I could scarce discover either his Eyes, Nose or Mouth, and the whole Head seemed a Mass of soft dough . . . On searching with my probe I found the Edges of the fractured Bones, forming an Arch, with part of the frontal and temporal Muscles lacerated. Having everything necessary for trepanning I made an Incision in the superior part of the Frontal Bone, first measuring with a string from the middle of the Chin to

17.   *Trephine with conical crown, c. 1730.*
(Royal College of Surgeons of Edinburgh)

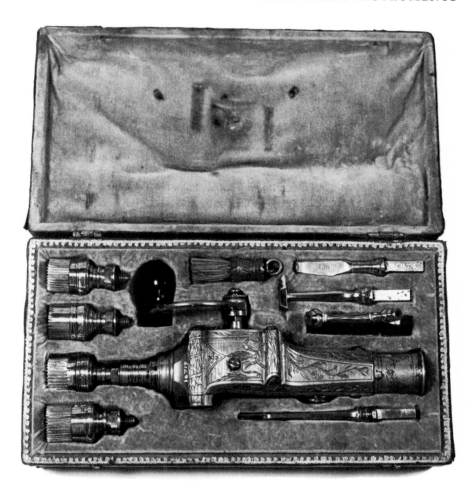

18. *Cased trephine set, c. 1720.*
15 by 20·5 cm.
(Museum of Historical Medicine,
Copenhagen)

the coronal Suture, lest I should injure the Sinus Longitudinalis of the Dura Mater. Having removed the scalp and Pericranium, I cut out a piece of the sound Bone, with about a fifth of the Fracture, on which issued out some extravasated Blood; it was through this Perforation that the Elevator was introduced . . . and the deprest or inward bent bones were raised up and restored to their natural situation, while the loose Fragments were taken away—(the Cure) was at last happily finished to the great satisfaction of his Parents and himself.'

The trephine of the ancient Greeks was a conical piece of metal with a circular serrated edge at the base making it into a form of saw which could cut a circular groove. A centre pin kept it in place while it was worked and we are told it was necessary to plunge it into cold water at frequent intervals because of frictional heat.

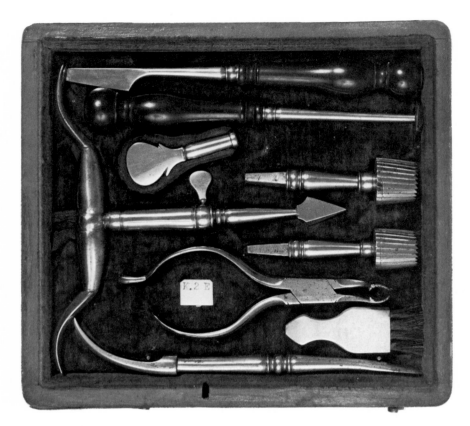

19.   *Cased trephine set, c. 1750. The handle of the trephine is fitted with an arrowhead perforator; just above it is the key for removing the centre pin. 38 by 17·5 cm. (Royal College of Surgeons of England)*

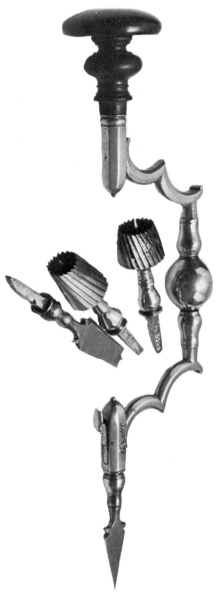

20.   *Trepanning drill and perforator, Petit-type, c. 1750. 15 cm.*
(Museum Boerhaave, Leiden)

Trephines in this country, first mentioned *c.* 1600, were circular saws for removing a disc of bone from the cranium, the saw having a slightly wider shoulder to prevent it sinking into the brain. Down the central shaft was a pin for engaging the instrument in the skull and it was then rotated either by a brace or drill-stock type of handle or, later, by a handle set at right angles to the shaft. John Woodall (1556–1643) (see Chapter 8) devised one of the early trephines in place of the brace trepan. Discs of up to 3·2 cm in diameter could be removed by this method. Scultetus describes trephines both with and without a central pin, called 'male' and 'female'. Samuel Sharp (1700–78) of Guy's Hospital (he wrote *A Treatise on The Operations of Surgery* in 1739) introduced a trephine from which the central pin could be removed by means of a key (pl. 19), and another, with a most elegant yoke-shaped handle is now at the Royal College of Surgeons (pl. 21). Another instrument, also in the Royal College of Surgeons, is Brambilla's (1728–1800) drill-stock trephine as in *Instrumentarium* of 1782, of beautifully turned steel (pl. 23). By 1798, Savigny could say that a trephine

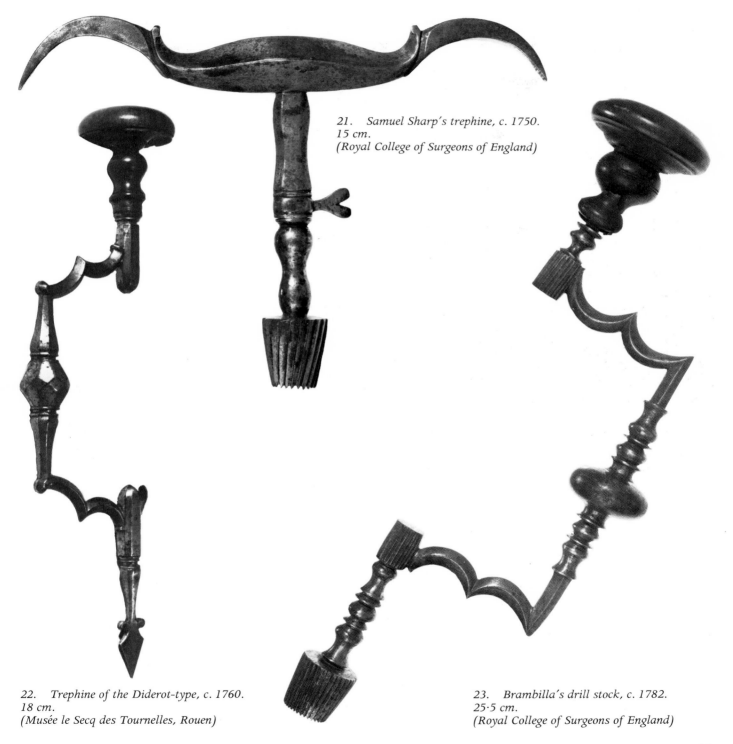

21.   *Samuel Sharp's trephine, c. 1750.*
15 cm.
(Royal College of Surgeons of England)

22.   *Trephine of the Diderot-type, c. 1760.*
18 cm.
(Musée le Secq des Tournelles, Rouen)

23.   *Brambilla's drill stock, c. 1782.*
25·5 cm.
(Royal College of Surgeons of England)

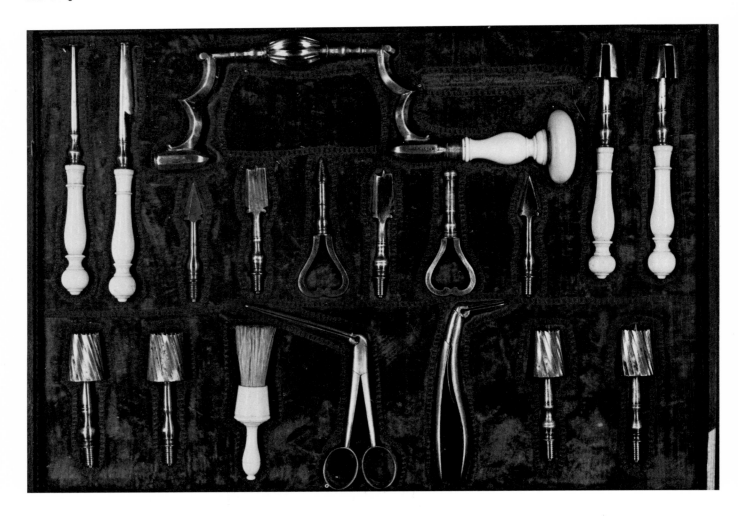

24. *Case of trepanning instruments, ivory handles, 1785. 38·7 by 17·8 cm. (Institute of Medical History, Vienna)*

used with a brace 'is now wholly laid aside in this country', and described an instrument that became standard, with small modifications, throughout the nineteenth century. In 1801, Benjamin Bell introduced teeth arranged in three groups of nine, thus allowing a gap to prevent clogging, and in 1817 the adjustable screw to raise or lower the pin was introduced from the Continent.

A mechanical trephine with a rotary handle like that of a coffee-grinder appeared *c.* 1830 but found little favour. Another interesting piece at the Royal College of Surgeons is a very elaborate trephine of *c.* 1790; this has side levers to extract the disc of bone after cutting (pl. 25). The great brain surgeon, Victor Horsley, who removed a tumour from the spinal column for the first time in 1887, evolved a trephine with a crutch handle *c.* 1870.

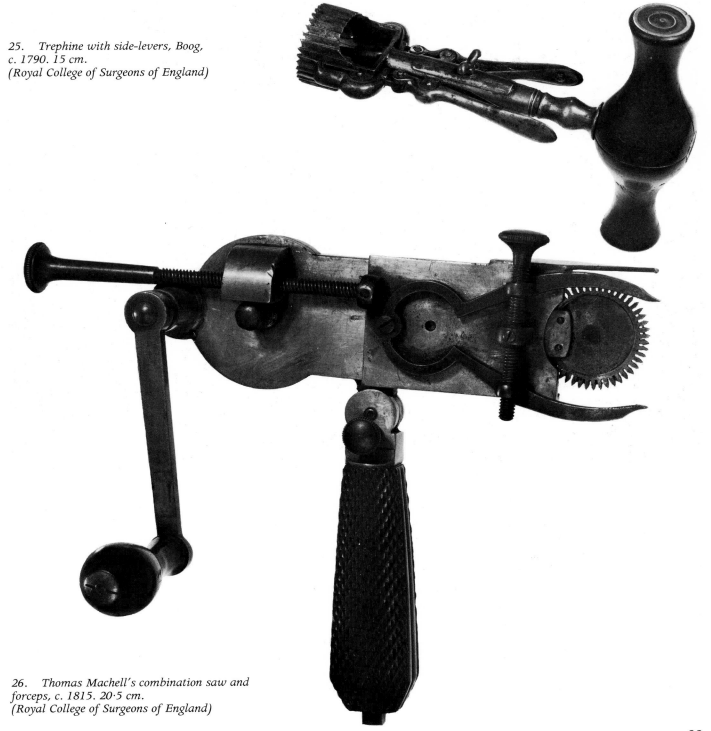

25.   Trephine with side-levers, Boog,
c. 1790. 15 cm.
(Royal College of Surgeons of England)

26.   Thomas Machell's combination saw and
forceps, c. 1815. 20·5 cm.
(Royal College of Surgeons of England)

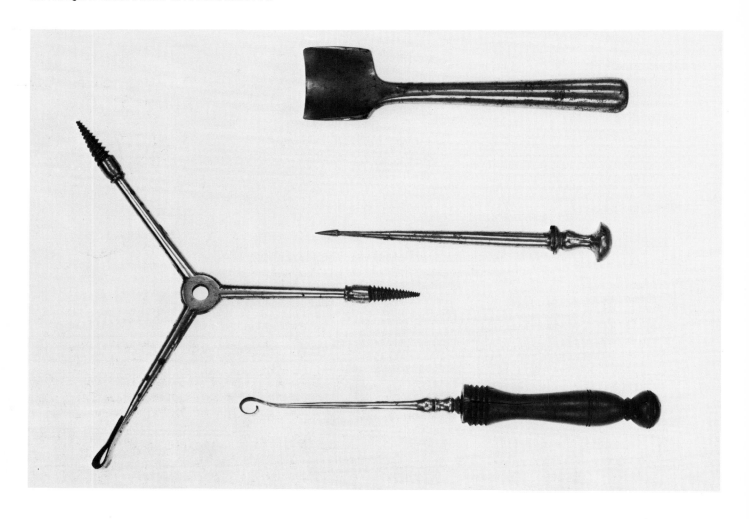

Cased trepanning sets of the early nineteenth century, mostly by Weiss such as the one in col. pl. I, usually contained the following:

2 or 3 Hey's saws;

2 or 3 trephines of varying diameter, all screwing into the same handle;

Cranium forceps, double ended, one fine, one broad;

Ivory handled brush for dusting the piece of skull removed;

Elevator for raising cut bone;

Scalpel for removing pericranium;

File or raspatory;

Lenticular for depressing the brain on removal of the piece of bone and trimming the edge of the perforation. This had a removable head for washing away the bone sawdust.

27. *Foliate bore for trepanning, bone scoop, setaceum screw, and hook. Prujean Collection, c. 1653. (Royal College of Physicians of England)*

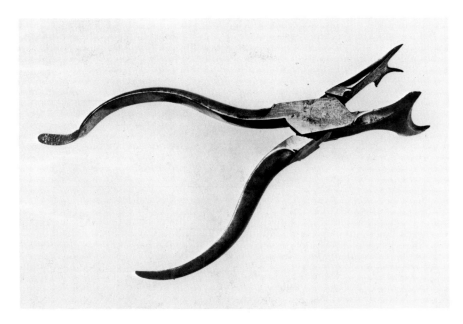

28. Samuel Sharp's forceps for removing circular pieces of cranium cut out by trephine, 1739. 15 cm.
(Royal College of Surgeons of England)

Visitors to the Wellcome Collection will see that the trephine set of *c*. 1750 there, contains all the above with the exception of the Hey's saws, with each piece noticeably larger and heavier. Alternatives to the trephine or skull saw were the 'cutting compasses' first introduced by Ambroise Paré (1509–90) in 1564 in which one arm of the compasses was engaged in the skull and the other, with a cutting edge, was driven across the cranium by means of a screw on the hinge. At the beginning of the eighteenth century came Petit's perforator, an arrowhead device for trepanning. With it, he invented an elevator of tripod form, for which the skull served as fulcrum. Samuel Sharp devised a cranium forceps with two curved blades at right angles to the shaft.

Thomas Machell, Surgeon of Walsingham, invented in 1815 a circular saw, worked by a handle with forceps attached—'the whole to supersede the use of the trephine, trepan, Hey's saw, bone nippers, rasp, mallet, chisel, etc.' It was very cumbersome and heavy and found little favour (pl. 26).

Not all the skull surgery performed at this time required the use of the trephine. Sir Astley Cooper (1768–1841) left a description of an operation to remove a cyst from the scalp of George IV. Asked what the tumour was called he said, 'a steatome, Sire'. 'Then', said the King, 'I hope it will stay at home and not annoy me any more.' For the operation, the surgeon was made a baronet and given an epergne costing 500 guineas.

35

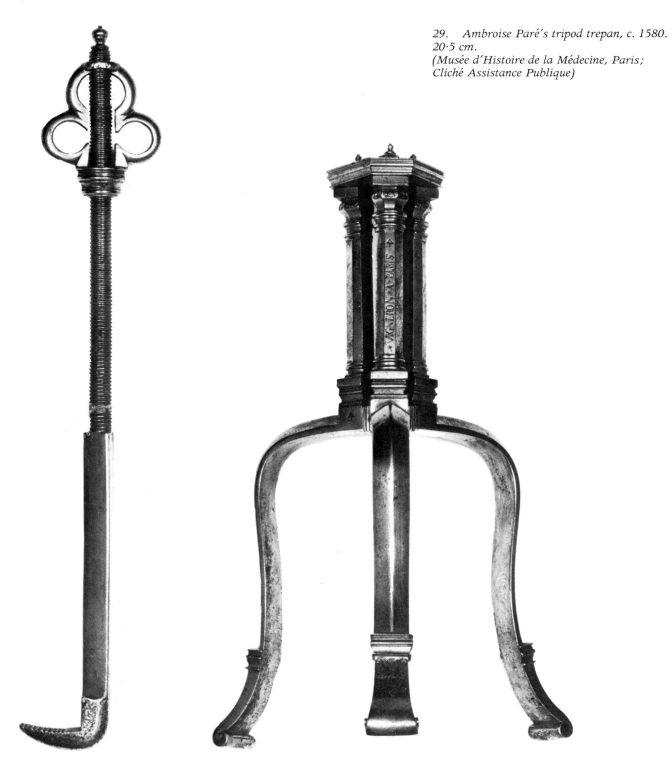

29.   Ambroise Paré's tripod trepan, c. 1580.
20·5 cm.
*(Musée d'Histoire de la Médecine, Paris;
Cliché Assistance Publique)*

30.   *Elevators, c. 1680. 15 cm.*
(Musée le Secq des Tournelles, Rouen)

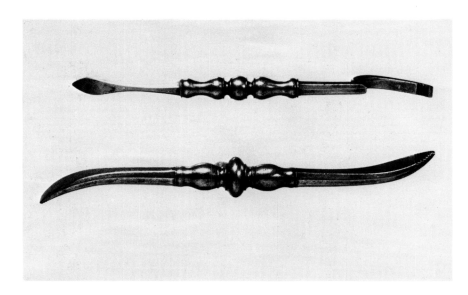

31.   *Instruments designed and made by*
Cornelius Solingen (1641–87). From left—
amputation pincers for fingers and toes, knife,
speculum for ear and nose, skull saw, forceps
and probed knife, c. 1675.
(Museum Boerhaave, Leiden)

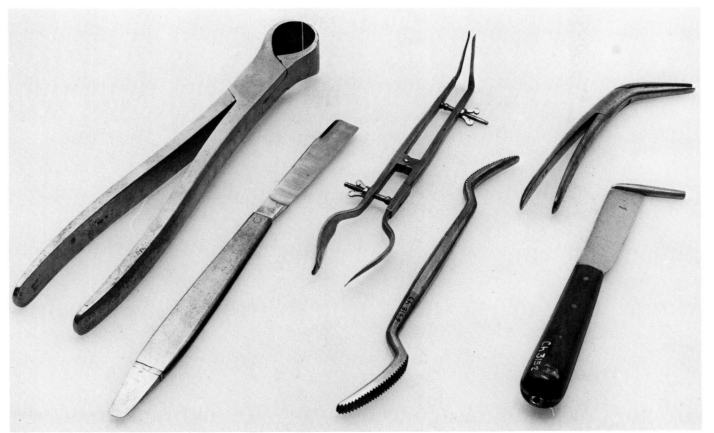

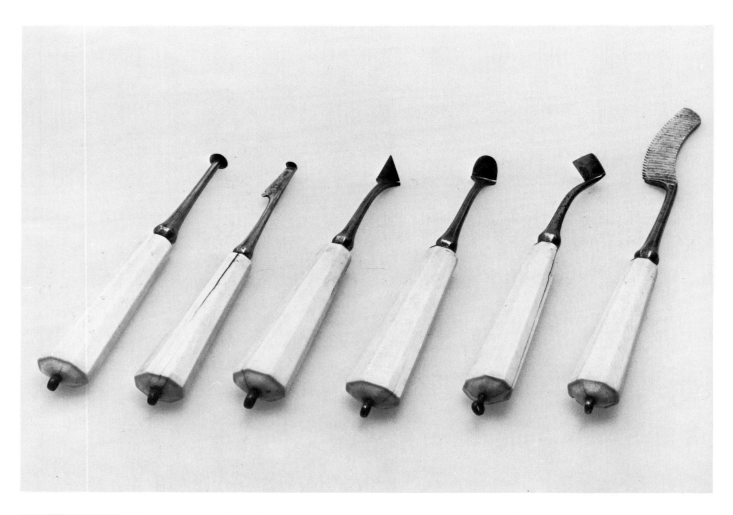

32. *Elevators, lenticulars, and a skull saw,*
c. 1750.
(Museum Boerhaave, Leiden)

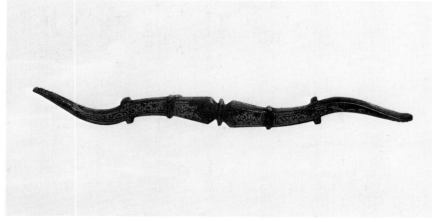

33. *Gold-plated steel elevator, c. 1750.*
15 cm.
(Royal College of Surgeons of England)

34. *Foliate bore for trepanning, c. 1780.*
radius 7·5 cm.
(Musée d'Histoire de la Médecine, Paris;
Cliché Assistance Publique)

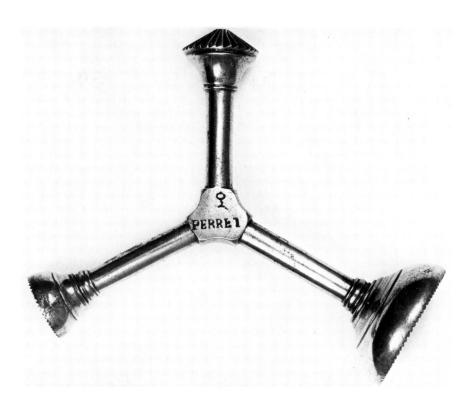

35. *Elevator on tripod, c. 1750. 20·5 cm.*
(Museum of History of Medicine,
Copenhagen)

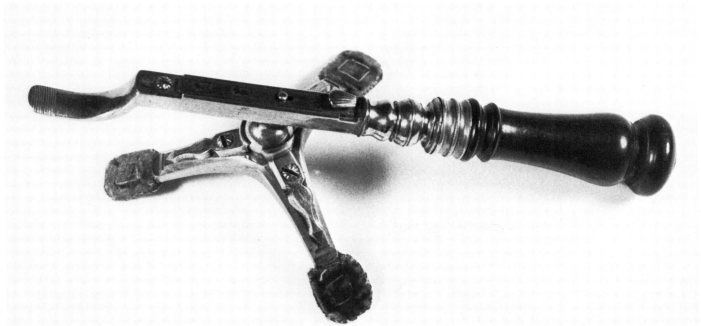

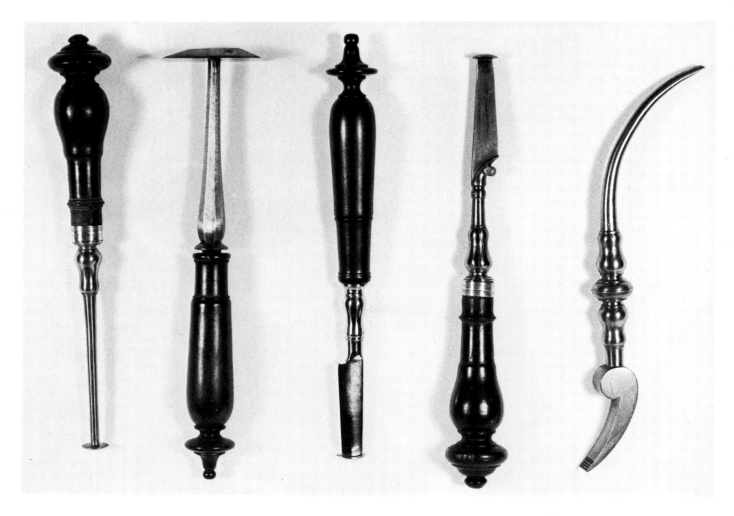

Phlebotomy instruments

36. *Group of lenticulars, c. 1780. 18 cm.*
(Museum of History of Medicine,
Copenhagen)

LANCETS

Phlebotomy or blood letting is one of the oldest forms of therapy, even practised by the ancient Greeks, and it is hard to find a single complaint or condition for which bleeding has not been thought the remedy, including obvious anaemia and debility. It was the most frequent and immediately suggested panacea, much as many people reach for the aspirin bottle today—though there was general agreement that it should never be done when the moon was on the wane, or during a south wind, and that there was no time so good as in early Lent. It is hardly surprising, therefore, that the most commonly found of all instruments is the lancet. The ideogram for physician in ancient Chinese was the same as the Egyptian—a lancet in the upper half and a bleeding glass in the lower. Caxton in 1474 probably made the first reference to a lancet in English: 'he did his vysage to be kutte with a knyf and lancettis'. The beautiful little cases in which they were usually kept are dealt with in Chapter 14. The lancets themselves are flexible razor-sharp pointed blades between 5 and 7·6 cm long, in folding guards of ivory, tortoise-shell, or mother of pearl. Their shape and size does not appear to have altered over the years and they can only be reasonably dated by their cases or makers (pl. 41). In the early nineteenth century an 'automatic lancet' was invented. This was a type of syringe, the head of which was released into the vein on a spring and the blood then draining into the glass bowl. These often had engraved silver mounts.

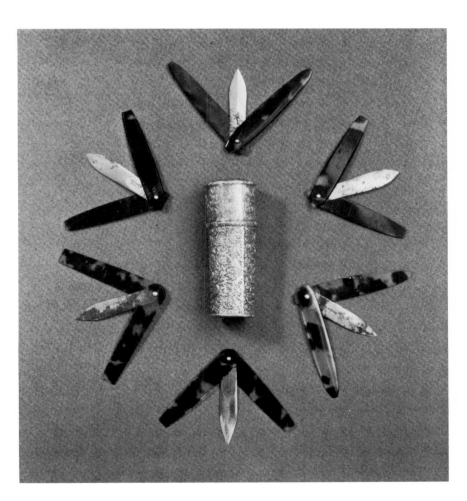

37. A German silver-gilt lancet case with six lancets in tortoise-shell guards, c. 1750. 6 cm.
(Simon Kaye Ltd, London)

41

BLEEDING BOWLS

These are the subject of endless and rather tedious controversy among collectors. It is generally accepted in this country that it is the one-handled shallow silver bowls which are known as bleeding bowls (pl. 38), and the two-handled ones that are referred to as porringers, whereas in the United States it is the other way about. The earlier ones were straight-sided, becoming slightly convex by the end of the seventeenth century. A bowl made in Norwich in 1689 for John Worrell, who was Master of the Norwich Barber Surgeons in 1693, would seem to be the only link between this type of bowl and the practice of phlebotomy, and far from proving the point that it was a bleeding bowl, it may well have been the basis of the misunderstanding that has persisted since. As Michael Clayton says, with some exasperation, 'one feels any receptacle might have been called into use on such occasions'—and as the majority date from 1625 to 1730, what were used from then until the practice ceased, towards the end of the nineteenth century? An exception to prove the rule is the pewter example marked in ounces (pl. 39).

38. Silver bleeding bowl, 1683. Maker's mark E.G. Diameter 10 cm. (S. J. Shrubsole Ltd)

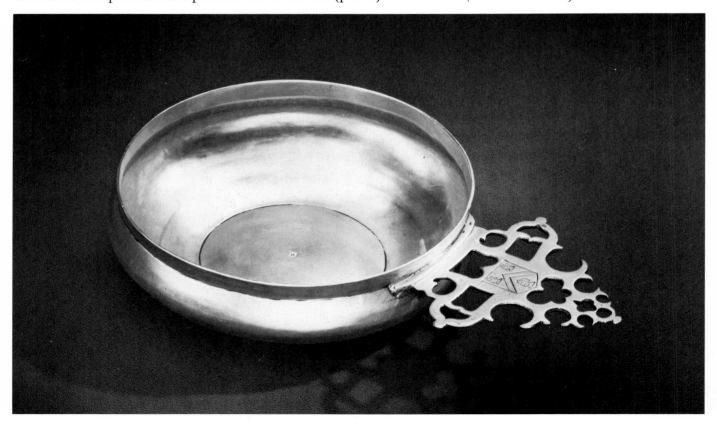

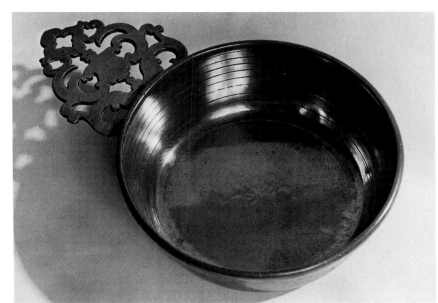

39. *Pewter bleeding bowl, measured in ounces, c. 1700. Diameter 10 cm. (Strangers' Hall Museum, Norwich)*

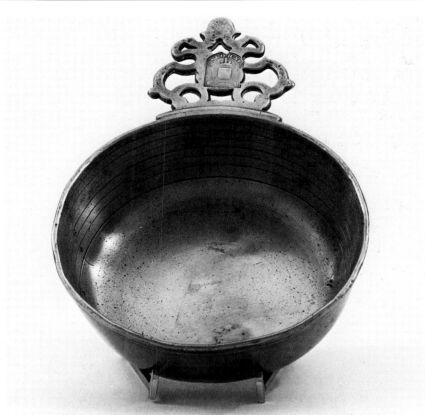

40. *Pewter bleeding bowl, c. 1745. 10 cm. (Division of Medical Sciences, National Museum of History and Technology, Smithsonian Institution, Washington D.C.)*

CUPPING INSTRUMENTS

A more sophisticated but equally ancient method of blood letting which enjoyed a revival during the seventeenth, eighteenth, and nineteenth century was that of cupping. The object of the practice was to draw blood to the surface of the skin, favoured parts of the body being the temples, behind the ears, and the base of the spine, but none escaped. Dry cupping was that practised when the skin was unbroken, and wet cupping after the skin had been scarified. The cups were dome-shaped, either glass or more rarely metal (pl. 41), and before being applied to the skin were warmed, creating a partial vacuum. The earlier ones were warmed over a flame or by burning paper inside them but during the nineteenth century valved cupping glasses appeared for use with a pump to withdraw the air (pl. 43). Maw's catalogue of 1868 shows a set of six of this kind, with syringe, for 13 shillings. A rare set in their original case was found recently. There are four flask-shaped cups, each marked in ounces, it was made by Weedon *c.* 1830.

42. A set of cupping instruments containing two pairs of cupping glasses, two-bladed scarificator, brass spirit lamp, ivory lancets. William Smith, 1805. Case 25·5 cm by 20·5 cm. (Simon Kay Ltd, London)

41. Three cupping glasses two c. 1800, one 1820. Silver lancet cases and lancets; from left—c. 1815 Taylor and Perry (for Evans); 1801; 1833 S. Mordan & G.R. Glasses 5 cm high, cases 5 cm long. (Simon Kaye Ltd, London)

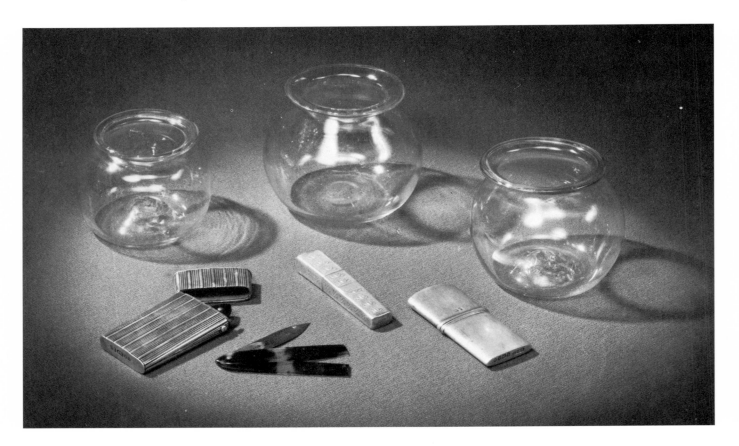

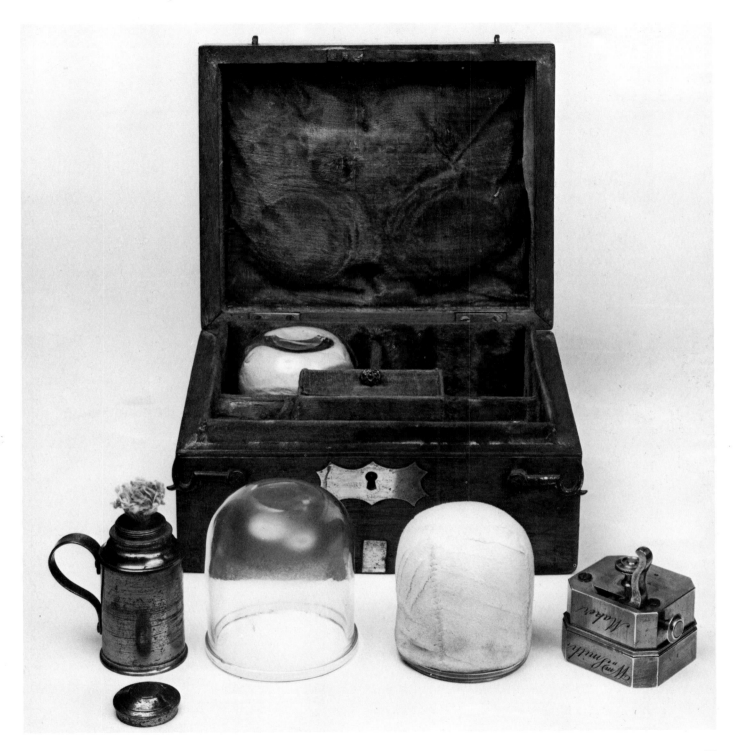

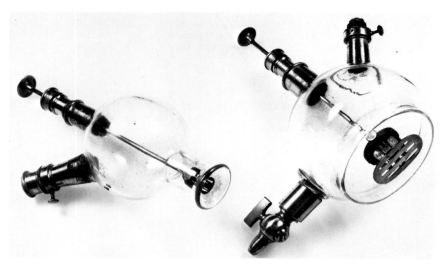

43. *Combined scarificator and cupping glass with valve as introduced by J. B. Sarlandiore (1787–1838), c. 1825. 18 cm.*
(Musée d'Histoire de la Médecine, Paris; Cliché Assistance Publique)

44. *Set of cupping instruments in cylindrical maghogany case, c. 1825. 18 cm.*
(Castle Museum, York)

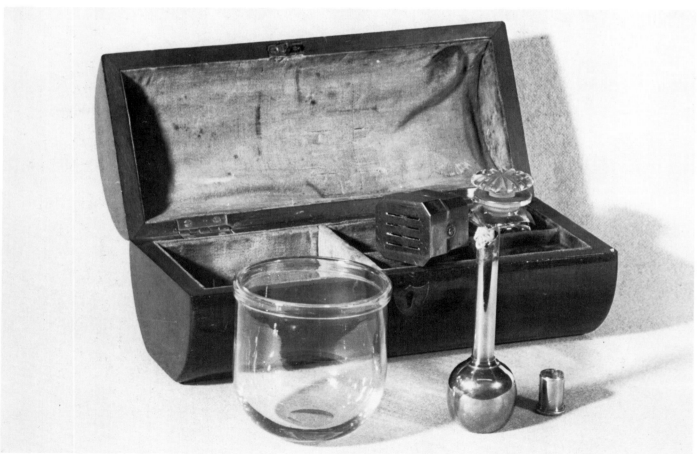

Cupping glasses are rarely found singly as they were made in nests of three and six, often fitted into a lined case with a scarificator and sometimes a lamp (pl. 44). They are made of stout flint glass with a folded rim to fit firmly over the surface of the skin with even pressure. Their size varies from 3·8 cm to 5 cm in diameter and they are of roughly equal height, Another type occasionally found is oval with a small opening on one long side. A mid-nineteenth-century variation for dry cupping was a hemisphere of glass with a rubber bulb on top which expelled air before application and then created considerable pressure on the blood vessels. It will be seen that all these receptacles were most useful to double their purpose as bleeding bowls.

45.   *Cased set of cupping instruments with valved glasses, c. 1860.*
(Division of Medical Sciences, National Museum of History and Technology, Smithsonion Institution, Washington D.C.)

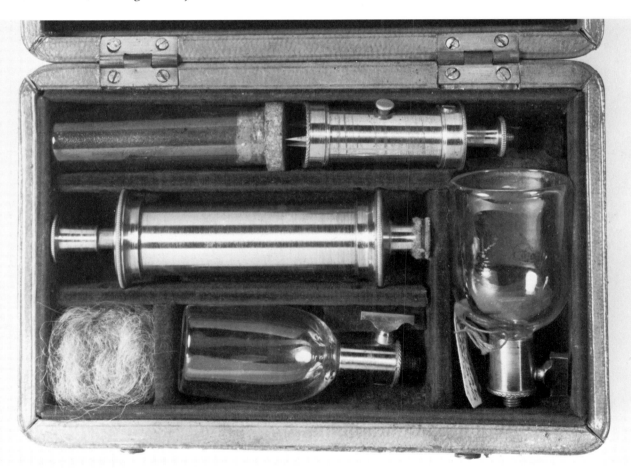

SCARIFICATORS

In the brothels of seventeenth-century London, a cupper was usually employed, who advertised his attendance: '2/6*d* by the old or the new way'. This referred to bleeding by the scarificator. The scarifier or scarificator is a highly ingenious instrument consisting of a square, brass, silver or silver-plated case with slots, from which protrude and move across, very sharp strong blades on the release of a trigger. It was developed in the late seventeenth century. The size varies from 3 cm to 6·3 cm square, and the number of slots from 2 to about 8. Since some are made with two blades per slot, there could be as many as 16 cutting the skin at one time. The blades are sometimes rounded and sometimes pointed, and the depth to which they are required to cut can be regulated by a screw at the base by the lever. The early ones were prettily decorated and look much as if they might be musical boxes (pl. 46). Another early type (not much made after the early years of the nineteenth century) was the single-bladed scarifier, occasionally called a Spring Fleam or Schnapper; this was invented by a German *c*. 1680. It was sometimes made with a curved guard, presumably for bleeding the finger, but the early type was for straight-forward venesection (pl. 47). They were occasionally used in dentistry (see Chapter 9). Early eighteenth-century examples have been found in steel, the cases chased and engraved with delicate scrolls and foliage. Later, as brass became the usual material, the decoration became less frequent with even a little engine-turning seeming opulent. Groups of scarificators are in pls. 46–48.

46.   *Scarificator in brass case, c. 1680.*
9 cm.
(Germanisches Nationalmuseum, Nuremberg)

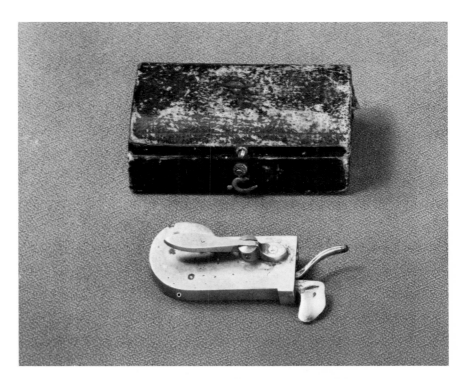

47.   Single-bladed scarificator, above
c.1780, single-bladed scarificator, below
c.1700, both with original cases. Length of
cases 6·4 cm.
(Simon Kaye Ltd, London)

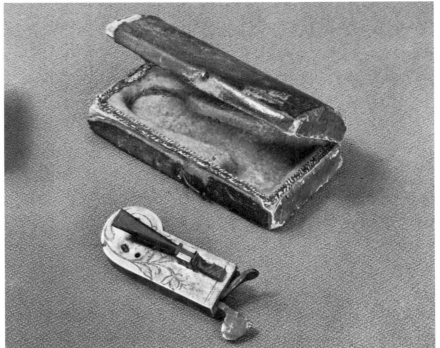

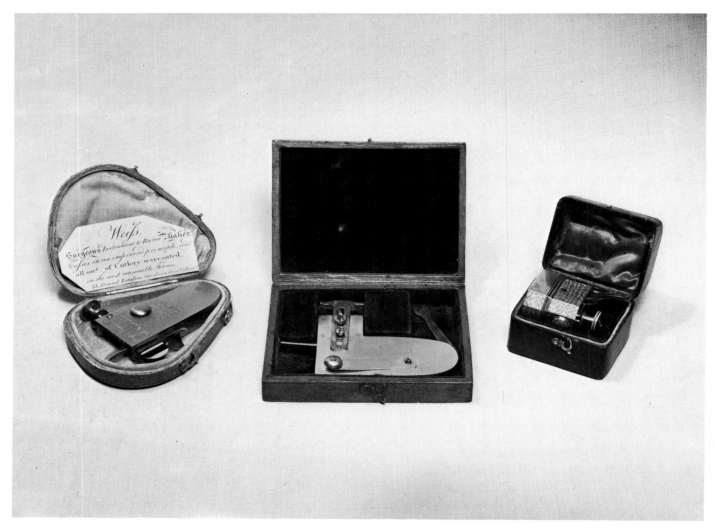

48.   Single-bladed scarificator, c. 1800,
Weiss; Single-bladed scarificator, c. 1830;
three-bladed scarificator c. 1830, H. Bigg.
7·5 cm, 7·5 cm, 3·8 cm.
(Simon Kaye Ltd, London)

Colour plate
Cased set of trepanning instruments
containing three trephines, elevator,
raspatory, cranium forceps, ivory brush,
scalpel, three Hey's saws, lenticular, c. 1820.
Weiss. Case 15 cm by 20 cm.
(Simon Kaye Ltd, London)

PLATE I

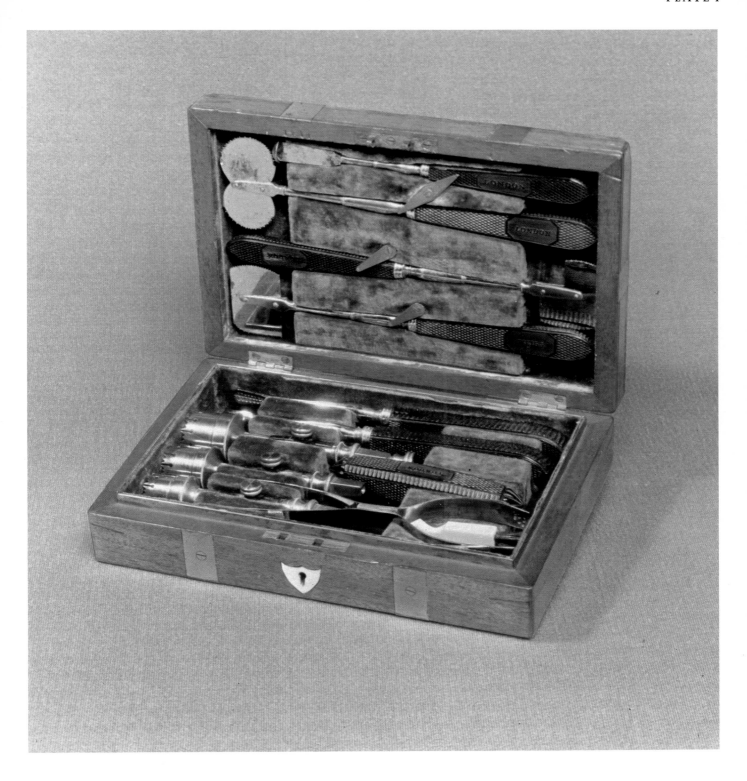

PLATE II

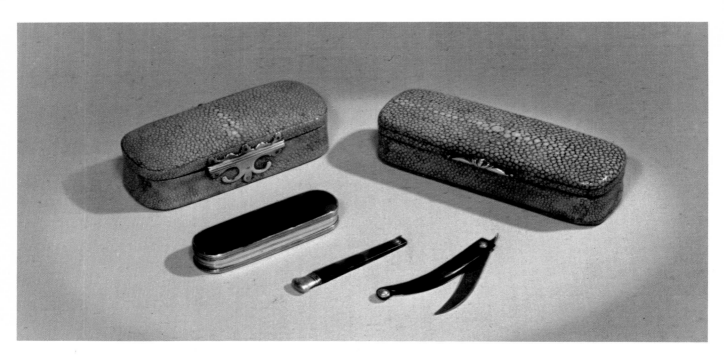

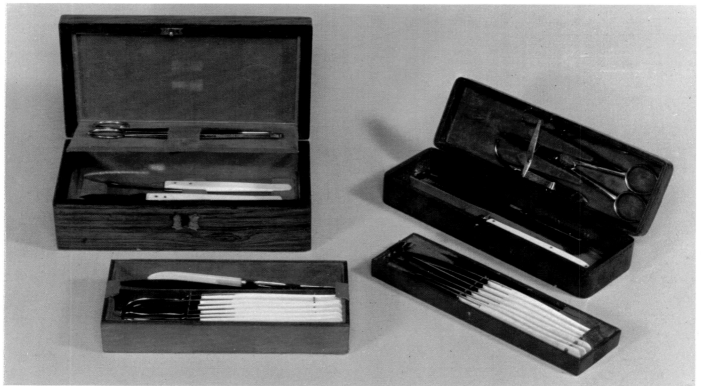

CHAPTER THREE

Knives, directors and forceps

Aulus Cornelius Celsus (25 B.C. – A.D. 50) gives us the first description of an amputation in the translation by Gerard of Cremona (A.D. 1114–87).

> 'When the malady gets the better of our medicines the limb must be amputated . . . but one remedy, expediency and not safety, is the paramount consideration. We are therefore to make an incision with a knife between the sound and morbid parts down to the bone, with this qualification, that we are never to cut opposite a joint and always to include some of the sound part rather than leave any of that which is diseased. When we come to the bone the sound flesh must be retracted so as in some measure to denude it; then it must be divided with the saw close up to the sound flesh. The end of the bone is then to be smoothed where the saw has left any asperity and the integuments brought over it, which in this operation, ought to be left loose enough to cover the entire stump as far as possible.'

Given that amputation is a mercifully uncommon occurrence today, this has remained sound advice since it was written.

The circular method, as in this description, contested the three-flap method for popularity across the centuries with now one, now the other, gaining ground. Infection was accepted though not fully understood, and adherents of the three-flap method, by which the limb was cut up to the point of severing the bone leaving three flaps to be sewn together over it, thought there was less risk of infection this way and less strain in the suturing. William Clowes (1540–1604), Surgeon to Queen Elizabeth I, writing of his experiences in amputating, said he needed only three instruments–a specially sharpened saw, a double-edged knife, and a scalpel. James Yonge (1646–1721) wrote in 1679 a very full description of this type of operation, but in 1693, John Moyle (d. 1714) in *The Sea-Chirurgeon* adhered to the circular method. John Atkins (1685–1757) advised speed in amputation, 'the men meeting their misfortune with greater strength and resolution than when they have spent the night under thought and reflection'. William Northcote (d. 1783) advised in 1770 the need for three assistants, one to hold the patient at the back, one to hold the arm and one to hold the hand and assist with

Colour plate
Above: Two silver-mounted shagreen instrument cases c. 1720. Tortoise-shell and silver case with two folding scalpels, possibly Scottish, c. 1790 Lengths of cases 14 cm, 15·5 cm, 10 cm.

Below: Two pocket-cases of instruments for minor operations; left, c. 1840, Ferris, Bristol; right c. 1875. Hawkesley. Lengths of cases 15·5 cm.
(Simon Kaye Ltd, London)

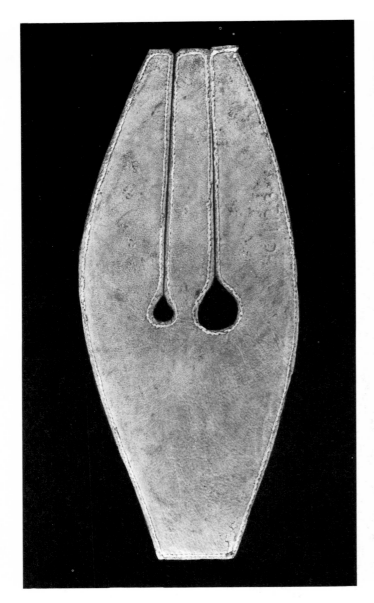

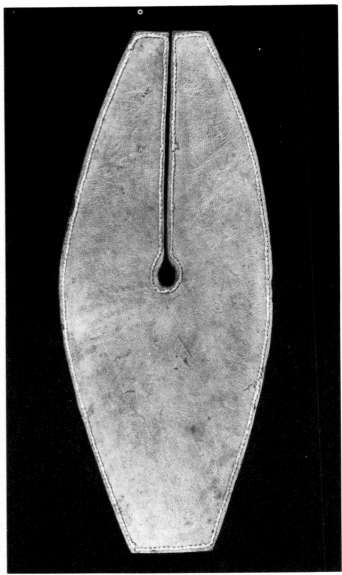

the tourniquet. During the Napoleonic Wars the same controversy pertained. The Germans and Russians were accused of causing agony to their patients with the circular method and making the fitting of artificial limbs difficult. Dominique Larrey (1766–1842), Surgeon-General to Napoleon and the inventor of the Flying Ambulance, did much to advance the art of amputation. He was a

1. *Very rare leather retractors, mid-eighteenth century. 38·5 cm.*
(Royal College of Surgeons of Edinburgh)

2. *Very rare leather retractors, mid-eighteenth century. 38·5 cm.*
(Royal College of Surgeons of Edinburgh)

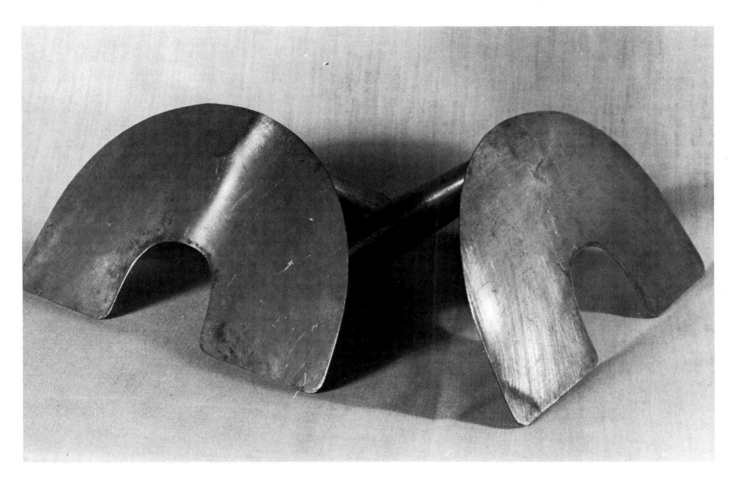

3. Metal retractors for use in amputation, c. 1800. 12·5 cm.
(Royal College of Surgeons of Edinburgh)

man quite out of tune with his age in point of honour and integrity, and his devotion to duty earned him the respect of many nations of soldiers. Napoleon, writing in his Will and leaving 100,000 francs to Larrey, said, 'He is the most virtuous man I have ever known'. Amputating right on the battlefield, and frequently under gunfire, he found he had a greater success rate than if he waited until the wounded were brought back to hospital. By this means, the wound was still numb from the impact of the cannon and infection had not had the chance to set in before the operation. Many of his cases just got up and walked away. Larrey was a firm believer in the bone being sawn off higher than the flesh but did not care for the three-flap method. He managed a circular operation that took both points into account, a feat clearly needing some dexterity, and his methods were widely copied. Muscle retractors to enable the bone to be severed higher are shown in pls. 1–3.

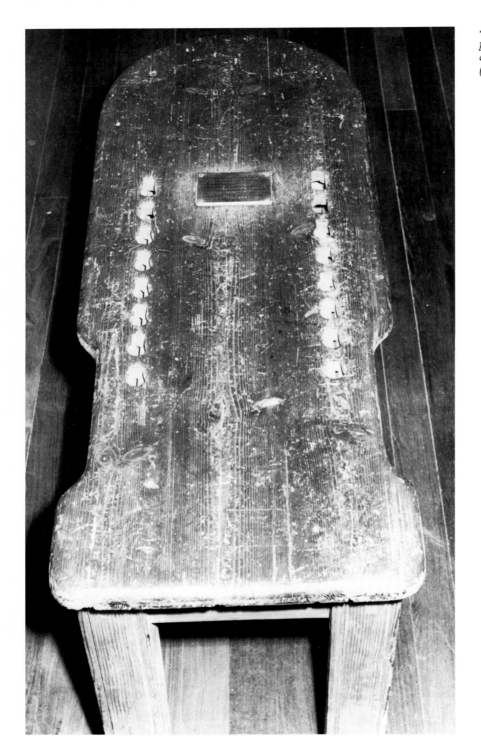

4. *The operating table on which was performed the first operation under anaesthesia on 21 December 1846. (University College Hospital Medical School)*

The man who advanced amputation most in this country was Robert Liston (1794–1847), Professor of Surgery at University College Hospital, and he performed the first operation under anaesthesia there on 21 December 1846 (pl. 4). He held the reputation as 'the fastest man with a knife in England'—so necessary if the patient were not to die of pain and shock. He was a giant of a man with great physical strength, his arms and hands likened to Hercules, who loved the job and operated with great zest and relish, often cutting notches on his knives for each operation in which they had been used. He was said to be a fearsome sight when operating as he held the knife between his teeth while he tied the ligature on the blood vessels. He would amputate a thigh single-handed, compress the artery with the left hand, using no tourniquet, and do all the cutting and sewing with the right hand. One man was so terrified at the thought of his impending operation he went and hid in the lavatory. Liston strode after him, cut open the lock with his amputation knife, hauled him out, strapped him down, and cut for stone in two minutes. He was once said to be so anxious to break his own record for speed (and bets were placed on his performance) that in amputating a leg he took off one of the patient's testicles and two of his assistant's fingers at the same time.

However, on that fateful Monday in 1846, he made his entry into the operating theatre announcing: 'We are going to try a Yankee dodge today, gentlemen, for making men insensible.' The patient, a butler, who had a suppurating leg ripe for amputation, was wheeled in, pale and terrified. The inhaler was applied and after his initial fright, the man soon relaxed and became insensible. Liston gave the sign that he was to begin—so that he might be timed, as usual—and after, some said 28, some 25, seconds, he had tossed the leg into the sawdust, with the patient apparently still sleeping gently. Liston announced to his audience with true Victorian drama, 'The Yankee dodge, gentlemen, beats mesmerism hollow.' *Gratias Deo.*

Amputating knives

Guy de Chauliac (1298–1368), author of *Chirurgia Magna* which influenced surgery for centuries, mentions amputating knives, as does John of Arderne ((1307–90). The latter alleged he had designed many instruments, particularly for surgery of anal fistula, but there is no precise record nor any known surviving example. His advice on the number of instruments needed in a case lists scissors, speculum, needle, lancet, razor, and scalpel, but no mention of a

55

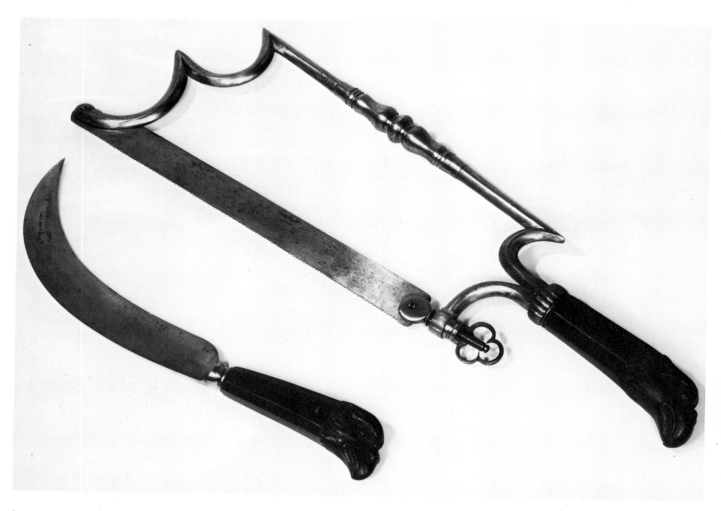

5. *Amputating knife and saw of Cornelius Solingen, c. 1670. 35·5 cm. (Museum Boerhaave, Leiden)*

larger amputating knife. However, John Wryghtson of Oxford, in 1350, depicts an amputation knife with a short blade curving inward a little at the tip. But a century later we find the shape of the blade changed to a bold curve, cutting on the convex edge.

Ambroise Paré (1509–90) was the first of the great military surgeons and served, successively, Henry II, Francis II, Charles IX, and Henry III of France.He was a Huguenot and was so well-loved that Charles IX hid him during the massacre on the Feast of St Bartholomew in 1572. He was a good and gentle man and took for his motto 'Je le pansay, Dieu le quarit'. ('I dressed his wounds, God healed him'.) Paré was the first writer on surgery to employ 'the common tongue' rather than Latin. He described two knives he used while operating, one he called his incision knife and the other a

56

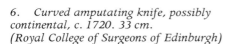

'crooked knife for dismembering', the blade of which is crescent-shaped, cutting on the inside. Pls. 5 and 6 show some varieties of curve which these early broad-bladed knives enjoyed over the next 250 years, the elaborate handles of wood, ivory, bone, *lignum vitae* beautifully finished.

Important changes were introduced in the early eighteenth century involving narrower blades, sometimes double-edged, and with less curve as the century progressed. At this date most handles were of ebony or *lignum vitae*, octagonal in section and pistol ended. In 1788 Loder advocated a knife with an almost straight edge

6. *Curved amputating knife, possibly continental, c. 1720. 33 cm. (Royal College of Surgeons of Edinburgh)*

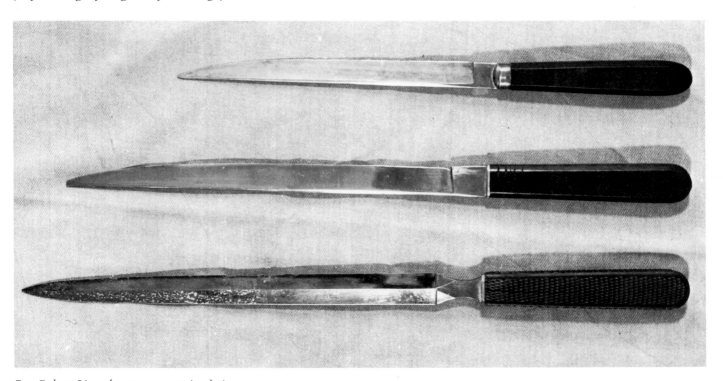

7. *Robert Liston's own amputating knives, c. 1830. 48 cm. (University College Hospital Medical School)*

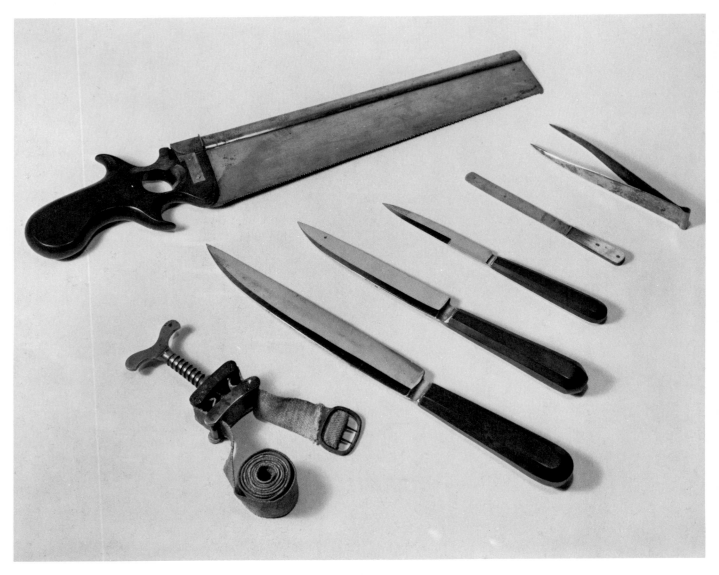

8. *Amputation saw, Liston knives, tourniquet, tweezers, and spatula, c. 1830. (College of Physicians of Philadelphia)*

which he found to be effective, and in the same year Benjamin Bell showed a similar one in his *System of Surgery*. Savigny in 1798, made a bid to keep the spine as narrow as possible but Sir Astley Cooper (1768–1841) of St Thomas' Hospital (and later of Guy's) preferred a broad back with a chequered ivory handle. A patient who had an amputation of the hip joint performed by Sir Astley said, after the 35-minute operation, that it was 'the hardest day's work I have ever had'. Sir Astley replied that it was almost the hardest he ever had.

As large a man as Robert Liston, both in physique and personality,

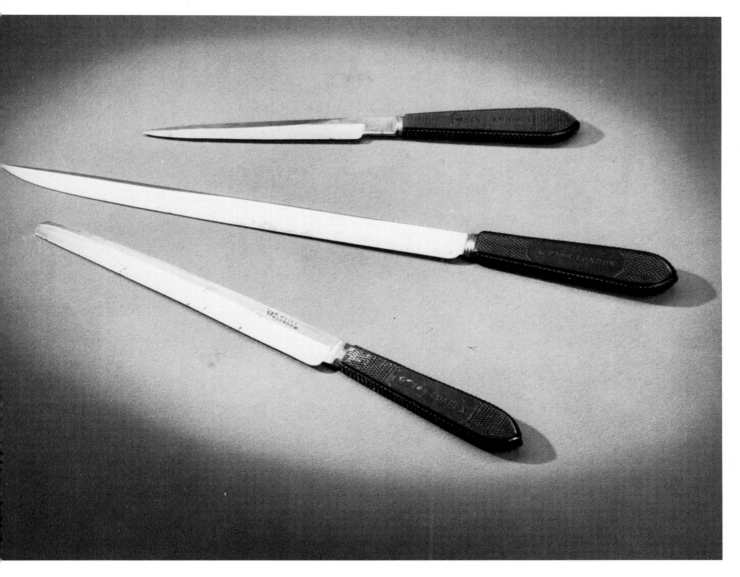

9. *A group of Liston knives, c. 1830, Weiss.*
(Simon Kaye Ltd, London)

clearly needed large knives. He designed, for the circular operation which he favoured, amputating knives with blades up to 37 cm long and 3·2 cm deep. They ended with a dagger point, the spine sharpened for the last 5 cm. These knives were designed to cut through the skin, the thick muscles, tendons, and tissues of the thigh, each in one sweep. The skin was cut by the 'tour de main', and the deep tissues by the 'tour de force'. The surgeon grasped his knife so that it would allow him to sweep right round the limb in one circular movement. 'The form and size of the instrument', wrote

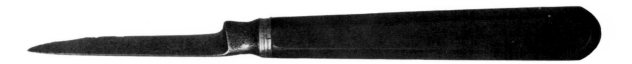

10. *James Syme's own ankle knife, c. 1850.*
15·2 cm.
(Royal College of Surgeons of England)

Liston, 'ought always to be in proportion . . . to the excision. If an extensive incision is necessary, an instrument possessing sufficient length of edge must be employed so that the parts may be separated smoothly and quickly.' Liston insisted that for greater dexterity the handle should be perfectly smooth rather than of the grooved and chequered type so popular for half a century. Some Liston knives are in pls. 7, 8 and 9. James Syme (1799–1870), Professor of Surgery at Edinburgh, was another of the great nineteenth-century surgeons and carried out the first hip dis-articulations in 1823. He devised a particular method of amputation of the foot and a knife for it. Syme's amputation knife is short, stout, and small in size (pl. 10); it is still used today for smaller joints involving cartilage. It was said of him that 'he never wasted a word, a drop of ink, or a drop of blood'.

For smaller operations and First Aid, knives were provided from the eighteenth century onwards in small pocket cases of instruments (see col. pl. II), often containing, among other items, as many as six assorted knives for differing purposes. In the mid-nineteenth century many of these were sometimes combined in one piece by folding each blade into a tortoise-shell guard like a multi-bladed penknife.

Maw's catalogue of 1868 lists a set of three amputating knives fitting into one spring-socket handle. For the all-purpose requirements of the Field-Surgeon, the same catalogue starts with a portable set of amputating instruments mounted in chequered ebony handles with silver ferrules consisting of: large saw, straight finger saw, one each Liston's large and small amputating knife, catlin (a small double-edged knife for cutting between two bones), tenaculum, sliding artery forceps, spiral tourniquet, needles and silk, in mahogany case—all for £4. A more elaborate set could be £10. Over the years, amputation sets of this type started with dozens of different cutting devices, then gradually dwindled to just a few, but with the addition of many haemostatic clamps of one sort or another.

For sharpening knives, Coxeter made for Liston a special steel or setting instrument which can be seen at The Royal College of Surgeons though this was not considered by other instrument makers, suitable for the purpose.

11. *A scalpel/bistoury with interchangeable heads. Quixall, c. 1800. 12·5 cm. (Castle Museum, York)*

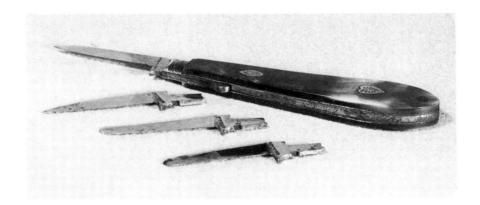

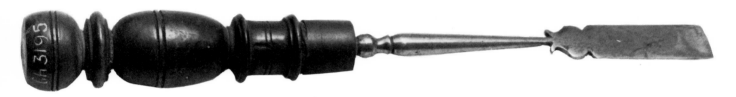

12. *A seventeenth-century chisel used for amputation. 38·5 cm. (Museum Boerhaave, Leiden)*

SCALPELS

The smaller surgical knife, the scalpel, used for incision and a multiplicity of purpose from dilating a wound to extracting foreign bodies, was known to the Romans as *scalpellus*, a small, light knife. Steel was the material used for the blades, though the finely worked handles were often silvered or gilt; sometimes the metal of the blade continued down between two plates which were screwed either side of it to form the handle, as is often done today. It will be seen that the range of scalpels varies little, apart from the Roman ploy of combining two instruments in one. The point of application as regards depth and angle of approach has obviously always necessitated difference in edge, size, point, and shape.

Handles of wood or bone appeared in the fourteenth century and John Wryghtson knew of a double-ended scalpel with a wooden handle between. In the sixteenth century the blades became more leaf-shaped and a hundred years later René-Jacques Garengeot (1688–1759) was again depicting a double-bladed instrument with only an ornate collar connecting the two. Fabricius shows a longer-bladed scalpel with an inside cutting edge and Heister's scalpel of 1740 has a scimitar blade. At the end of the eighteenth century the handles of wood or ivory became chequered to give a firmer grip, and terminated often in a spatula end. Nineteenth-century surgeons preferred shorter blades either

61

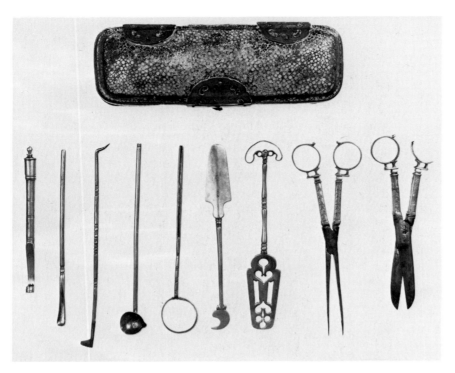

13. *Shagreen case and instruments, c. 1672.*
There is a drawer in the base of the case.
Length of case 12·7 cm.
(Royal College of Surgeons of England)

straight or only slightly curved. Handles were very thin and flat with tortoise-shell now frequently used. Double-bladed scalpels with two very fine blades parallel, such as that on pl. 10 (p. 160, Chapter 8), were devised by G. G. Valentin of Berne (1810–83).

BISTOURIES

A bistoury is a knife with a long cutting edge of uniform breadth. The blade may be straight or curved and the point blunt or sharp; it is for cutting the internal organs of the body and often only one section of the blade is sharp. Percivall Pott devised a curved and guarded bistoury for fistula-in-ano and many surgeons, notably Sir Astley Cooper, designed special hernia bistouries. These often had a concealed second blade for accuracy in fine cutting in a confined area.

Cased bistouries are often found with one or two spare blades, pointing to the necessity for extra sharpness.

14. *From top to bottom: two-edged saw, two early skull saws, bone brush, lithotome, probed knife, amputation fork for use in amputation of the breast, mid-eighteenth century.*
(Museum Boerhaave, Leiden)

62

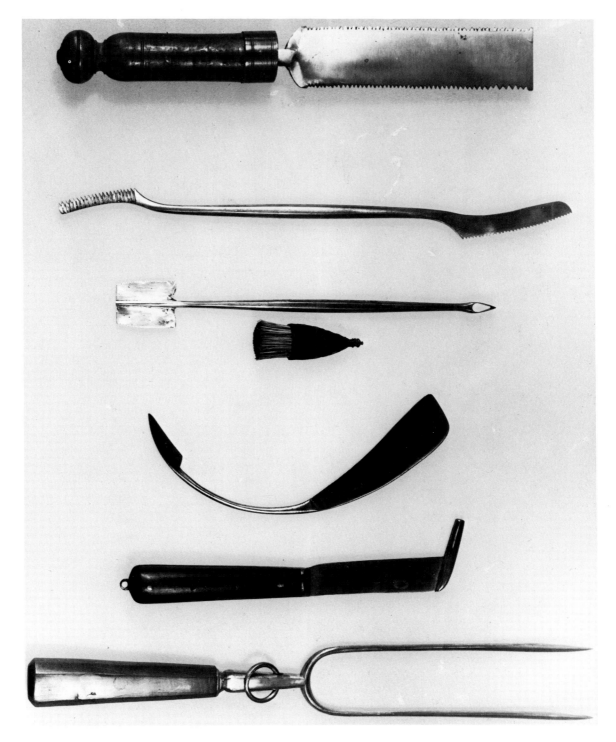

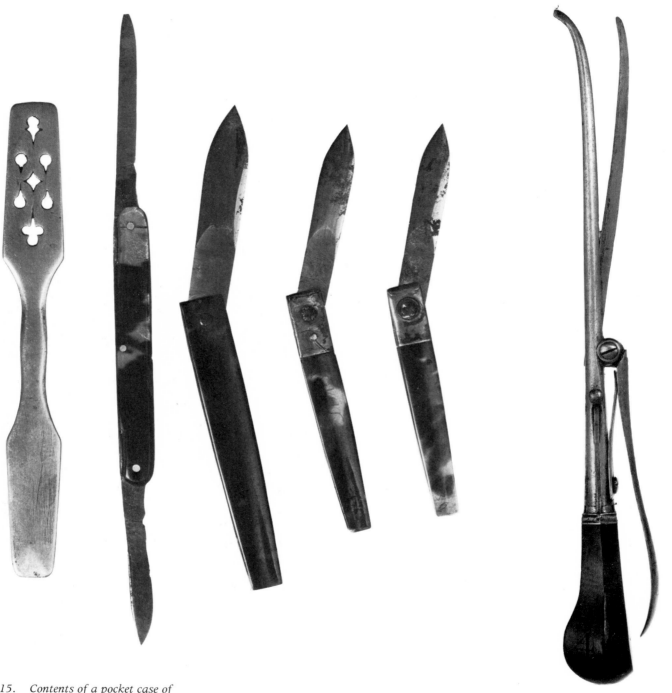

15.   Contents of a pocket case of
instruments, dated 1731.
(Royal College of Surgeons of England)

16.   Frère Côme's bistoury cache, c. 1760.
(Royal College of Surgeons of England)

Forceps

The forceps is one of the earliest known surgical instruments for which the original model was obviously the human hand when the thumb and index finger are used for gripping. Surgical forceps for different purposes have been found at Pompeii in which the alignment of the fine-toothed jaws cannot be excelled today, and the Danish Bronze Age people had toilet forceps or tweezers. Nowadays, surgical instrument makers manufacture over 1000 different forceps.

The term forceps appears to have been first applied to an instrument with long blades as distinct from those with short blades which were usually called pincers. Early medieval examples of omega-shape with a simple hoop and either fine-pointed or broad-bladed jaws were of bronze or silver, but few survive. The

17. Steel and ivory haemorrhoid forceps with rack, Hajek, c. 1840; Steel and ivory rectal dilator, c. 1780. 18 cm, 20·5 cm. (Simon Kaye Ltd, London)

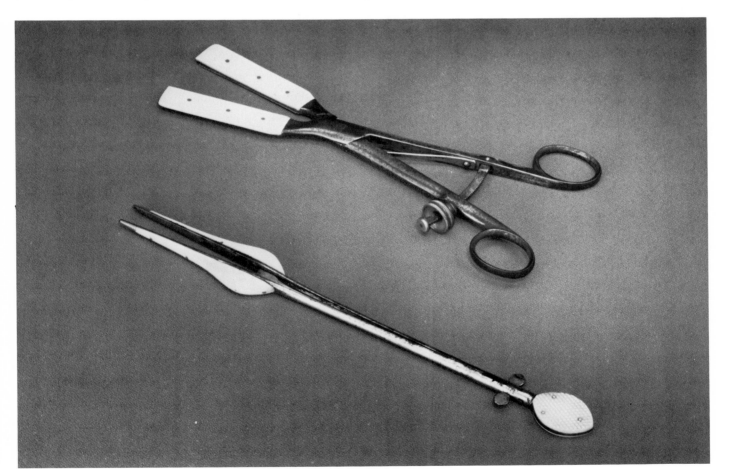

invention of printing meant that illustrated medical books became available and new instruments were easier to copy. Andreas della Croce (1500–1575) showed several new types, mostly of the tweezer variety for epilation, removing bandages or extracting fishbones from the throat, and a broad-bladed forceps with widely bent legs for fixing haemorrhoids (pl. 17). From Paris, in 1598, came Jacques Guillemeau's (1550–1613) forceps with finely-toothed jaws for use in trepanning. Ambroise Paré (Guillemeau's father-in-law) shows bullet forceps with curved blades and was the first to devise a type of haemostatic clamp to arrest haemorrhage which he called the *Bec de Corbin ou de Perroquet*, to be used instead of the pitch or boiling oil hitherto applied following an operation. This crows-bill had long serrated jaws and was held closed by various methods—sliding clamps, a rack, or spring-action. By the time of Scultetus (1595–1654) it was possible for him to describe fifteen different forceps including the 'deceitful' forceps 'for dilating hollow places'. Fabricius Hildanus (1560–1634) showed a forceps with spoon-shaped jaws for removing foreign bodies. There is a very heavy bone-holding forceps *c.* 1653 in the Prujean Collection at the Museum of London, each concave jaw containing three strong teeth (pl. 5; p. 277). Lorenz Heister (1683–1758) in Germany was the first to use bow-handles on forceps. These went out of fashion during the nineteenth century but returned *c.* 1870.

Juan Alexand Brambilla (1728–1800), a famous Austrian military surgeon, introduced many new types. Mostly with fine jaws for epilation, removing splinters, or ocular surgery, they all have flat wide legs and appeared in England *c.* 1780. They are undoubtedly those first invented by Baron de Wenzel (1728–1800).

In the eighteenth century came the first slot-slide needle-holding forceps, giving greater accuracy though later superseded by pincer type needle-holders. Jean-Louis Petit (1674–1760) introduced forceps of the double tenaculum type and Jean-Jacques Perret of Paris introduced the first spring forceps with crossed legs in 1771. The Savigny catalogue of 1798 shows spring cranium forceps, double-ended for large and small pieces. In the same catalogue the first of the bone fragment forceps appeared; they had short, thick jaws and a slot-slide hold for removing fragments of bone during an operation. Paolo Assalini (1759–1849) published a treatise in 1810 describing his forceps (pl. 17) of which one leg was attached to the handle and the other operated on a spring by the thumb. This remained very popular until the end of the nineteenth century when it was largely superseded by the double tenaculum-type. However, the greatest event in the history of the forceps was the

PLATE III

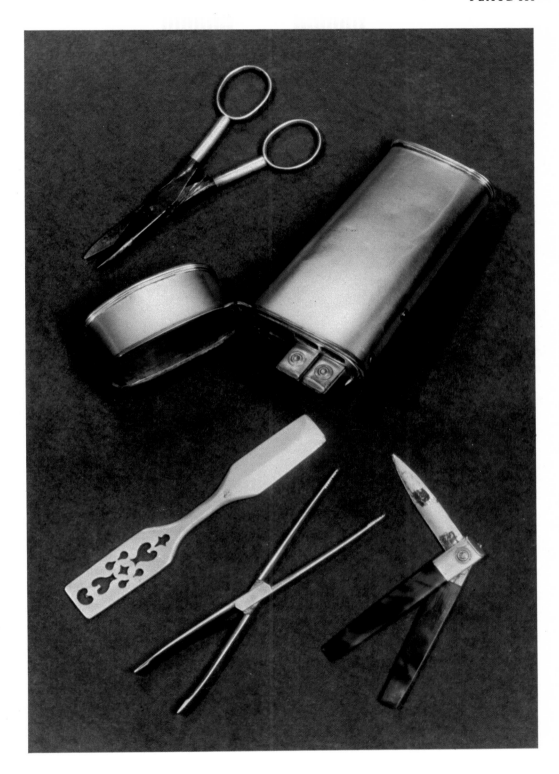

Silver etui containing three lancets, scissors, tweezers, spatula/tongue depressor and probe, c. 1750. Length of etui 13cm.
(Simon Kaye Ltd, London)

PLATE IV

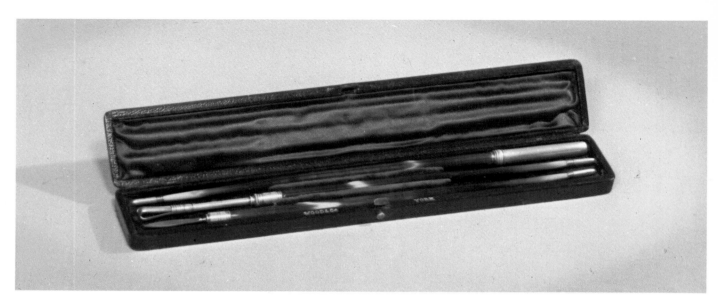

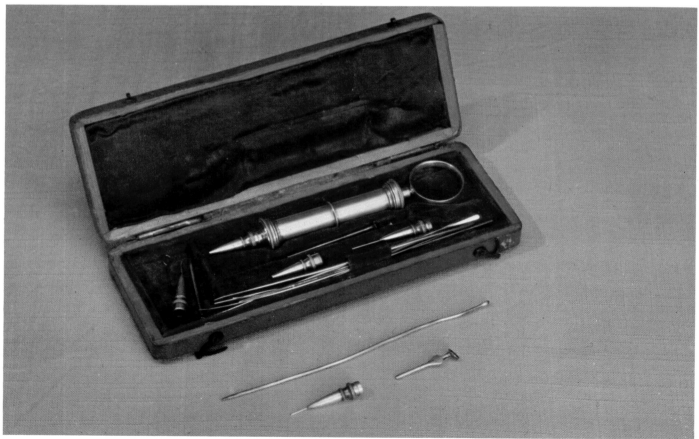

KNIVES, DIRECTORS AND FORCEPS

invention, *c.* 1840, of the cross-legged forceps by Joseph Frederic Charrière (1803–76) of Paris, which could act as a clamp and inaugurated a new era of artery forceps.

During the eighteenth century, there had been some reaction against ligatures and the use of forceps for bleeding arteries was preferred. P. J. Desault (1744–95), who is chiefly remembered for his introduction of the wire-snare or *écraseur* used in tongue excision, devised a method of placing the artery between two wooden palettes and compressing with cord. This was developed during the early nineteenth century by Percy and others, to produce many small compressors, mostly with a slot-slide grip. These went out of favour *c.* 1830 when Carl von Graefe (1787–1840)—the first to operate for cleft palate—introduced his artery forceps, which could be operated with one hand. These small instruments had tiny curved legs closed by their own resilience and opened by pressure on two discs, each attached to opposite legs by a small stem. Charrière's invention meant that his principle was applied to all types of forceps but most usefully to this artery forceps. In Germany it was called Dieffenbach's Bulldog forceps after J. F. Dieffenbach (1792–1847) of Berlin who introduced it there. The great advantage of this forceps was that the surgeon's hands were freed and a smaller number of assistants was needed to grip the blood vessels. Dieffenbach can be considered as the first practical plastic surgeon, and the children of Berlin sang a rhyme, of which a free translation has been made:

'Who knows not Dr Dieffenbach
The greatest doctor of today?
He, to make new ears and noses,
Cuts your arms and legs away.'

In 1848 Vidal de Cassis, a French surgeon, devised a variation of the Bulldog forceps looking much like a modern wire paper-clip, which became known as a *serre-fines* (once described to the writer as a seraphim).

Artery forceps differed from others in that they remained closed by some special device. Another of these invented by Charrière was the spring catch, a self-locking principle consisting of a small spring with knob, which engaged in a hole in the opposite leg when closed. Johann Fricke (1790–1841) devised a locking system with a pin running in a slot in one leg and engaging in the pin of the other.

Artery forceps of the tenaculum variety, in addition to Assalini's

Colour plate
Above: Cased set of porcupine quill and silver uterine instruments containing caustic-holder, swab-holder and curette, c. 1870, Wood, York. Length of case 25 cm.

Below: Cased ophthalmic syringe and probes similar to those of Dominique Anel, c. 1800. Case 12·7 cm by 5 cm.
(Simon Kaye Ltd, London)

18. *A group of forceps, clockwise: Assalini type, c. 1810, Weiss; harelip forceps as Thomas S. Smith c. 1870; Mayer-Meltzer tweezers, c. 1850; cranium forceps, c. 1820, Weiss; fenestrated forceps, c. 1850; combined torsion and suture-holding forceps, c. 1870, Wright. 10 cm. 12·5 cm, 10 cm, 12·5 cm, 10 cm, 10 cm.*
(Simon Kaye Ltd, London)

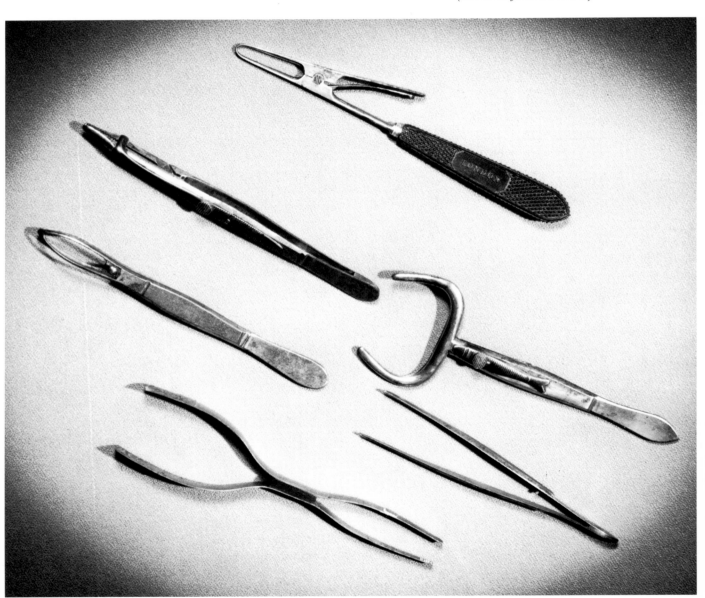

already mentioned, were those of Weir in 1820 which had a ring-slide, and of Karl Hueter (1838–82) in 1860 which were cross-legged. The latter were said to be used for circumcision and a wide variety of operations requiring suturing; they could be used as ligature-holders but had no wide popularity as excellent tenacula with a needle eye were then available. In 1847 a further advance was made with a torsion forceps with a spring catch, devised by Robert Liston, and in 1855 Thomas Wakley, son of the founder of *The Lancet*, introduced his fenestrated spring forceps (pl. 18); William Taylor's self-holding forceps followed in 1866.

Hare-lip operations were first described by Paré and have been performed frequently since, to achieve the perfection of today. Hiester in his *Chirurgeria* first describes special forceps for the operation. However, he records seeing an operation for hare-lip in Amsterdam performed on a child of 2 with 'a good pair of scissors and three crooked needles'. An identical method is described by Samuel Mihles in 1764. By the nineteenth century forceps were shown in most catalogues, firstly with long jaws at right angles to the legs, and later of the type designed by Thomas Southwood Smith (1788–1861). These appeared in the Maw catalogue of 1868 and are shown in pl. 18 looking like an old-fashioned mole-trap.

The use of the setaceum was an old form of treatment, the object of which was to form a fistula under the skin which was kept in a constant state of suppuration by the insertion of a foreign body—the whole operation to cause a counter-irritant and act as an outlet for foreign matter. It was first used in the twelth century, and by the sixteenth century special forceps were being used by Paré and others. They were flat-jawed instruments with hooped legs and a hole in each jaw through which a needle might pass. The legs were held either by a ring-slide, in the version by Ferrara, a Milanese surgeon, or by a screw in those by Petit and Magni. The setaceum or seton was much advised by Richard Wiseman (1622–76) and was fully described by William Salmon in 1699 in this way. 'Take up the skin with a perforated pair of forceps, nip it pretty hard to stultify it. Through the perforations of the forceps and the skin pass a needle red hot after which, with another needle, bring through the silken string or cord. Afterwards let the string be drawn every day sometimes to this side, sometimes to that, that the mattery part may hang out of the wound; the ulcer is thus kept open, as long as the need requires.' This treatment was an extension of the practice of deliberately keeping wounds open for the exit of 'laudable pus', based on the theory first derived from Galen and which lasted until Lister (pls. 19–22).

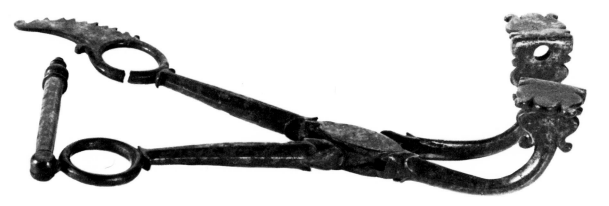

19. *Setaceum forceps as those of Scultetus,*
1672. 14 cm.
(Musée le Secq des Tournelles, Rouen)

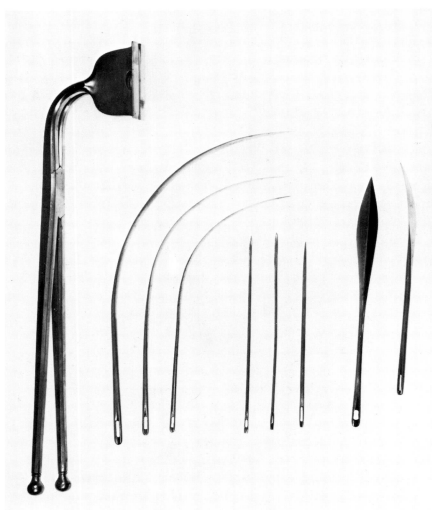

20. *Setaceum forceps and sutures, c. 1770.*
(Musée d'Histoire de la Médecine, Paris;
Cliché Assistance Publique)

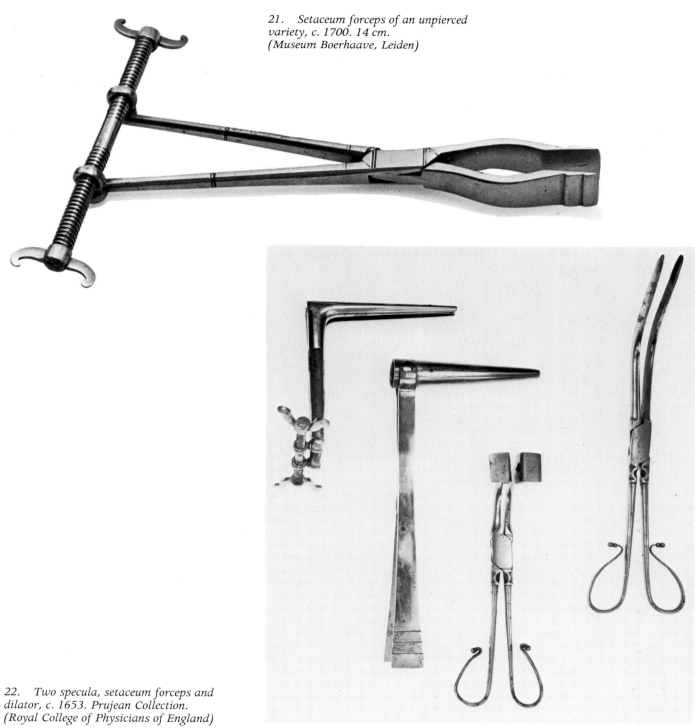

21.   *Setaceum forceps of an unpierced*
variety, c. 1700. 14 cm.
(Museum Boerhaave, Leiden)

22.   *Two specula, setaceum forceps and*
dilator, c. 1653. Prujean Collection.
(Royal College of Physicians of England)

By the nineteenth century treatment by setaceum became obsolete except for veterinary use (see Chaper 10) and setaceum forceps disappeared from the instrument makers' lists. Interesting examples are those illustrated by John Woodall and the one from the Prujean Collection (pl. 22).

As a general dating principle for forceps, the following may be of help:

Ring-slide and slot-slide dating back to 800 B.C.;
Screw-close on seventeenth-century forceps;
Charrière's spring-catch c. 1830;
Fricke's catch c. 1840;
Charrière's cross-legged forceps c. 1840.

23. *From left: aneurysm needle, c. 1840; surgical scissors, 1808, Eley Fearn and Chawner; two sutures, c. 1840; director and probe, c. 1860, Ferris, Bristol; early spatula and scoop, c. 1730; director and scoop, 1848, G. Clements (all silver). Needle 11·5 cm, scissors 15·2 cm. (Simon Kaye Ltd, London)*

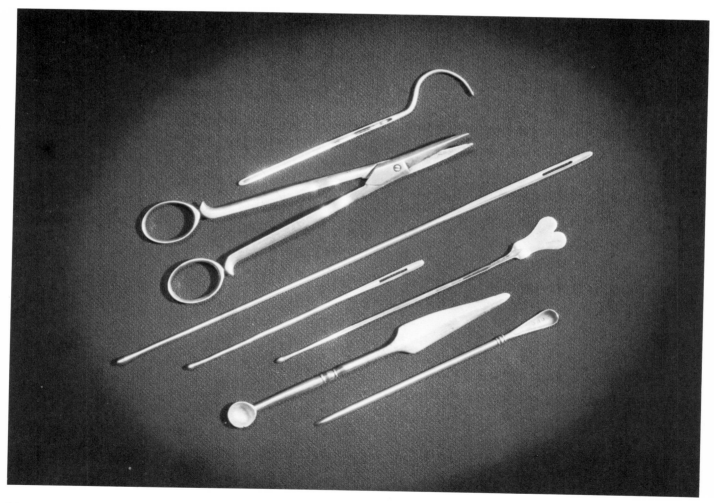

Surgical scissors

As we know them today, scissors are a comparatively modern instrument, the Romans and other ancient civilisations having used a proximal spring joint such as we have on sugar tongs. Scissors used for surgical rather than other purposes appear in seventeenth and eighteenth-century medical etuis, although those found separately are difficult to distinguish as such. In general the blades are shorter and certainly finer than general purpose scissors, although who is to say that any that performed the required function might not have been used? They were mostly silver with silver or steel blades (pl. 23). Left-handed examples have even been found. Dressing scissors with the blades at an angle of about 45° were not much used before the nineteenth century. Scissors used as an alternative to the scalpel and popularised at the Mayo Clinic in America do not come within the confines of this book.

Directors, probes, and sutures

Surgical directors, probes, and scoops, usually silver, date from the seventeenth century at least, and were often combined. Instruments of this type of combination were made by the Romans. They made a typical arrowhead spatula with probe or scoop at the other end which was used here, practically unchanged, through the eighteenth century (pl. 23). With a limited knowledge of anatomy and without the benefit of X-rays, much probing of wounds was done. In gunshot wounds it was particularly convenient to have the probe combined with a director so that the knife might reach the bullet as accurately as possible. These vary in length from 10·2 to 17·8 cm and have a fairly deep directing groove ending 2·5 cm from the probe head. Other directors end in a small scoop for cleaning foreign matter from the wound before and after surgery. These are comparatively delicate instruments and should not be confused with the very tough-looking steel bone gauges that were made in the nineteenth century. Hernia directors by the early nineteenth century, were wide and curved with a flat, serrated silver handle. From around 1800 aneurysm needles were made with a directing channel in the main, short shaft.

Probes were combined with sutures as well as directors and varied from the fine small ones in the etui in col. pl. III to the long ones, such as those on pl. 23, which were made of varying thickness and had a straight groove to carry the wire. In the nineteenth century there was a movement towards more flexible probes and they were made of finer silver and sometimes of whalebone.

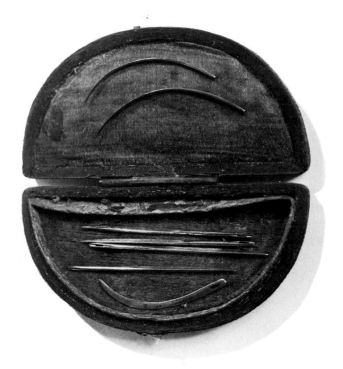

24. *Fishskin suture case, velvet-lined,*
c. 1800. Width of case 7·6 cm.
(Strangers' Hall Museum, Norwich)

Suturing of the outer layers of skin was mostly carried out with ordinary sewing needles though from the late eighteenth century one can find curved specialist needles in most large cases of instruments. Occasionally, too, there are small semi-circular needle cases found (pl. 24). Shrimpton and Fletcher were making ranges of suture needles from 1830 but those with a cutting edge did not appear until *c.* 1870.

CHAPTER FOUR

Lithotomy and urethrotomy instruments

'Urinary calculi vary exceedingly in their size, form, and tenacity. Some calculi do not equal a millet seed in size, while some have been found so large as to fill the entire cavity of the bladder. Mr Earle has described a very large stone which has been extracted but with a fatal result, by the celebrated Cheselden. Its weight was $18\frac{1}{2}$ oz. Circumference in the large axis was $11\frac{1}{4}$ in, in its short axis 10 in. Dr Charles Preston relates in the *Philosophical Transactions*, that he saw, at La Charité in Paris, a stone which weighed 51 oz. The patient died under the hands of the operator.'

So said the *Cyclopaedia of Practical Medicine* in 1833. The modern reader is not so much amazed that the patient died under operation but that he had not died previously. As a result of their poor and monotonous diet, our ancestors appear to have suffered from bladder stones to a far greater degree than we do today, so it is not surprising that it was one of the first conditions they tried to alleviate. Urate calculi have been found as old as 7000 years. For many centuries amputation and stone removal were the only operations from which one might, with luck, hope to recover. The Greek surgeon, Ammonius, crushed stones in the incised bladder with a blunt-ended instrument pressed against a hooked one— rather like a nineteenth-century bullet extractor. The Arabs described the breaking of calculi with a diamond-tipped probe, which they apparently demonstrated to Alexander the Great.

However, Hippocrates (460–375 B.C.), in the Oath, banned cutting for stone; the reason is not clear but possibly he did not wish his disciples to follow a practice of high mortality. The Romans advanced the study considerably. Pliny the Elder advised stone-sufferers to take infusions of peony-seed and the waters of an island near Sorrento. Both male and female catheters were known, as well as lithotrites. Many urological complaints were recognised as can be seen from the terracotta votive offerings that have been found. The first double-curved catheter made of bronze comes from the House of the Surgeon in Pompeii—an instrument not made again until Petit's, 1600 years later. Salerno was important in the study of

75

lithotomy, both under the Romans and in the ninth century when the medical school was founded.

As we know it, the catheter was first introduced c. 1100. John of Gaddesden (1280–1361), Prebendary of St Pauls and Physician to Edward II, is believed to have been the first to employ forceps in removing stone, Guy de Chauliac (1300–1367) required for lithotomy a razor, a large hollow hook, long forceps, thread, needles, cotton, linen, eggs, and red powder. The best age for lithotomy, he thought, was 14 years, and the best seasons were spring and autumn. He did not advise operating on apprehensive or complaining patients, 'And if serious complications develop, may God help us'. An enormous debt was owed to the anatomical studies of Leonardo da Vinci, and Ambroise Paré was so interested in anatomy that he kept an embalmed body in the house to study before an operation. François Roussel, in 1581, described the extraction of bladder stone by incision through the bladder-wall and a story is told of a blacksmith c. 1660 who performed the operation of perineal lithotomy on himself and successfully extracted a stone larger than a hen's egg, weighing 4 oz with no other instruments than a common knife and his fingers—a deed which may well compare with the most valiant in history.

From all the foregoing it can be seen that perseverance on the part of the surgeon and great courage on the part of the patient resulted in an early advance in lithotomy methods. Undoubtedly the excruciating pain of the condition alone could have resulted in consent to the operation, but the few successful cases must have encouraged others. Pepys's experiences are mentioned in Chapter 14, but it is worth recording that although he lived to give thanks for a successful outcome, he was given an unintentional vasectomy at the same time, apparently not an unusual occurrence. Queen Caroline, consort to George II, when operated upon for stone, bravely cried out in the middle of the proceedings not to spare her because she was a queen but to cut deeper if they felt the necessity. Speed, as with all operations, was of the essence—thus preventing much dexterity or delicacy of touch.

James Syme (1799–1870), Professor of Surgery at Edinburgh, used to practise by sharpening pencils and by shaving with his left hand. A French surgeon used to walk to and from his hospital carrying a lithotrite in his left hand, picking nuts out of his pocket with it, to keep his fingers in practise. The precise nature of bladder stones is not often understood by those unfamiliar with them, and those imagining a piece of chalky substance should visit the Hunterian Museum at The Royal College of Surgeons—there they

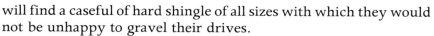

will find a caseful of hard shingle of all sizes with which they would not be unhappy to gravel their drives.

A patient of 1811 described his operation for stone in this way: 'My habit and constitution being good, it required little preparation of body and my mind was made up . . . I was prepared to receive shock of pain of extreme violence and so much had I overrated it, that the first incision did not even make me wince . . . The forcing up of the staff prior to the introduction of the gorget gave me the first real pain.' The operation was thought to have lasted 10–12 minutes. 'With respect to the pain, I am persuaded that if it were possible to concentrate what I have often suffered in one night into the same space of time it would have been less endurable . . . Upon the whole, should I be again similarly afflicted I should not hesitate in again submitting myself to the same mode of relief, provided I could place myself in equally capable hands.'

Catheters

The Roman catheter was introduced into the urethra with a plug of wool at the end, attached to a thread. When it was firmly in the neck of the bladder, the wool was extracted and the urine followed as with a syphon. Paré, who would appear to be the first to inject caustic by means of a catheter, had his made curved for a considerable part of their length. He used wax candles and tapers lubricated with astringent ointment and lead sounds smeared with quicksilver 'and kept in day and night as long as the patient can endure'. Fabricius described catheters of silver, copper, and brass, though he preferred horn. Another, he wrote, was of cloth impregnated with wax and mounted on silver. Turquet de Mayerne (1573–1655), Physician to James I, passed bougies of wax or horn of increasing size and then rigid catheters of pewter or lead before applying caustic. It is small wonder that it was often difficult to obtain the patient's consent. In 1640, Covillard recommended catheters of rushes, wax, or lead, and Garengeot (1688–1759) illustrated a catheter traversed by a metal wire ending in a small button which filled the orifice during introduction.

Experiments with flexible catheters were made at the end of the seventeenth century (pl. 1), sometimes covered in parchment to prevent tearing of the mucous membrane, but most surgeons used a

1. *Cornelius Solingen's flexible spiral catheter, 1706. 30·5 cm.*
(Royal College of Surgeons of England)

77

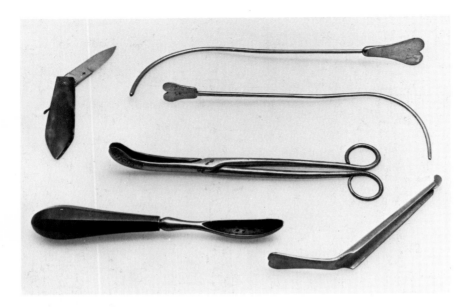

2. *Early eighteenth-century lithotomy instruments: lithotome, probes, stone forceps, scoop, and gorget.*
(Museum Boerhaave, Leiden)

rigid silver one. After the introduction of rubber in 1735, a jeweller named Bernard invented a rubber-covered catheter, but it was very unsatisfactory as it was sticky in hot weather and had no elasticity when cold: flexible rubber catheters were not successful until Dominique Larrey (see Chapter 3) used them in 1812. In 1831 John Weiss introduced his first flexible metal catheter. This was of finely overlapping and jointed sections which makes one fear for pinching of the urethra.

Throughout the eighteenth century catheters were almost entirely of silver, and not until *c.* 1840 did they appear of silver-plate or steel. Nevertheless, Robert Liston, writing in 1846 in his *Practical Surgery*, says, 'Some practitioners have carried fashion so far that many even of the catheters and sounds are to be found fitted with wooden handles, chequered and grooved.' Liston insisted that the handles of all instruments, where delicacy of touch was necessary, should be perfectly smooth. It is manifest, however, that only where catheters were concerned, did many agree with him.

Naturally, catheters were made in different sizes, though cased sets of three to twelve are only mid-Victorian. It is interesting to note that although varying sized male catheters are found from the early eighteenth century, the female urethra was apparently thought to be of uniform size, and the entirely straight form for females only became slightly curved by about 1830 (pl. 3). Catheters, both male and female, are among the most commonly found instruments and those in silver are often fully hallmarked.

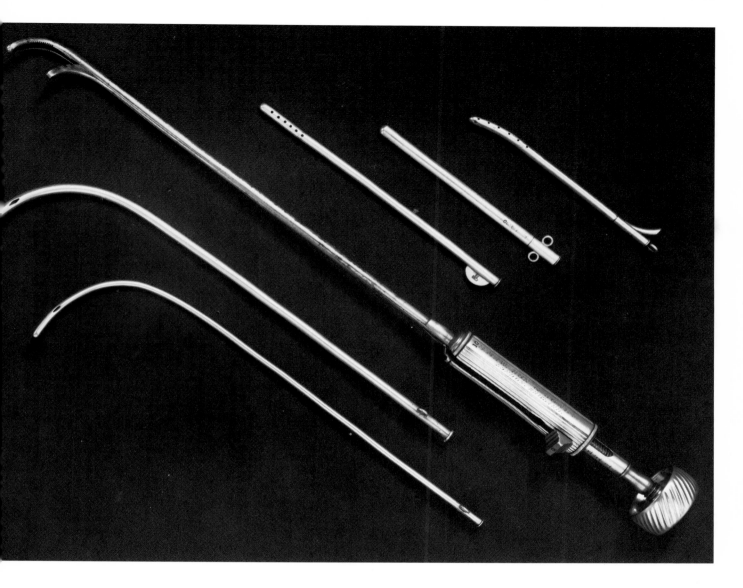

3. *From left: two male catheters in silver, 1836, G. Clement, and 1842, George Adam; a lithotrite, silver handle, c. 1860, Maw; three female catheters, c. 1790 Charles Watts, c. 1830; and double channel c. 1860. Lithotrite 35·5 cm.*
(Simon Kaye Ltd, London)

By 1823 Jean Amussat (1796–1856) had shown that the male urethra was not right angled and that its curves could be straightened. He introduced a straight male catheter but it was not popular and in 1854 Gely of Nantes said that the curve of the urethra was much larger than had been thought and catheters were made with a huge curve; after this, rubber catheters were being produced more satisfactorily and the curve became less necessary.

Much favoured were catheters with two eyes, and these were widely used until *c.* 1860. The caustic used in cases of urethral stricture and ulcers was usually silver nitrate, as recommended by John Hunter and others; Wakley's caustic potash produced complications and the method was discarded. Those with one eye at the end of the neck were for applying caustic at the neck of the bladder. Double-channel varieties (pl. 3) were for injecting the bladder in a continuous stream and had a stopcock on a chain attached to the end—now usually missing. Others were of the forcing-rod, or probe, type. The Prujean Collection includes some of this type with a firm T-shaped handle, the sound well-curved and deeply grooved. Nineteenth-century examples had a measure in inches at the base to show how far penetration of the urethra had been achieved. A very rare and unusual catheter was found recently that might be described as trans-sexual. It unscrews into parts to adjust the length, and has an interchangeable male or female end according to the patient; it is in silver and dates from *c.* 1850.

In 1836, a urethrometer was invented in Bordeaux, consisting of strips of metal which expanded when released in the urethra—the prototype of an instrument much copied later.

CATHETER GAUGES

Victorian gauges in silver or silver-plate might often pass the collector by unnoticed. They are of two types. The first is a plate approximately 10 by 6·5 cm, pierced by a series of holes, inscribed with numbers. These are not unlike what used to be sold as a knitting-needle gauge, and would have gauged the size of a particular catheter. The second kind, which fairly brings tears to the eyes, is a graduated silver probe inscribed with numbers at intervals, and would have been inserted into the urethra to decide the size of the catheter needed.

Lithotrites and other stone-extracting and crushing instruments

Bartolomeo Senarega (d. 1514) recorded in 1510, a surgeon removing stones 'as big as an egg' with 'a slender iron instrument with another instrument twisted into a hook to remove the stone'. The presence of the calculus would first have been proved with a sound; a grooved sound would then have been introduced and a broad knife would have cut down the groove. Two conductores or directors might then be inserted into the open wound preparatory to the passage of the dilator. Forceps could now be introduced to grasp the stone, great care being taken not to crush it. Paré shows a complicated instrument with a rack between the handles for

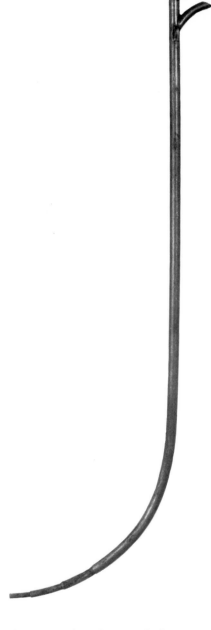

4. *Telescopic male catheter, Whicker & Blaise, c. 1856. 25·5 cm. (Royal College of Surgeons of England)*

80

extracting stone, but did not perform the operation himself. Fabricius (1560–1634) claimed to have invented many instruments for lithotomy, principally a four-pronged dilator, showing his ingenuity. Covillard, in the seventeenth century advised crushing by forceps and removing the pieces with spoon and curette.

The year 1697 marked the arrival in Paris of the most spectacular figure in the history of lithotomy, Frère Jacques (1651–1714). He does not appear to have been a member of any religious order but assumed the monks' habit and made a living as an itinerant lithotomist. His method was to use an ungrooved sound and a long wide bistoury before introducing the forceps. He devised a cutting forceps with a knife-blade between the jaws, a four-bladed forceps, and the fondamental. He had considerable success in Paris, but when 25 out of 60 patients died he was forbidden to operate. Later, the authorities relented on condition that he used a modified method. In 1703 the Marechal de Lorges summoned 22 patients to his mansion and watched Frère Jacques operate on them. Each operation was successful so the Marechal underwent it himself— and died. The Hague presented Frère Jacques with two gold sounds to mark his work in lithotomy—one of the first known instances of presentation instruments.

William Cheselden (1688–1752) was the surgeon in this country chiefly responsible for building on Frère Jacques's experience and advancing lithotomy here. He had a special interest in operations for stone as his Master, Ferne, held a licence for the work at St Thomas' Hospital. He was called to account by the Barber–Surgeons in 1714 for dissecting malefactors in his own house without permission, but in 1723 he achieved respectability by publishing his *Treatise of High Operation for Stone*. His speciality was in having reduced the time required to extract stone from one hour to less than one minute and was based on Frère Jacques's method. It became famous throughout Europe and has hardly been improved upon today; his fee for stone extraction was £500. Cheselden was surgeon to Caroline of Anspach and did much to make the profession acceptable. A man of many talents, he designed the original Fulham bridge in 1729.

Many strange instruments were devised to extract stone and ensure that no part of it was left in the bladder. Some had a kind of fishing net attached to forceps or an ox-bladder on guides. There was a curious Danish invention, like a sling on whalebone, but it was probably only an experiment and not used.

In 1819, John Elderton described a two-bladed instrument for crushing stones or filing them away if too hard. 1822 saw the introduction of Sir Astley Cooper's stone-holding forceps which

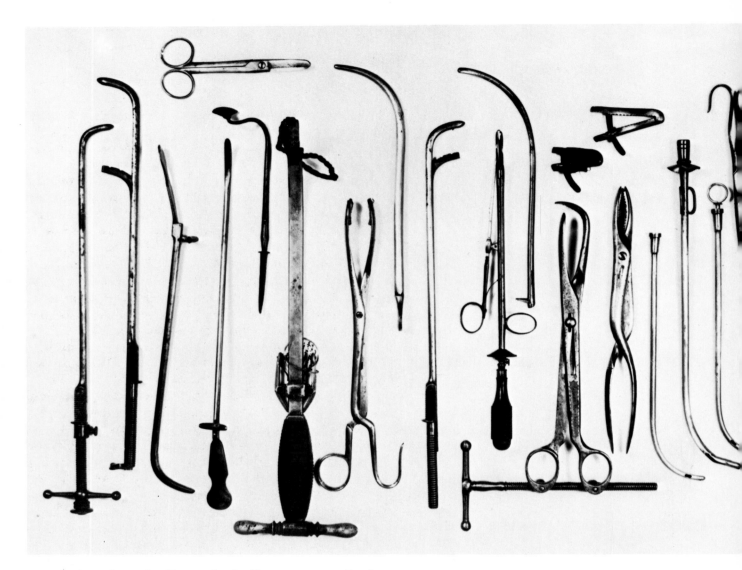

was designed on the lines of a bullet extractor. In the same year Leroy d'Etoilles (1798–1860) devised a drilling-type instrument with a basket cage for grasping the stone; it had retractable claws curving inwards towards a fixed blade. All through the early nineteenth century great strides were made in the study of lithotomy in France and by 1823 a stone was successfully crushed *in situ*. By 1853 both Robert Liston and Sir William Ferguson were experimenting with a rack and piston type lithotrite.

Although there is mention of lithotrites even by the Romans, a screw lithotrite for extraction was introduced by John Weiss in

1831 in terms which suggest that it was very *avant-garde*. He took the opportunity of cautioning the profession against plagiarism by instrument makers. His name, he said, had been forged upon spurious items in England, Ireland, and America, and only instruments bought direct from Weiss or his agents could be depended upon. This gives an insight into the good name and reputation the firm must have enjoyed, but uncovers an impossible trap for the collector, the copied pieces presumably being alike in appearance and contemporary in date.

The screw lithotrite was much like a split catheter, the two inner lips of the split having teeth. After drawing off the water from the bladder 'the better to grasp and confine the stone', the lithotrite, obviating the need for cutting, might be inserted and the jaws opened to the required size of the stone by means of the screw handle. They could then be locked by a slide-lock and the stone extracted. A beautiful precision-made example by Maw is in pl. 3. The silver handle is fluted and embellished, and it will be seen that it is sized and numbered. This instrument was also used to crush the stone while still in the bladder, and the quality of the workmanship suggests that it was well up to the task. This is undoubtedly an example of the screw lithotrite invented by Sir Henry Thompson in 1860 which has remained the prototype for this type of instrument. There was another variation for dealing with the problem of stones too large to extract which took the form of a lithotrite with a fine saw between the jaws, operated by a lever in the handle.

Many mid-century lithotrites have screws of such complexity that their use must have entailed much practice. One interesting example was introduced by Sir William Ferguson (1808–77) who was Professor of Surgery at King's College and Surgeon to Queen Victoria. This needed a key to be inserted into the main screw shaft to lock it. For a man who was known to use singularly few instruments for an operation, this seems complicated. However, it was said of him that he had 'the eagle's eye, the lion's heart, and the lady's hand', so perhaps these qualities combined to deal with it. For soft calculi, a different type of instrument was evolved; on insertion into the bladder, three claws were released from the end of the instrument which, on grasping the stone, were pulled back until they held it tight and the lithotrite was then withdrawn. Sir Astley Cooper (1768–1841), of St Thomas's and Guy's, and Surgeon to King George IV, introduced yet another variation; the handle was attached at an angle of 45° and a lever working on a rack held the split jaw.

Two other instruments expressly for crushing stones are in the

5. A group of early nineteenth-century lithotomy instruments. (Pitt Rivers Museum, Oxford)

Maw 1868 catalogue. One is a fairly crude device, presumably like that of Ammonius, consisting of a long piece of metal, spoon-ended with the bowl serrated. Attached to this is a threaded slot through which passes a pointed screw with handle, to be screwed down on to the bowl. The second is in the form of serrated beaked forceps, the two ring handles of which are connected by a screw which therefore forces them together and the jaws of the forceps likewise.

An instrument for extracting foreign bodies from the urethra—possibly fragments of calculi that have not been completely passed—was introduced in France by Leroy d'Etoilles and made in this country by Maw at least. It is quite straight, as an early female catheter, and has a small perforated head at a slight angle. Presumably a slight vacuum could be produced in the end by withdrawing the inner tube and any extraneous matter adhered to it by suction.

Lithotomy forceps have generally had strongly serrated and slightly concave jaws, one ring handle for the thumb and an open loop for the fingers. However, the seventeenth-century Prujean Collection has several with two bent-back ring handles and the firm jaws folding one slightly over the other (pl. 6). Lithotomy scoops, again, were boldly made and this set includes an interesting one with a hook for the finger at the base of the handle. Later scoops, such as Erichson's, appeared in the nineteenth century and took the form of an open oval loop of metal.

Lithotomes and other lithotomy knives

Generally speaking, knives used in lithotomy were about 15 cm long with a short, strong blade and a reinforced spine which curved forward to the base of the cutting edge and, at the tip, formed an extra guarded point. However, there were many variations. Claude Nicholas le Cat (1700–1768) invented several instruments including an urethrotome, a knife, with a short, thick blade which was grooved to take a second knife, the cystotome, a thick blade with a curved cutting edge. William Cheselden had a lithotome with a short scimitar-shaped blade. About 1730, the lithotome cache with a retractable blade was introduced. In 1748 came a lithotome 24 cm long, very like the curved bistoury with concealed blade used in operating for hernia. The origin of the lithotome cache is the subject of some dispute. A bistoury with hidden blade had been invented much earlier, but this was the first time it had been applied to lithotomy.

6. *Lithotomy forceps and scoops, c. 1653.*
Prujean Collection.
(Royal College of Physicians of England)

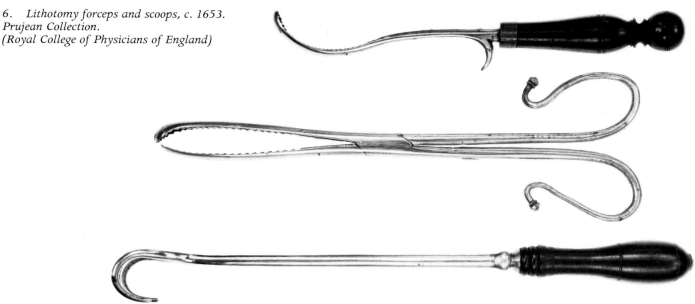

In the second quarter of the eighteenth century, gorgets were introduced; semi-tubes for the passage of the lithotome. John Caesar Hawkins of St George's Hospital and surgeon to George II invented a cutting gorget with one sharp edge in 1753, which speeded the operation considerably. In the later eighteenth century, many new instruments were invented which only served to make things more complicated. Dupuy of Bordeaux used a thin knife inside a catheter (pl. 7), and in other cases, catheters were fitted with a cutting edge. A more practical invention was a toothed bar in a forceps to keep the blades from closing once the stone was grasped.

Neil Arnott (1788–1874), the inventor of the water bed, performed a novel operation for stricture on the Captain of a boat to China, and later designed two instruments for the purpose with retractable blades. By *c.* 1825 several surgeons were devising lithotomes with blades that cut forwards from behind.

Urethrotomes, for the splitting of strictures, known on the Continent from the sixteenth century, are more difficult to identify. The first description of puncture for urethral strictures was by François Tolet (1651–1724) in 1686, who used a strong trocar and tapering cannula with a fine, double-edged bistoury. Frère Côme's (1703–81) *soude à dard* of *c.* 1750 took the form of an open-ended male catheter with two ring handles which carried a very sharp, curved trocar. Leeches were often used as a form of treatment for stricture and were introduced on the end of a leech tube.

85

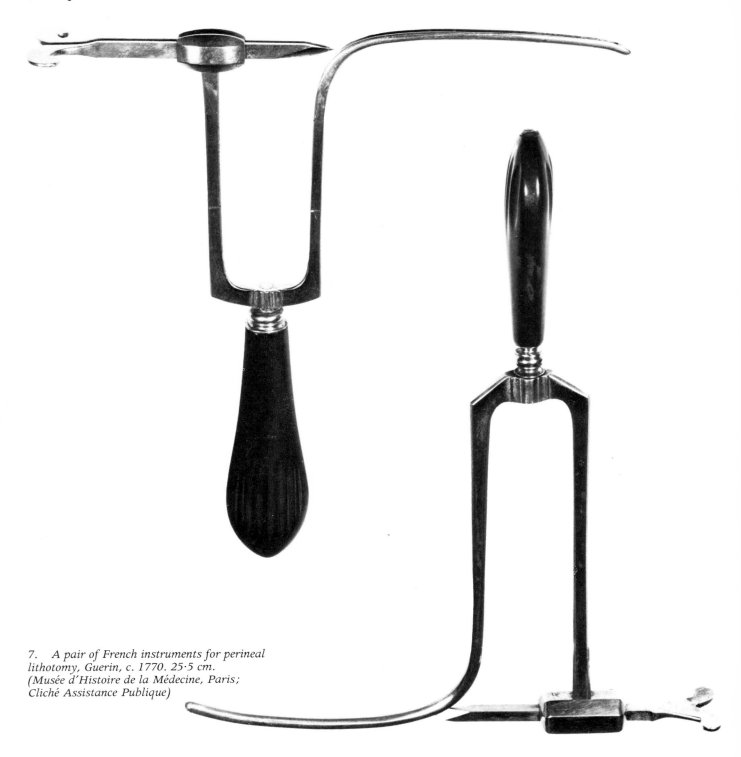

7.   *A pair of French instruments for perineal
lithotomy, Guerin, c. 1770. 25·5 cm.
(Musée d'Histoire de la Médecine, Paris;
Cliché Assistance Publique)*

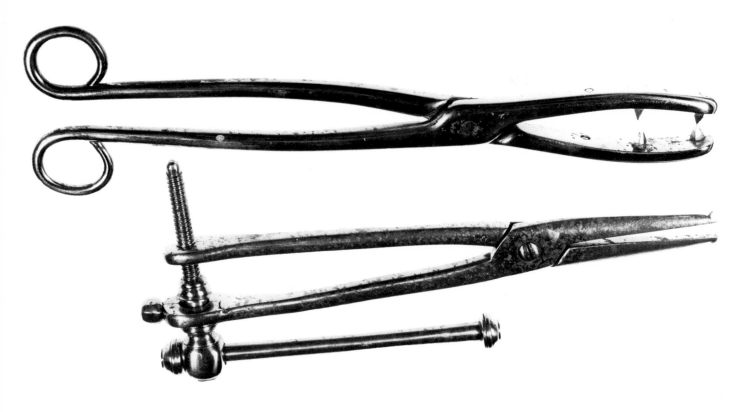

8.   Claude-Nicholas le Cat's stone
extractors, c. 1750.
*(Musée d'Histoire de la Médecine, Paris;
Cliché Assistance Publique)*

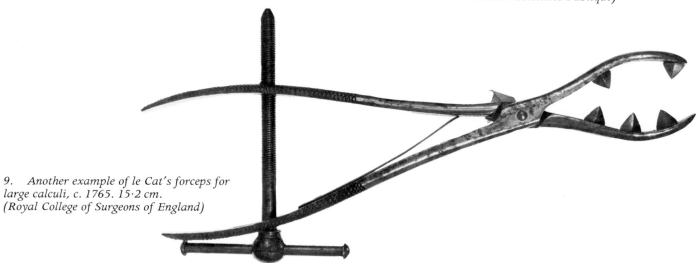

9.   Another example of le Cat's forceps for
large calculi, c. 1765. 15·2 cm.
(Royal College of Surgeons of England)

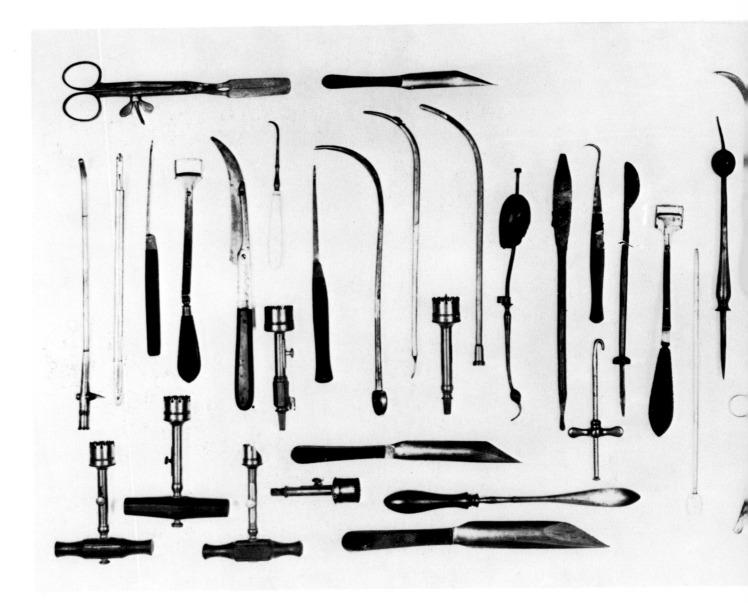

10. *A group of early nineteenth-century instruments, mostly for trepannation and lithotomy. Top left is a haemorrhoid forceps.*
(Pitt Rivers Museum, Oxford)

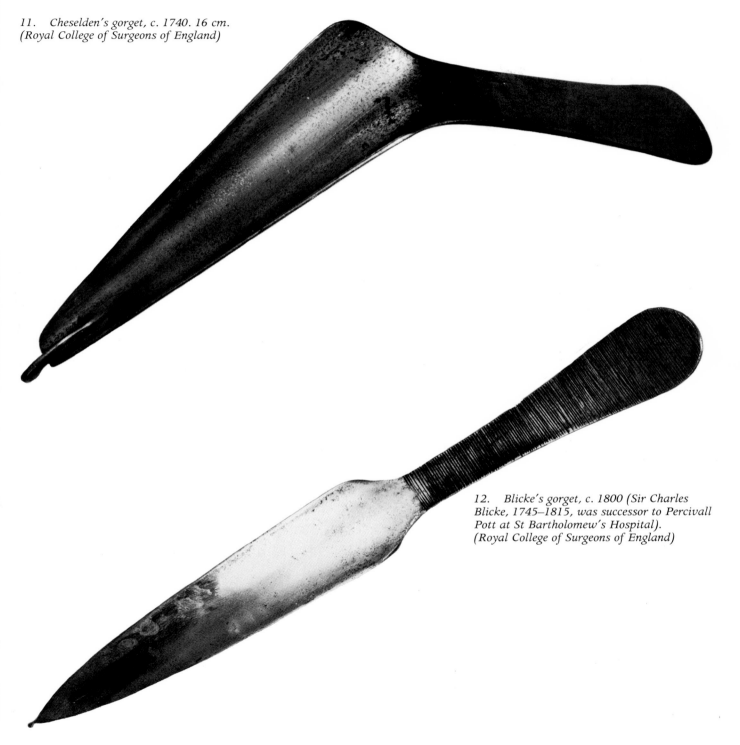

11. Cheselden's gorget, c. 1740. 16 cm.
(Royal College of Surgeons of England)

12. Blicke's gorget, c. 1800 (Sir Charles
Blicke, 1745–1815, was successor to Percivall
Pott at St Bartholomew's Hospital).
(Royal College of Surgeons of England)

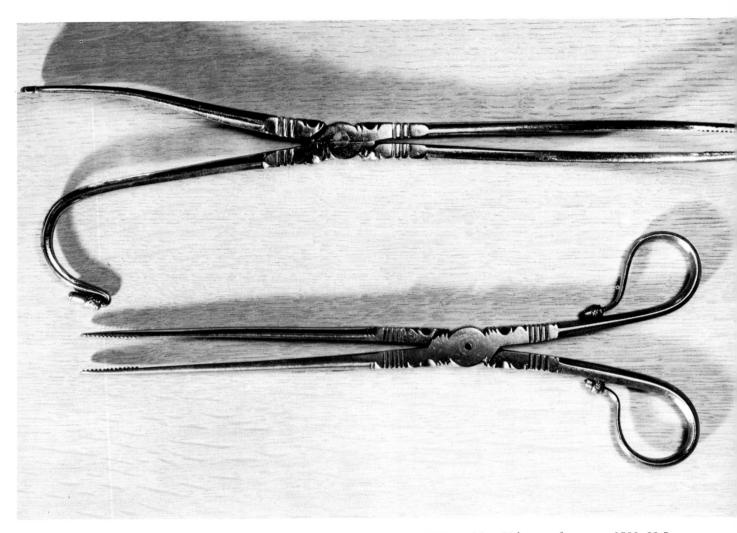

13. *Lithotomy forceps, c. 1580. 38·5 cm.
(Germanisches Nationalmuseum, Nuremberg)*

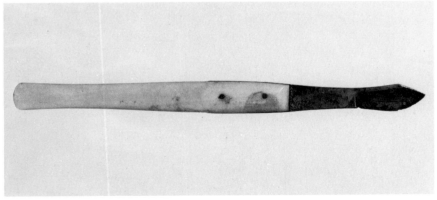

14. *Cheselden's short convex lithotomy
knife, c. 1750. 12·5 cm. (Presented to the
College by Robert Liston, who used it.)
(Royal College of Surgeons of England)*

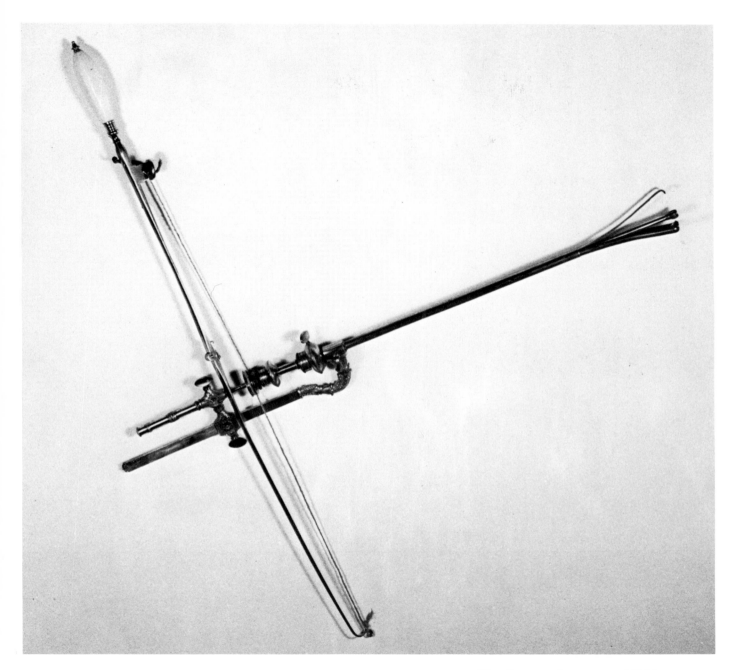

15. Bow type instrument of 1826 to remove
stone by drilling; the drill was pushed
forward by bow. 30·4 cm.
(Museum of Historical Medicine,
Copenhagen)

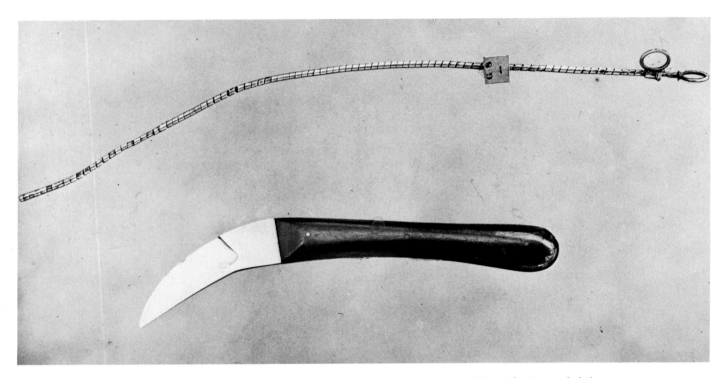

16. *John Hunter's lithotomy instruments,*
c. 1780.
(Royal College of Surgeons of England)

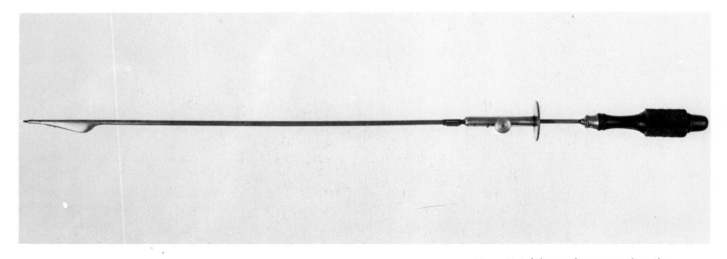

17. *Civiale's Urethrotome, Charrière,*
1849—'cutting from behind forwards'.
30·5 cm.
(Royal College of Surgeons of England)

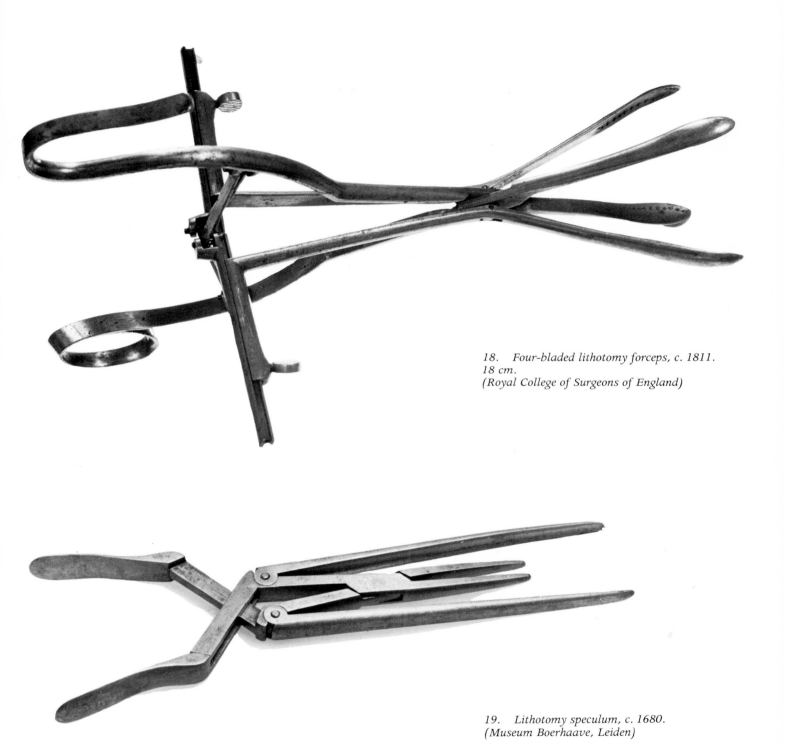

18. *Four-bladed lithotomy forceps, c. 1811.*
18 cm.
(Royal College of Surgeons of England)

19. *Lithotomy speculum, c. 1680.*
(Museum Boerhaave, Leiden)

93

Dilators

Dilators for both the male and female urethra, first invented by
Fabricius (see p. 81), were on the principle of a catheter which,
the handle being unscrewed, split into three to four parts and
extended at will. Some have an index on the handle, by the
nineteenth century, marking the extent of the dilation. A different
type of urethral dilator is in the Prujean Collection and is on the
same principle as a Victorian glove stretcher; pressure on the lower
arms of the X forcing the upper arms to open.

In 1822 dilators were invented that were catheters with inflatable
ends of varnished silk, and in 1834, Leroy d'Etoilles introduced a
spiral-tipped bougie for dilation. Thomas Wakley (1795–1862), son
of the founder of *The Lancet*, made a special dilator for use with
urethral stricture in 1851.

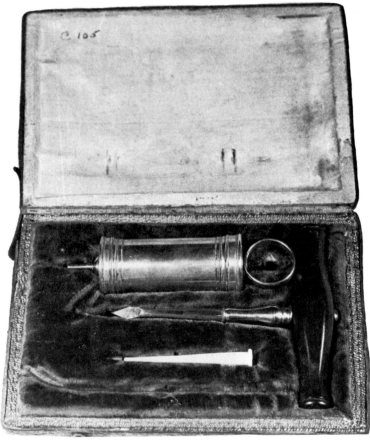

20.   *Cased set of instruments for anal fistula, c. 1780.*
(Museum of Historical Medicine, Copenhagen)

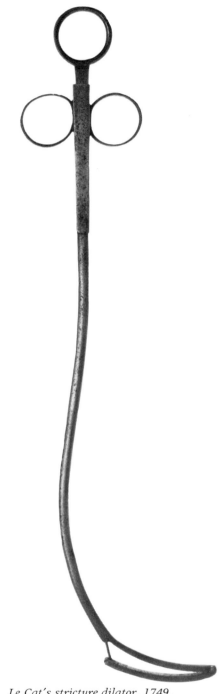

21.   *Le Cat's stricture dilator, 1749.*
20·5 cm.
(Royal College of Surgeons of England)

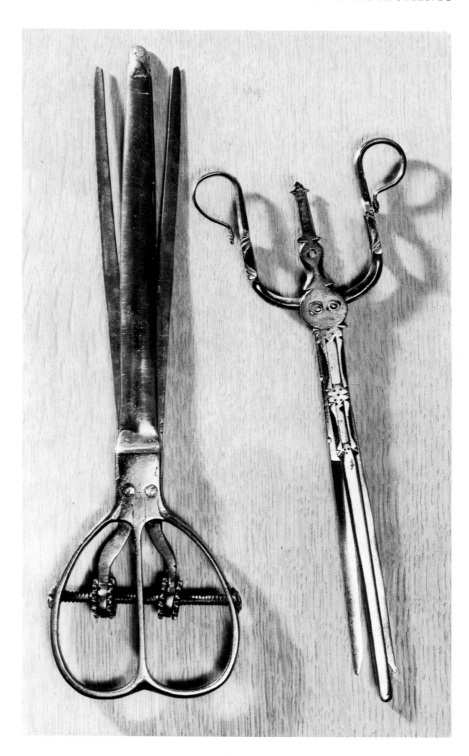

22.   *Two dilators with bistoury cache.*
c. 1680. 25·5 cm.
(Germanisches Nationalmuseum, Nuremberg)

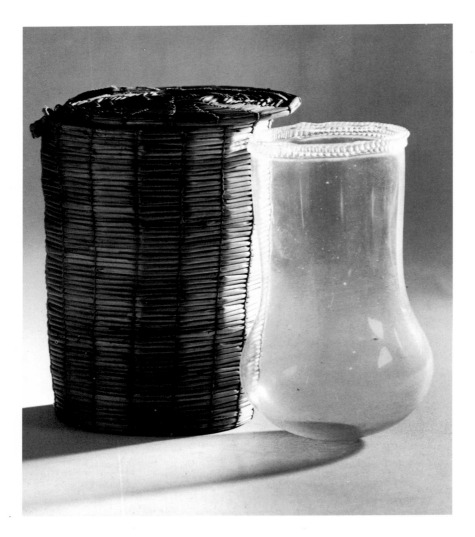

23.   Uroscopy glass and basket case, c. 1700.
Height 12·5 cm.
(Germanisches Nationalmuseum, Nuremberg)

Uroscopy vessels

Uroscopy was the study of health through the condition of the urine. It was therefore necessary to have the use of transparent vessels and there are illustrations of these as early as 1576 in a manuscript at Marburg. However, it is unlikely that any can be found whose purpose may be relied upon. Methods were open to abuse and in the sixteenth century the Royal College of Physicians protested at the practice and passed a statute forbidding treatment being given without seeing the patient. In Germany, however, the practice pertained and an early eighteenth-century vessel from Nuremberg is shown in pl. 23.

CHAPTER FIVE

Ear, nose and throat instruments

The connection between the ear, nose and throat was understood by both the Greeks and Romans, but the diseases that afflicted them attracted very little attention until the nineteenth century. The extraction of foreign bodies from the ear and the removal of polyps from the nose was always attempted. Apart from this, Roger of Salerno said in 1170 that he had performed a successful operation for goitre; but since he described the use of strips of bacon for draining wounds, one is doubtful; in 1770 Jean-Louis Petit opened the mastoid for the first time and about 1800 Sir Astley Cooper first perforated the ear drum for relief of inflammation. These were isolated advances and generally speaking quack medicine dealt with most E.N.T. conditions until the nineteenth century.

Aural forceps

John of Gaddesden (1280–1361) recommended that discharge from the ear should be sucked out through a tube—a duty naturally delegated to one of the lowest orders. This practice would only later develop into the use of a trocar (see p. 108) but he would certainly have used forceps for removing a foreign body from the ear. Medieval forceps for this purpose were basically unchanged throughout the sixteenth and seventeenth centuries. They were all variations on the hair pin type—two fine parallel legs ending in a long, prettily turned and chased finial the jaws being pointed and straight. The eighteenth century saw a simplification of design and a greater use of silver; the finial reduced to a mere ball or sometimes replaced by a small scoop. By the early 1800s the very slender legs were being placed at a slight angle to the finger-piece and could double as nasal forceps, the jaws having been reduced almost to a pin-head, or made slightly larger and serrated. One forceps for the purpose appears in Maw's catalogue for 1868 and has two fine inward-curving jaws meeting together on the slot-slide principle. Lister used both a single and double-ended curette for the purpose though, obviously, this called for considerable skill. Patients had, no doubt, to suffer the attempts of several amateurs to extract the body before resorting to the doctor, as the following extract from *The Cyclopaedia of Practical Medicine* 1883 suggests:

'In some cases considerable ingenuity is required to extract the foreign body from the ear. In one instance a small ivory ball had been detached from the top of a pen-holder in the care of a little boy. Syringeing had done no good and the forceps failed to grasp it and only pushed it in further. At last it was extracted by bringing the point of a small brush, dipped in glue, in contact with its surface, allowing the glue to harden, and then removing brush and ball together. This is a hint that might be of service in difficult cases. The case is recorded of a nurse who, having failed to remove a button from a child's ear, actually tried to push it out the other side. We need hardly say that not only could such a thing be impossible but such treatment is highly dangerous.'

1. *Cased set of instruments used to perforate the ear drum by Kølpin, c. 1790. (Museum of Historical Medicine, Copenhagen)*

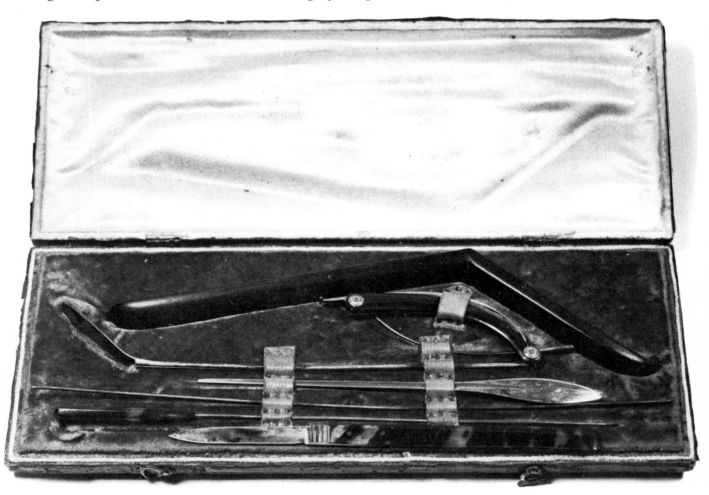

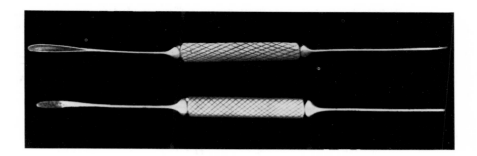

2. *Two double aural curettes, c. 1860, said to have belonged to Joseph Lister. 14 cm. (Wellcome Collection)*

Aural specula and auriscopes

The aural speculum was invented by Fabricius (1560–1634), city-surgeon at Berne, but in 1764, Samuel Mihles speaks of examining the ear 'by the help of a lighted candle and a convex lens, to direct the conveyed Rays to the bottom of the Ear.'

Small trumpet-shaped specula for the ear, usually made of silver or Old Sheffield Plate, were in use from the latter part of the eighteenth century. Victorian catalogues list them in sets of three, 4 cm high, with graduated sizes of aperture. Wilde (father of Oscar) introduced a straight-sided speculum with a circular aperture whereas most others had a concave side, those of Turner and Yearsley having an oval aperture. An exquisite cased speculum made of platinum and gold, probably a presentation piece, is illustrated in pl. 6. A dilating speculum appeared in the early nineteenth century; the two halves of the trumpet attached to a sprung handle from which the pressure was applied. From the early nineteenth century, the rapid development in viewing instruments with better lighting techniques brought about a major change in surgery.

The auriscope, invented by John Brunton (1836–99) in 1862, was a great step forward. The article describing it appeared in *The Lancet* in 1865. It was first made in brass and later of steel, and complete sets can still be found. Several sizes of speculum are included and these can be attached to the auriscope which works on a periscope principle; the light from a candle or lamp is concentrated by funnel and then reflected on a plane mirror with a central perforation.

Others introduced an auriscope or illuminator, following Brunton, though none enjoyed the popularity of his. Jordan's Ear Illuminator, which cost £1.2s.0d in the Maw Catalogue of 1868, was a simple device whereby a lighted taper on an elevator was brought level with the junction between the broad aperture of the speculum

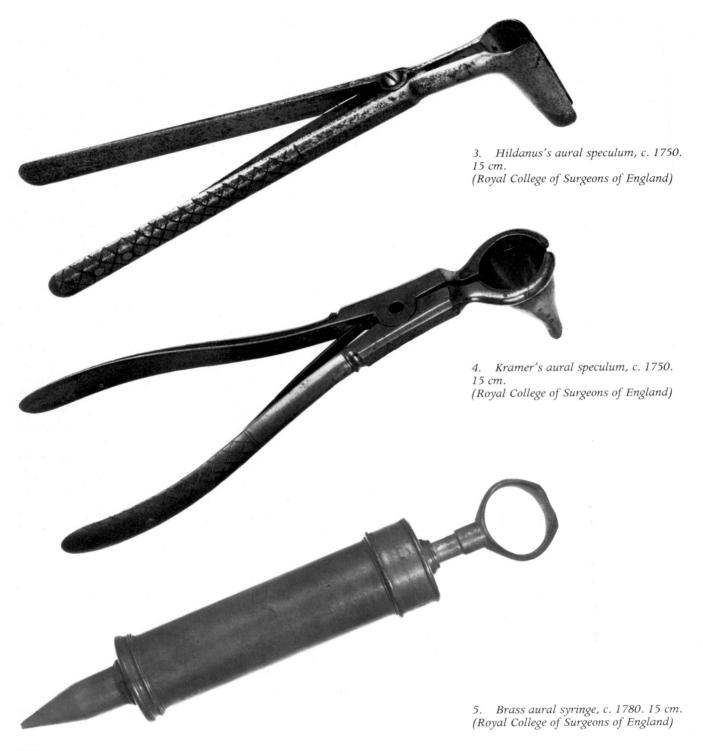

3. *Hildanus's aural speculum, c. 1750.*
15 cm.
(Royal College of Surgeons of England)

4. *Kramer's aural speculum, c. 1750.*
15 cm.
(Royal College of Surgeons of England)

5. *Brass aural syringe, c. 1780. 15 cm.*
(Royal College of Surgeons of England)

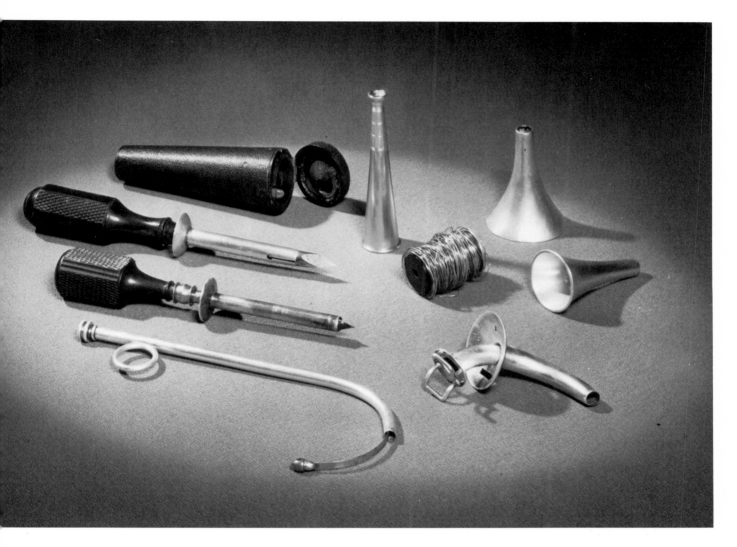

6. *A group of ear, nose, and throat instruments: a gold and platinum aural speculum with case, c. 1865; 2 silver aural specula, c. 1840, Mayer; 2 trocars and cannulae, c. 1860; a nasal polyp-remover, silver, spring-action, c. 1860, Mayer & Phelps; a silver tracheotomy tube and spool of silver wire, c. 1850. 5·8 cm, 3·8 cm, 12·7 cm, 12·7 cm, 5·8 cm. (Simon Kaye Ltd, London)*

and the magnifying lens to which the doctor's eye was applied. Ear channels for use in syringeing appeared *c.* 1840 and had either a steel spring to clip over the head or a strap that tied or buckled.

Another ear forceps occasionally found is the ear-piercing forceps. Lorenz Heister (1683–1758), the first German university professor to teach surgery, did not consider such a frivolous purpose beneath his notice and introduced a series of these in the early eighteenth century. Heister's forceps held the lobe of the ear between two flat parallel blades with a circular aperture in them. By the nineteenth century, ear piercers had become so common that catalogues seldom bothered to illustrate them, though they were usually listed.

Polyp removers and other nasal instruments

The ancient Greek method of removing nasal polyps was to attach four linen threads to a tight ball of sponge with the other ends passed through the eyehole of a tapering metal rod. This flexible rod was then thrust up the nose and into the mouth. The whole lot was then pulled through, the sponge dragging the polyp with it. Other methods, almost as crude, continued across the centuries with small success. Most involved the use of forceps but William Cheselden (1688–1752) in the eighteenth century advised a ligature twisted round the polyp, which avoided subsequent haemorrhage. In 1784, Bell introduced a special forceps with holes in the jaws to carry the ligature and assist in tying it. In the early nineteenth century the spring canula was introduced by Bellocq and others. It took the form, usually in silver, of a slightly curved, short catheter. On release of the spring, operated by unscrewing the handle, a pierced button was projected some 7·5 cm forward in a downward curve. This instrument was first used in curing epistaxis but was afterwards used extensively with polyps (pl. 6). In mid-century, polyp-removing forceps were introduced, mostly bow-handled, with curved serrated jaws and, occasionally, a rack.

Nasal specula appeared in the nineteenth century distinguished from those for the ear by the less exaggerated flare of the trumpet and the slightly smaller length. Duplay and others devised a speculum and dilator which worked on a spring ratchet, c. 1865.

Tracheotomy instruments

An operation for tracheotomy was first mentioned by the Arabs c. A.D. 1000, advising 'a canula of silver or of gold'. Hippocrates wrote of cases where, when suffocation was imminent, 'one should introduce a canula into the throat along the jaw bone so that air can be drawn into the lungs'.

Diphtheria was first studied seriously in France by Pierre Bretonneau (1771–1862) and he used tracheotomy in its cure. His pupil Armand Trousseau (1801–67) developed his methods considerably and performed the operation in Paris both for diphtheria and croup. Trousseau's dilator, a pincer-type forceps with short curved legs, was much favoured as was that of A. Bardelieu (1819–95) which was cross-legged so that pressure on the finger-piece made it act as a dilator for the tracheotomy tube.

Knives used in the operation are distinguished by a short arrow-shaped blade on a curved shaft. This, too, was the usual shape for the tracheotomy trocar.

Tracheotomy tubes are a frequent find for the collector and are usually of silver or silver-plate. The earlier tubes were circular in section and only slightly curved; the inner tube having one, two, or three rings for withdrawing on its outer aperture (pl. 6). An article in *The Lancet* appeared in 1853, 'Tracheotomy—a new method of Performing the Operation', which featured a double-channel tube which was oval in section and of heavier build than previously. *Circa* 1860 came tubes with a split outer tube which could be introduced quite flat and only opened on insertion of the inner

7. *Speculum for the mouth, as Paré's, c. 1700.*
(Museum Boerhaave, Leiden)

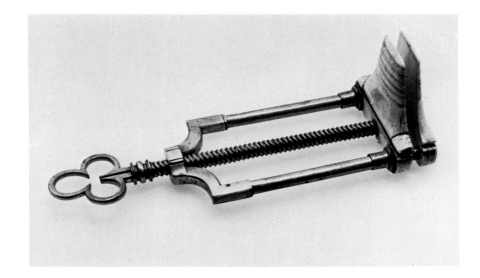

8. *Oesophagus pincers, c. 1700. 15·2 cm.*
(Museum Boerhaave, Leiden)

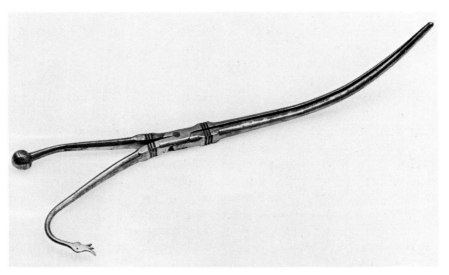

103

tube. This type usually had a larger, complicated throat piece. One of these illustrated by Maw in 1868, is said to 'allow the patient free motion of the head'.

Tongue depressors

Little interest in looking down the throat occurred before the seventeenth century, and so-called tongue depressors of an earlier date are more likely to have been spatulae, although who is to say what tool might not have been used? John Woodall (1556–1643) illustrates a widespread 'speculum linguae' reminiscent of a fish-slice with similar piercing. That in the Prujean Collection is the same with the interesting addition of a screw device which acts as a gag to hold the mouth open. For use with it, no doubt, is a beautifully

9.   *Tongue depressor, c. 1760.*
(Musée le Secq des Tournelles, Rouen)

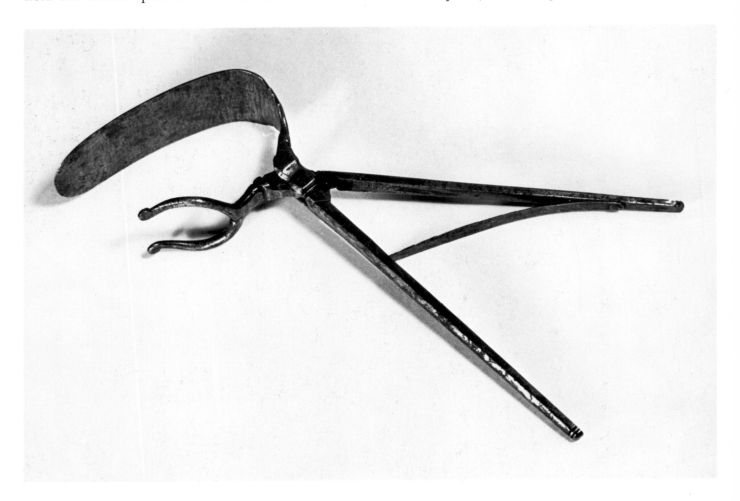

tooled and decorated uvula forceps. Eighteenth-century examples were heavy blunt silver blades approximatley 10–13 cm long of almost uniform width. Often they were perforated with a decorative design, such as that in pl. 13 (p. 62), or pierced at the handle end for the insertion of a cord or ribbon. By the first quarter of the nineteenth century, hinged tongue depressors had been introduced; often with a wider and sometimes with a serrated blade. As the century progressed, more elaborate examples were made with decorated handles, curved, or even right angled shafts, and occasionally, slightly spoon-shaped blades. Another nineteenth-century variation was to make tongue depressors with a small throat spoon at the reverse end. They were almost always of silver or silver-gilt, but plated examples were made in the latter half of the century, and ivory and tortoise-shell are not unknown.

10.   A group of tongue depressors: plated, hinged, c. 1860; silver, hinged, and inscribed, 1843, Hutchinson, Sheffield; plated, c. 1850; silver, 1802, Charles Watts. 10 cm. (Simon Kaye Ltd, London)

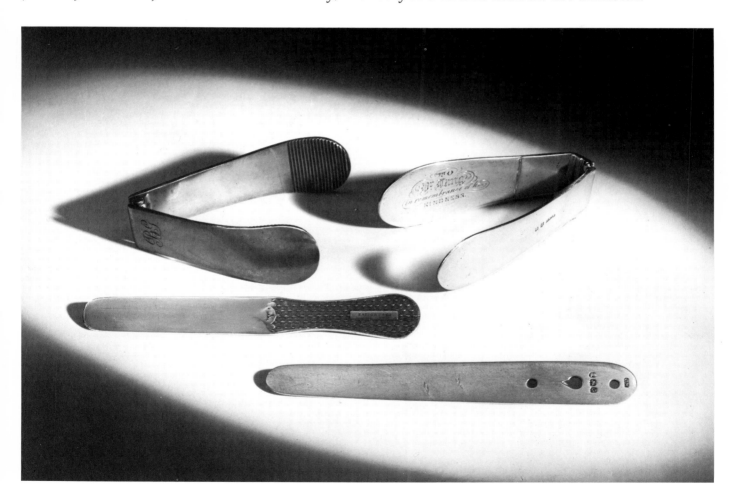

Tongue depressors were a favourite presentation piece from a grateful patient and are frequently found with an inscription engraved on them, or, at least, the doctor's name (pl. 10).

A complicated mouth gag, as opposed to a tongue depressor, was invented by William Ferguson in the mid-nineteenth century.

Laryngoscopes

A type of laryngoscope was made by Avery and Weiss in the 1840s, but was not satisfactory. It consisted of a short candlestick with an adjustable arm supporting a concave mirror with speculum and head harness. The first adequate laryngoscope, as we know it today, was invented by Manuel Garcia, a singing master, in 1854 to enable his pupils to see their throats 'in action'. This was the first time that

11.   Cased laryngoscope as introduced by Lennox-Brown, c. 1870, Coxeter. Mirror 10·5 cm.
(Simon Kaye Ltd, London)

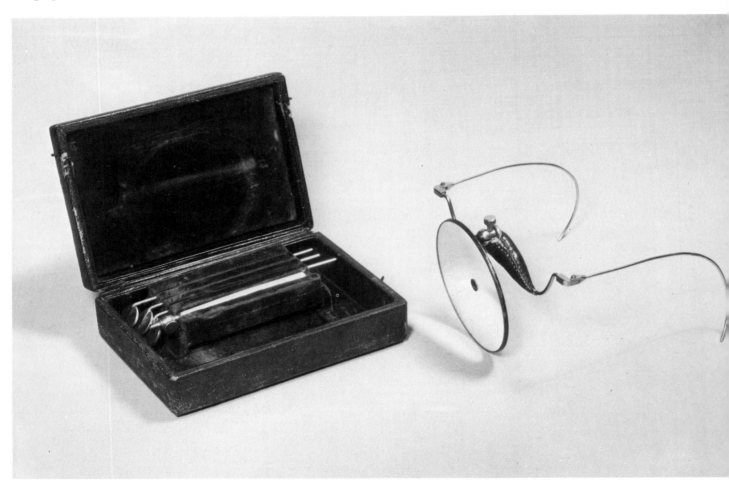

the larynx could be studied properly and laryngeal polyps removed with any degree of success. Garcia's instrument consisted of a circular concave mirror with a central hole attached to a tongue depressor which was adjustable to the handle. For use with it was a set of rectangular polished steel mirrors set at an angle on long rods about 13 cm long. A later development attached the concave mirror to the nose piece of a pair of spectacles (pl. 11), and the Maw catalogue of 1868 lists an instrument that doubled as a laryngoscope and ophthalmoscope.

Tonsillectomy instruments

An operation for tonsillectomy described by Celsus *c.* A.D. 40, was by the modern method of dissection, but from then until the present century the method in use was the guillotine. Early illustrations show tonsillectomy knives for the right and left side of the throat which would seem to indicate the frequency of the operation. Heister (1683–1758) advised a specially concealed lancet. 'An

12. Concealed tonsillectomy lancet as described by Heister, 1745; silver-gilt caustic-holder and applicator, c. 1850. 15 cm, 13 cm. (Anthony Finch, London)

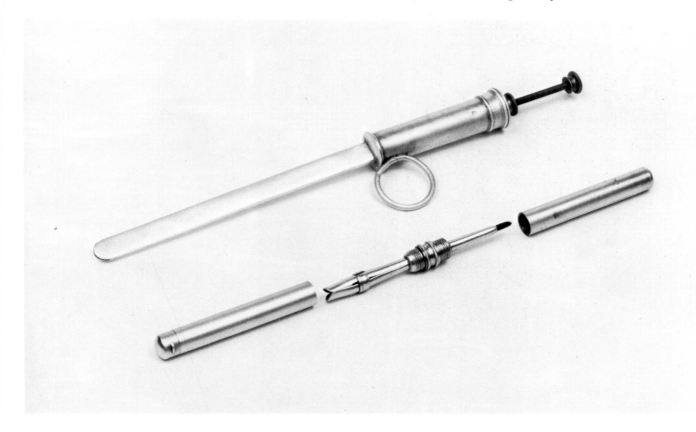

instrument maker of Amsterdam showed me a new instrument for opening suppurated tonsils, the inventor of which is unknown to me . . . which appears like a spatula and in which is contained the lancet' (pl. 12). Guillotines and forceps were listed in the catalogues from the early nineteenth century and were in two sizes, for adults and children. Tonsil-guillotines are easily recognisable by means of the two parallel sliding rings, one with cutting edge, and between them, worked by pressure of the finger on the handle, is a retractable two-pronged lance (pl. 13). Unlike many other instruments, the earlier examples tend to be lighter while those of a later date become complicated and cumbersome with elaborate finger pieces. Cased sets with various spare attachments were made c. 1860. by Charrière and others, but simple steel and brass guillotines have survived from at least ten years earlier.

Trocars

Trocars, used to relieve many conditions, mainly of a dropsical nature, became so frequently associated with ear, nose, and throat surgery that they have been put in this chapter. The term appears not to have been used until the eighteenth century although the instrument as such was known to the Romans; a bronze example has been found at Pompeii. Albucasis, the Arab surgeon of Cordoba (936–1019), mentions a simple exploring needle with a groove mounted on a handle. By the seventeenth century Scultetus described in more detail the instrument then in use; 'a little round

13. *Tonsil guillotine, c. 1860, 22 cm. (Museum of Historical Medicine, Copenhagen)*

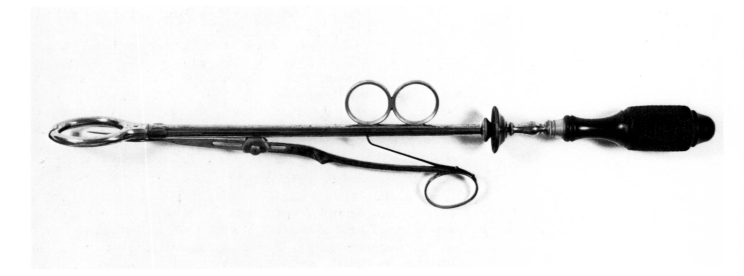

needle with three points and a pipe with shoulders with which the navels of dropsical persons and the scrotum, in waterie herniae are opened to let out the waters.' In addition, Scultetus suggests an alternative in the form of a round needle and a small pipe by which the 'navel of hydropsical persons can be perforated in safety'.

The term trocar seems to have been used for the first time in 1706 and would appear to have been derived from the French *trois-quarts*, a three-faced instrument consisting of a perforator in a tube or cannula used for withdrawing fluid from a cavity. They are frequently mentioned for draining the lachrymal sac and nasal ducts. From the middle of the century trocars of many sizes and forms and for varying purposes were made. Heister shows a flat type, while others preferred a perforator of prismatic shape with convex surfaces. By the end of the eighteenth century, most cannulae had a circular shield at the handle-end and the instrument was either curved or straight according to purpose (pl. 6), relief of dropsy and hydrocele still being the most frequent. Up to this point silver was the material used but in the 1780s Andrée introduced a steel cannula split into two parts and united at the base by a screw. This idea was later modified by Savigny who split the cannula on one side only.

Percivall Pott (1715–88) used a trocar in the mid-eighteenth century with a rectangular guard to the cannula and a prismatic point to the perforator, while Benjamin Bell favoured the split cannula type. By 1842, Sir William Ferguson had introduced an exploring trocar for tapping in hydrocephalus. By the mid-nineteenth century, syphon trocars were made with a stopcock and india rubber bag attached, particularly Spencer Wells's for the emptying of ovarian cysts.

However, by now trocars for use in tracheotomy and draining the larger nasal cavities were made, and one occasionally finds sets of three for the former operation, of graded size and curve. A nineteenth-century innovation was the very fine exploring trocar used a great deal for draining abscesses and pockets of suppuration. The innovation took the form of a case, usually of ivory or *lignum vitae*, the cover for the perforator screwing into the handle. The handle, however, was hollow and contained the cannula which could be removed on unscrewing a cover at the base. The Maw catalogue for 1868 introducing this novel device said 'It often occurs after an operation, that the Trocar is put away without being wiped dry, and the consequence is, that when required again for use, it is found so rusty as to be utterly useless; the plan of having two separate compartments (one for the Trocar and one for the

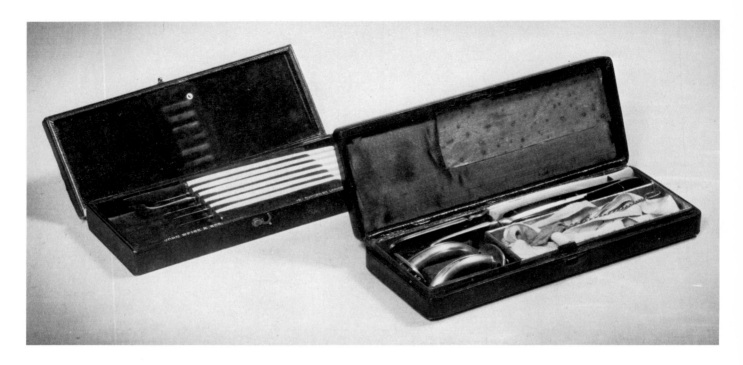

14. *A cased set of ophthalmic instruments, c. 1855, Weiss. Case 12·7 by 5·8 cm. Cased set of tracheotomy instruments, c. 1860, Ferguson.*
(Simon Kaye Ltd, London)

Cannula) entirely removes these objections; the Cannula may be put away without being wiped, and yet not interfere with the Trocar.' That this might be published one year after Lister's first treatise on antisepsis well illustrates the tardiness of its acceptance.

A variation on this type was that introduced by Henry Herbert Southey (1783–1865), younger brother of the poet, and Physician-in-Ordinary to King George IV. The Southey trocar contained, no less than four cannulae in the handle compartment, so that another was readily available when it was desirable to leave one inserted in the body for draining purposes.

CHAPTER SIX

Obstetrical and gynaecological instruments

During the Middle Ages it was not only beneath the dignity of surgeons and physicians to take an interest in midwifery but no man, other than the most cloistered celibate was considered pure enough even to discuss the subject. To approach it could only have been for reasons of prurience or lust. Midwives used the methods of the farmyard justified by superstition, some of which still persist. Practices were so bad that in 1580 a law was passed in Germany forbidding swineherds and shepherds from attending women in labour. The first book on the subject had been published there in 1513, *A Rose Garden for Pregnant Women and Midwives*. Others followed, each astonishingly inaccurate; from Switzerland, in 1544, came *A Very Cheerful Booklet of Encouragement Concerning the Conception and Birth of Man and its Frequent Accidents and Hindrances*, which was in no sense either cheerful or encouraging, followed by *The Byrthe of Mankind* in 1555. A Dr Werff of Hamburg then became interested but realised he could only learn by witnessing births; as a man he would never be admitted to one, so he dressed himself as a woman and attended the next confinement in the district. After a while the ruse was discovered and there was an immediate storm of protest, resulting in Werff being burned to death.

Paré was the first to help the situation with his book *De Generatione* published in 1651 and by establishing a school for midwives at the Hôtel Dieu in Paris. There, he taught the turning of the child *in utero*. Malnutrition resulted in many women being so warped and twisted by rickets that a normal delivery was impossible; countless women died undelivered and countless babies were stillborn. Craniotomy was the only remedy and Paré shows in his book several fearsome crotchets and perforators to that end. His son-in-law and successor at the Hôtel Dieu, François Moriceau, wrote in 1668 a description of a craniotomy whereby the crotchet was fixed to the child's head and the body was then extracted. As he says, either the child was already dead or would have died from lack of delivery, so the compelling need was to save the life of the mother. However, the hacking to pieces of the

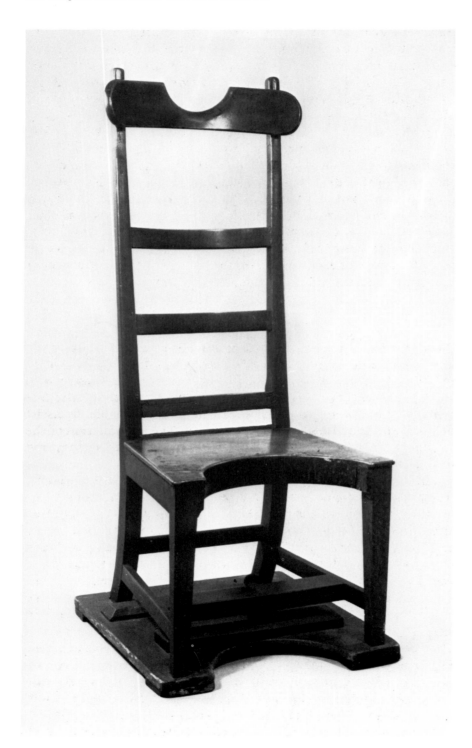

1.   *Obstetrical chair, c. 1750.*
(Royal College of Surgeons of Edinburgh)

OBSTETRICAL AND GYNAECOLOGICAL INSTRUMENTS

child and removal of forward-born limbs often destroyed the mother too so that the very presence of the surgeon was feared by women, which in itself perpetuated the stronghold of the mid-wives. This slackened a little when Louis XIV employed Jules Clement (1648–1723) to attend Madame de Montespan, giving him the title Physician-Accoucheur, thus making a man's presence acceptable, at least in fashionable circles. In this country, the Barber–Surgeons' Company had started granting licences for its members to practise midwifery c. 1600, though it provided no teaching in the subject and antagonism pertained for a long time to come. Many broadsheets were published against doctors attending births, accusing them of bawdiness and indecency of touch, and the midwives, who were licensed by the bishops, were often chosen for their character rather than their skill and experience. It is open to doubt if many modern women not conditioned to bearing great pain could survive the kind of experience recorded.

Forceps

The invention of obstetrical forceps must be regarded as one of the most important events in medical history. Although it is now known that the Arabs had invented a device for the purpose c. A.D. 1000, the knowledge was lost, and in Europe until the seventeenth century there were no mechanical methods available to assist delivery and the idea was completely new. The introduction of the forceps was made more dramatic for being cloaked in secrecy and held as a prized heirloom by one family.

The Chamberlen family came to this country from France as a result of the Huguenot rising. The father and two of his sons set up in practice here and achieved some standing despite repeated altercations with authority regarding their qualifications to do so. Dr Peter Chamberlen of the third generation, who studied at Padua as well as at Oxford and Cambridge, managed to find acceptance and was present at the birth of Charles II. He proposed the setting up of a corporation for the training of midwives, but this was turned down when the rumour became common that he 'used instruments of iron'. This is the first mention of specific instruments. Dr Peter Chamberlen then ran true to family tradition and fell foul of the Physicians and the Barber–Surgeons and retired to Essex where it is probable he continued his midwifery. His son Hugh, who was a doctor in London during the Plague, visited Paris in 1670 and offered to sell Jules Clement (see above) the 'Family secret' for 10,000 crowns, but the offer was refused. Although his son Hugh

113

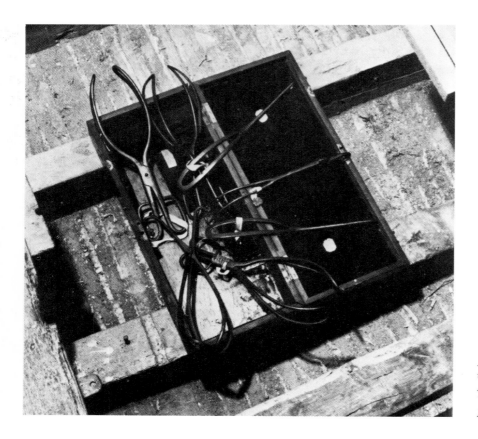

2. Chamberlen forceps and vectis, where they were found in Woodham Mortimer Hall, Essex, 1813.
W. Radcliffe's Milestones in Midwifery, *Bristol, 1967*

the Younger (1664–1728) achieved a tomb in Westminster Abbey, father Hugh was the most unpopular of this little-loved family.

> 'To give you his character truly complete,
> He's doctor, projector, man-midwife and cheat.'

He eventually fled the country in 1699 to Amsterdam where he is said to have sold his secret. Amsterdam, therefore, became the centre for knowledge of the forceps which gradually leaked out. The full secret was only discovered in 1813 when a cache was found below the floorboards at Woodham Mortimer Hall in Essex, the last home of Peter Chamberlen, who died there in 1683. In it, apart from various personal objects such as 'my husband's last tooth', were three sets of instruments, each consisting of a forceps, a fillet, and vectis. There was a fourth forceps but of such a crude design as to suggest it was probably the first experimental pattern. The other forceps consisted of two curved metal levers which could be united at the end by a hinged joint (pl. 2).

114

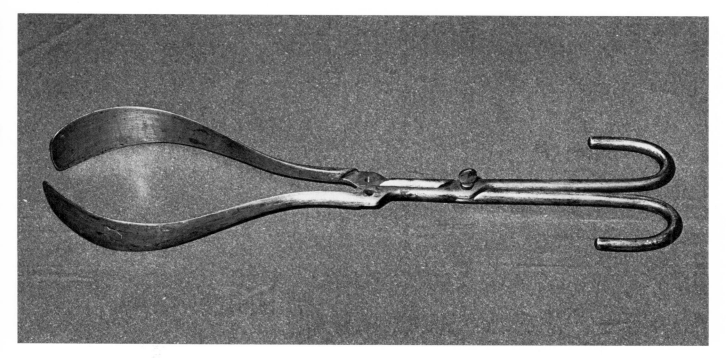

3. Dusée forceps with alternative joints, c. 1735, as described by Alexander Butter in 1733. 30·5 cm.
(Department of Obstetrics, Edinburgh University)

It was from Amsterdam, therefore, that the first publication on the Chamberlen forceps came in 1747. John Peter Rathlaw, who wrote it, devised his own improvements; more curve and fenestrated blades for a better hold.

John Palfyn (1650–1723) of Ghent worked on his own invention based on the rumour of Chamberlen's forceps and produced two curved steel spoons in round wooden handles. He was virtually the first to take into account the full pelvic curve, though his forceps failed when exhibited in Paris in 1720, as they had no lock. However, they were developed into the *tire-tête* used by Gregoire the Younger in Paris. There, again, Dusée had an obstetrical forceps (pl. 3), but his was found to be too large. A description was published in London *c.* 1735 by Alexander Butter of a forceps with solid curved blades, but having a lock for the first time so that the blades might be inserted one at a time and the two withdrawn together.

Meanwhile, certain doctors, significantly all from Essex, were using an obstetrical forceps; either, presumably, from a leak in the Chamberlen family at Woodham Mortimer Hall, or working on their own idea of a rumour. Edmund Chapman published an account of his version in 1733, obviously of the Chamberlen type, as he describes losing the screw from the hinge at a delivery. William

115

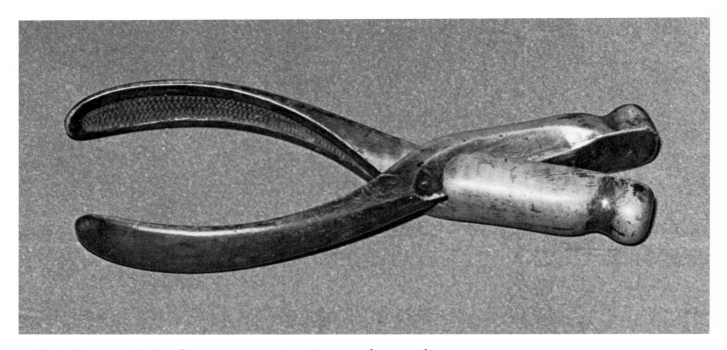

Giffard first used the forceps in 1726. His was shorter than Chapman's but was still with a screw. Benjamin Pugh described his in 1750 as having wooden, notched handles and a new improved pelvic curve. However, by this time, others had the same idea—André Levret (1702–80) of Paris in 1751, and, most notably, William Smellie in London.

William Smellie (1697–1763) has become known as the father of English obstetrics. He was born at Lanark but served his apprenticeship in London at the height of the unparalleled orgy of gin drinking. Infant mortality was of appalling proportions, only one out of five survived the fifth year and it was considered a miracle to save the life of the mother; the child was rarely expected to live. The loss of so many babies was of great concern to Smellie and despite his coarse manner, uncouth accent, and, apparently, enormous hands, he appears to have been a man of singular humanity, of goodwill to patient and student alike, with an unselfish devotion to both their interests. He was a lifelong friend of Smollett with whom he trained and who edited all his written works.

Breech births became his speciality and although early on he mentions using a crotchet and fillet, clearly he was seeking a better instrument. He writes that he had procured 'a pair of French forceps . . . but found them so long and ill-contrived that they but no means

4. Smellie's wooden forceps, c. 1745. 25·5 cm. (Department of Obstetrics, Edinburgh University)

116

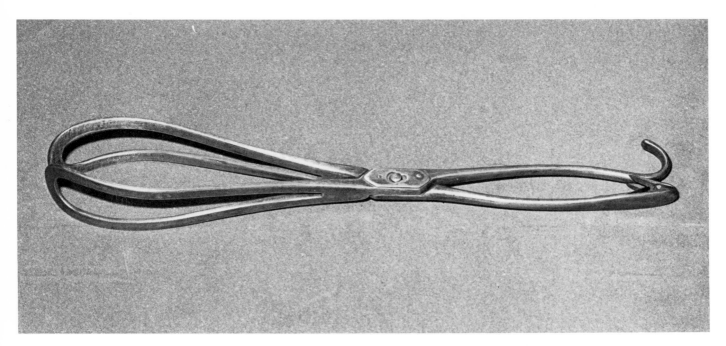

5.   *Gregoire forceps, 1746. 30·5 cm.*
(Department of Obstetrics, Edinburgh
University)

answered the purpose'. He came from Scotland to London and Paris to find better but was disappointed in both places. 'Here I saw nothing was to be learnt'. However, at the lectures of the two Gregoires in Paris he did see a 'machine' or 'phantom', a basket work model of the pelvis covered in black leather for demonstration purposes, which impressed him. In 1739 he set up in London as a practitioner and became a teacher of midwifery in 1741. In his first year he took into his house as boarder and pupil the young William Hunter. His first lectures (mornings for women, afternoons for men) and demonstrations were on 'machines', but he soon found this inadequate so he took the unheard of course of demonstrating on living patients and delivered poor women free. This would seem to be the first time students were allowed to see patients other than as spectators at an operation. (For the Romans, however, it was apparently the custom as the poet Martial, tongue in cheek, recounts: 'I was feeling seedy, Symmachus, but you came to the rescue promptly with five score students trailing in your wake. A hundred hands, ''cold as paddocks'' in the North winds, were laid upon me. I had no ''temperature'', Symmachus, now I have.')

Smellie did not entirely abandon his ingenious machine (see Chapter 14), however, and there are records of its immense versatility. There were six artificial babies with pliable craniums and the pelvis contracted and dilated. The intricate use of forceps

117

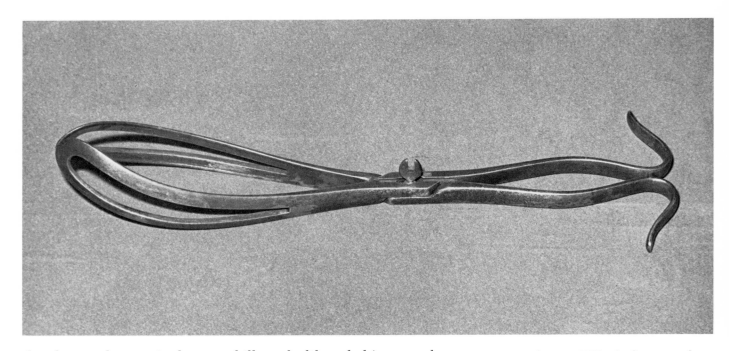

that he taught required great skill, and although his name has become associated with it, he was always at pains to stress that it must never be used unless absolutely necessary. 'As in other parts of surgery, it requires more skill to prevent than to perform an operation.' He did everything possible to prevent the necessity of craniotomy or evisceration which was all too common in cases of difficulty. Deliveries took place under cover of a sheet that stretched from the mother's shoulders and had its end tied round the doctor's neck so that the only part of her he ever saw was her head. The forceps, if used, was introduced without the knowledge of the patient as, if anything went wrong, it was sure to be the forceps that would be blamed. There are many records of this deceit, the usual one being for the doctor to have one blade in each of his breeches' pockets and return them there after use, in the meantime being careful never to let the metal clink together. (It was 1840 before Astley Cooper could amputate a breast and actually see what he was doing.)

The first forceps Smellie devised was of wood with flat blades (pl. 4). This he found unsatisfactory and later had it made of steel covered in leather. Leather, he felt, was kinder to the touch and, like wood, did not clink. He instructed that the leather be renewed after every delivery for fear of venereal infection, though he had no knowledge of the causes of puerperal fever. Later, others used

6. *Levret forceps, 1751, the first to apply the pelvic curve, 30·5 cm. (Department of Obstetrics, Edinburgh University)*

118

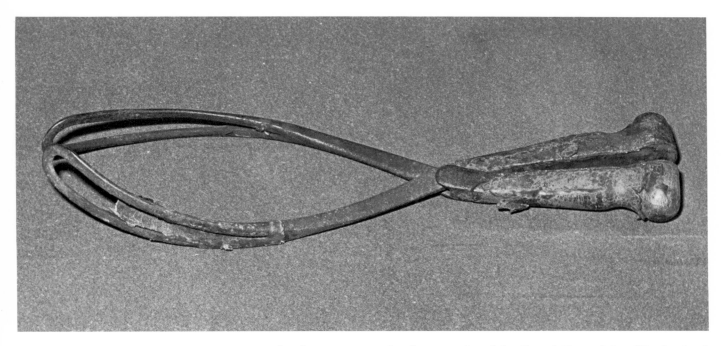

7. *Smellie's curved forceps of 1753, showing remains of leather covering the fenestration. 30·5 cm.*
(Department of Obstetrics, Edinburgh University)

leather to cover the fenestration (pls. 7 and 8), and Smellie devised many types applying the pelvic curve and both shortening and lightening the instrument. His principal contribution was the lock, known as the 'English lock' abroad and 'Smellies's lock' at home, which was copied everywhere. Previously, both Pugh and Smellie had used notched wooden handles—developed from the Palfyn type—to take tapes which bound them together before withdrawing. The notches remain on obstetrical forceps even today, though their purpose was abandoned with the invention of the lock. Smellie had his forceps made by Best of Lombard Street, and after experimentation used two types—a short one for normal deliveries and a long one for the aftercoming head in breech births. It was the Chamberlen family who invented the forceps but Smellie who taught its use and gave Britain pre-eminence in midwifery.

John Burton (1710–71), the founder of York Hospital, was a bitter opponent of Smellie and claimed to have delivered women where Smellie had failed. 'My forceps are better than any yet contrived', he said, though it is doubtful if anyone else ever used them. They were modelled on the lobster's claw, the curved blades hinged on a single shaft, opening when the handle was depressed, and able to lock into any position by means of a screw (pl. 9). Burton was the first to place women on their side during delivery—a practice dismissed by the French as 'pruderie Britannique'. He was pilloried

119

by Smellie's great friend Smollett as the original Dr Slop in *Tristram Shandy*, at whose birth he is described using forceps and breaking the boy's nose—though he did manage to avoid the other catastrophes suggested. This unpleasant man was, curiously, one of Boerhaave's pupils (see Chapter 1). It was said of him that he was 'unlovely in his person and indelicate in his anecdote'.

Antoine Dubois (1756–1837) in Paris, *c.* 1790, invented forceps with a blunt hook (used for the thigh in breech births) in one handle and a perforator in the other, while John Evans *c.* 1780 made a forceps with a space between the shanks some way after the lock so that the finger might be inserted for a better grip in traction—a device still featured today. In addition he added a screw-rack to the handle to fix the hold so avoiding overcompression of the skull. John Aitken of Edinburgh, who published his treatise in 1784, had

8. *Leather-bound forceps with adjustable curve, c. 1760. 33 cm. (Department of Obstetrics, Edinburgh University)*

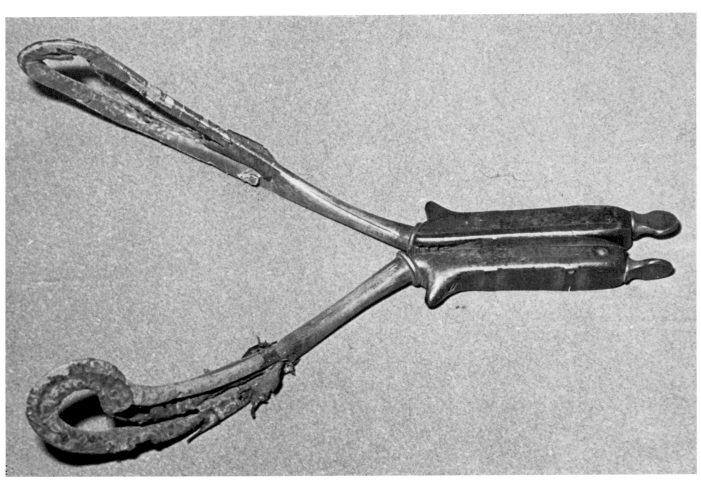

the same idea which was carried out for him by Archibald Young of Edinburgh. R. Wallace Johnson (a pupil of Smellie) produced forceps as early as 1769 with a perineal curve, whereby the handles were bent slightly backwards, an idea much built on later. Folding forceps of the Smellie type were introduced to Edinburgh in 1793 by Professor A. Hamilton and were very popular while forceps were still carried in the pocket—a practice only discarded post-Lister. On the Continent a similar idea had been devised in 1791 by Matthias Saxtorph. Arnold van der Laar of The Hague produced a forceps in 1771 with a slot for tapes in the fenestrations so that the pull came straight from the blades, another idea still used. John Leake even invented a three-bladed forceps. In all, Johannes Mulder was able to describe and illustrate fifty different types by the end of the eighteenth century.

9. Burton's forceps, c. 1760. 30·5 cm. (Department of Obstetrics, Edinburgh University)

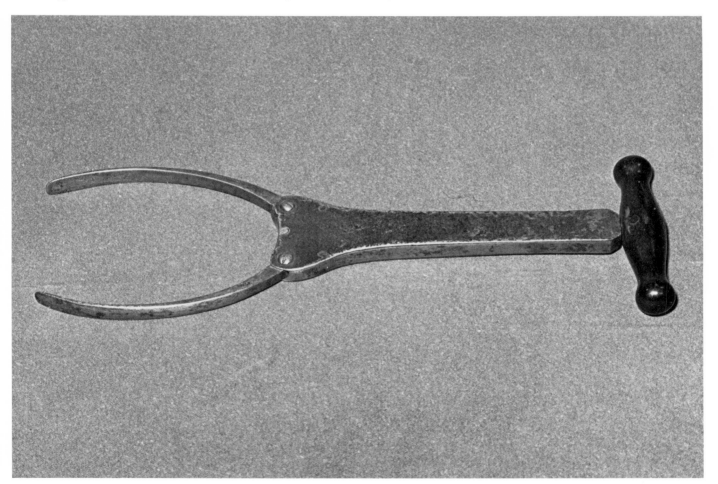

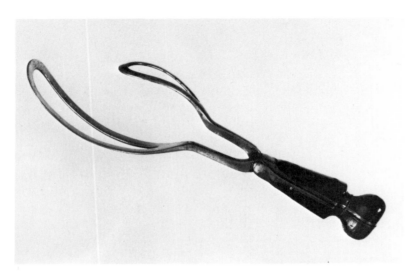

10. *David Davis's asymmetrical forceps,*
1825. 30·5 cm.
(Royal College of Surgeons of Edinburgh)

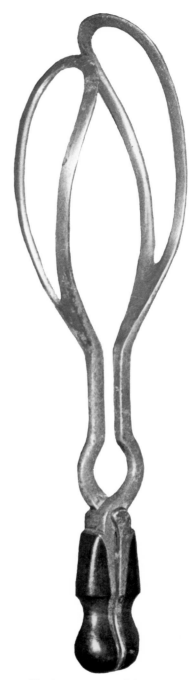

The next century saw the introduction of new patterns but few radical changes. In France a pulley tackle was invented for traction by Pros of La Rochelle; an elaborate screw traction apparatus with a cross-bar against the woman's buttocks. In Britain, however, the great reluctance to use forceps unless compelled by necessity to do so, as taught by Smellie, had gained ground to an exaggerated extent, gaining for British obstetrics a reputation for dilatoriness. William Hunter (1718–83), brother of John Hunter, whose magnum opus was *On the Human Gravid Uterus*, was the chief opponent of the use of the forceps. He would frequently pull from his pocket his own, covered in rust saying 'where they save one, they murder many'. His influence was so great that masterly inactivity was carried to dangerous lengths. In 1819 Princess Charlotte, daughter of the Prince Regent, was left in labour for 52 hours. As a result the mother and baby died and Queen Victoria eventually came to the throne—the accoucheur, Sir Richard Crofts, went out and shot himself.

Although François Roussel in 1581 describes six Caesarian operations it was not until 1793 that the first operation of this kind was performed from which the mother, though not the child, recovered. Carle von Graefe (1787–1840) did much to improve the operation in Germany, but the forceps was still pre-eminent in

11. *Radford asymmetrical forceps,*
Manchester, 1825. 30·5 cm.
(Department of Obstetrics, Edinburgh
University)

122

saving lives. When the use of the long-curved forceps was at last introduced at the Rotunda in Dublin, the craniotomy rate was halved.

James Young Simpson (1811–70), who at the age of 28 was elected Professor of Midwifery at Edinburgh, made his the most sought after course in the land. He was the first to use chloroform in obstetrics, although he was a bitter opponent of the introduction of antisepsis. Together with Robert Lawson Tait (1845–99) he was principally responsible for the separation of obstetrics from gynaecology and for making advances in both, James Marion Sims the American surgeon (1813–83), becoming the greatest exponent of their work.

12. *Smellie's forceps; John Palfyn's forceps; Hendrik Roonhuyze's lever, c. 1760. (Museum Boerhaave, Leiden)*

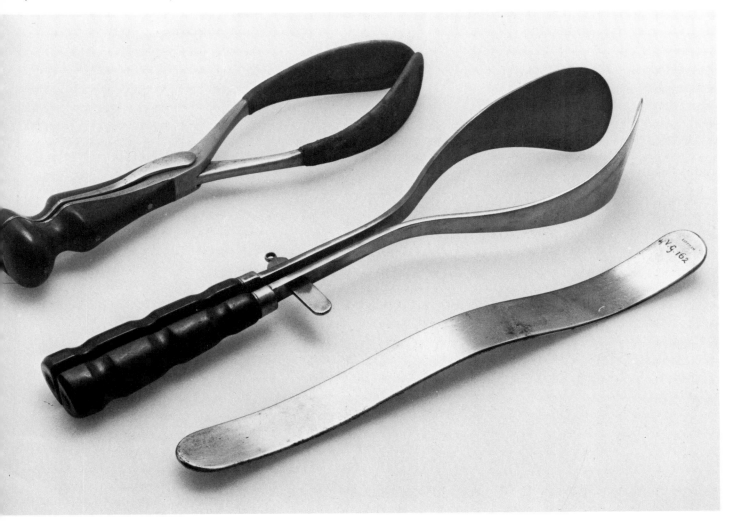

Craniotomy instruments

Perforators were a variety of instrument used to pierce and empty the skull in craniotomy. They were often very complicated and appear in early illustrations as being on the boring principle with a screw mechanism. La Motte is reported to have used an ordinary pair of scissors and Smellie extended this idea to evolve his own perforator of scissors with a stop on the outer edge of each blade to arrest them at a convenient depth for opening the skull (pl. 13). This became the prototype for all subsequent perforators and as late as 1868, Maw's catalogue illustrates one very similar. John Freke of St Bartholmew's Hospital (1688–1756) invented probe-pointed scissors as a perforator and actually made them himself. A singular character—it is he who presides in Hogarth's *The Reward of Cruelty* (see pl. 5; p. 8)—he even carved the wooden chandelier which still hangs in the Stewards' Room at St Bartholomew's Hospital. A perforator as part of a forceps has already been mentioned, although Professor Pajot told his students, 'Remember, Gentlemen, that this hook and this perforator have been put here to remind you never to use them.' Nineteenth-century perforators did include the quill or lance type that was inserted blunt, thus causing less damage. Instruments of this latter type were also used to induce premature labour.

The crotchet was essentially a sharp hook to give a hold on the head either before or after craniotomy. This and the blunt hook used both for craniotomy and breech delivery had been in use fully a century before Smellie. He made several improvements; he gave it a cephalic curve so that it could be fixed high on the head, then made it a double instrument combining it by means of his own lock to a blunt hook. A simpler variation on this was an instrument he made with a crotchet at one end and a blunt hook at the other. In almost unchanged form this was used in breech deliveries right through the nineteenth century (pl. 21).

Craniotomy forceps were hinged with a screw and the short thick blades were serrated for a heavy grip in crushing the skull. Their design altered little until they became obsolete (pl. 15).

The basilyst, the last of these deliberately destructive instruments, was mostly used on the Continent and was for dismembering the body of the child either before or after craniotomy. A long curved steel guard concealed a sharp blade that swung out on pressure from a thumb piece attached to the handle (pl. 18). It is difficult to imagine it being used without damage to the mother. However, it continued to be made until the late nineteenth century.

124

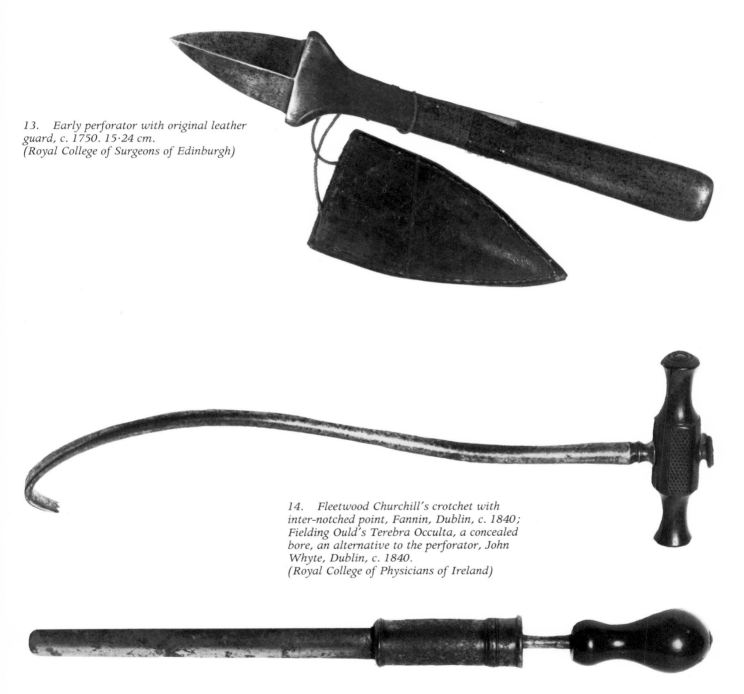

13.   Early perforator with original leather
guard, c. 1750. 15·24 cm.
(Royal College of Surgeons of Edinburgh)

14.   Fleetwood Churchill's crotchet with
inter-notched point, Fannin, Dublin, c. 1840;
Fielding Ould's Terebra Occulta, a concealed
bore, an alternative to the perforator, John
Whyte, Dublin, c. 1840.
(Royal College of Physicians of Ireland)

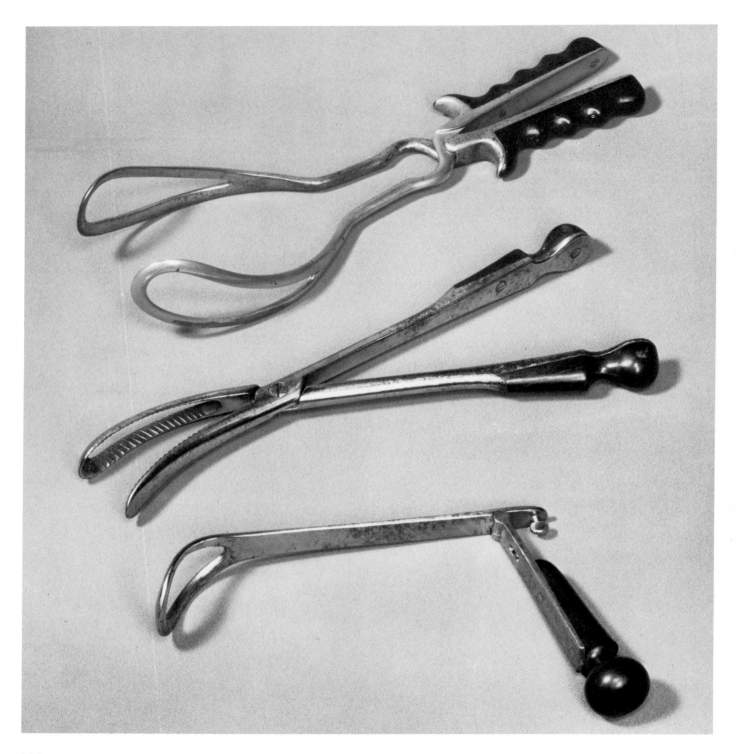

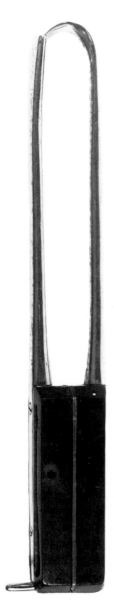

15.   Anderson's forceps, c. 1850; Murphy's craniotomy forceps, c. 1850; Lowder's vectis, c. 1820, Evans. 35·6 cm, 30·4 cm, 25·4 cm. (Simon Kaye Ltd, London)

16.   Combined hook and crotchet of Jean Civiale (1792–1827), c. 1850. 30·5 cm. (Museum of Historical Medicine, Copenhagen)

Fillet or lack

This was a very early device—a ribbon-like loop of material used as a noose to provide a hold for traction. By the mid-eighteenth century a hollow ribbon was threaded with a fine strip of whalebone but by the nineteenth century it was possible to make a sufficiently flexible metal fillet.

Lever and vectis

The lever was a flat strip of metal used to prize out the infant's head, obviously causing much damage (pl. 20). It was very popular in the mid-eighteenth century in Holland but its use was overtaken by that of the vectis. It is known that the Chamberlen family had a vectis though Francis Sandes, or Sandys, is generally credited with its invention *c.* 1740. Whether he had the idea from them or if it was original is not known. It is a special form of hook with an ovoid fenestrated blade to be applied to the infant's head. Its use and design were perfected by Dr William Lowder for breech births. It had three purposes; to be used as a lever, or as a tractor hooked either over the head or under the chin. Lowder introduced a hinge on the shaft and taught his students to use it between the blades of a forceps (pl. 15).

Vaginal specula and dilators

The vaginal dilator and speculum as used by the Romans clearly evolved from the idea of the human hand with the fingers closed in a cone-shape for introduction, and the spread outwards for exploration. This expanding blade type of instrument later developed side by side with the tubular (see trade-card at the top of p. 319).

A four-bladed bronze version was found at Pompeii, a piece of engineering complexity no less than 33 cm in length. Dilators used through the Middle Ages were a simplified version of this. Three blades, triangular in section and blunt-ended, are at right angles to a frame with simple screw mechanism. Guy de Chauliac, writing in 1363, mentions an 'instrument called speculum, which is provided with a thumb-screw' though gives no other description. However, Hans von Gersdorff (1477–1551) in 1526 and Jacob Rueff (or Ryff) of Zurich (1500–*c.* 1569) in 1554 both had a speculum matricis which they recommended for use by midwives. Rueff, indeed, clearly intended that a looking-glass should be used in conjunction with his. Later, a definite development took place, as shown by Paré in

127

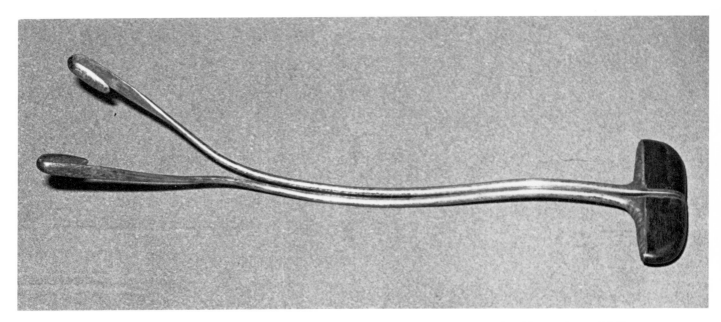

17. *Double crotchet, c. 1860.*
(Department of Obstetrics, Edinburgh
University)

18. *Ferguson's basilyst, Soyez, Paris,*
c. 1835. 25·5 cm.
(Simon Kaye Ltd, London)

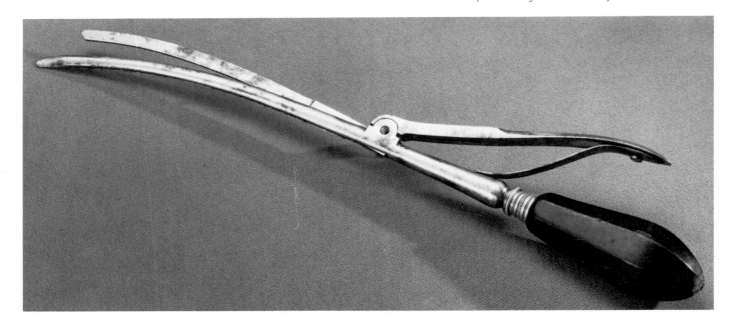

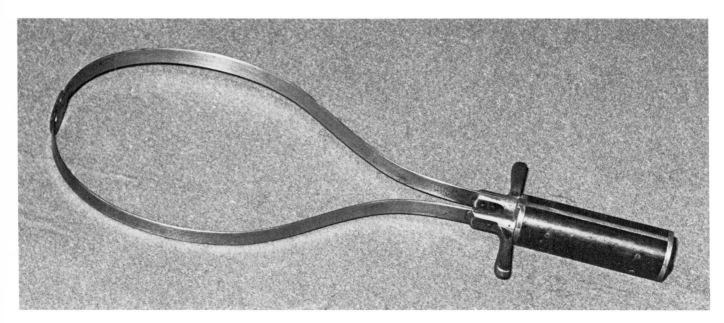

19. *Spring fillet, c. 1810.*
(Department of Obstetrics, Edinburgh
University)

20. *Early wooden vectis, c. 1740. 25·5 cm.*
(Department of Obstetrics, Edinburgh
University)

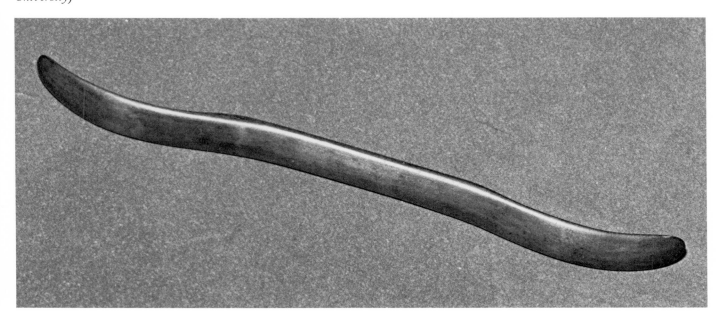

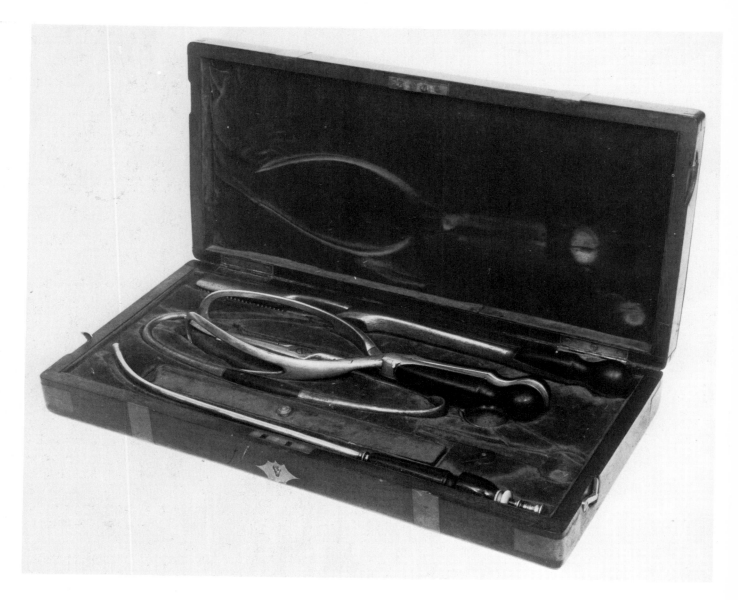

1579, whereby the screw was worked by a winch. Down to the seventeenth century, both Fabricius and Scultetus were depicting three-bladed dilators. During the eighteenth century bi-valve specula, as used today, came into use. Among them was that of Heister in 1753 and Brambilla in 1782.

The tubular speculum is probably of equal antiquity to the bladed type, the Talmud explaining the use of such a rod, possibly a hollow bamboo stem. Metal tubes of a cylindrical shape were used

21. *Cased set of obstetrical instruments, Evans, c. 1850, containing: cephalotribe, short forceps, perforator, blunt hook and crotchet, catheter, perforating trocar and cannula, space for scissors. 45 by 30·5 cm. (National Army Museum, London)*

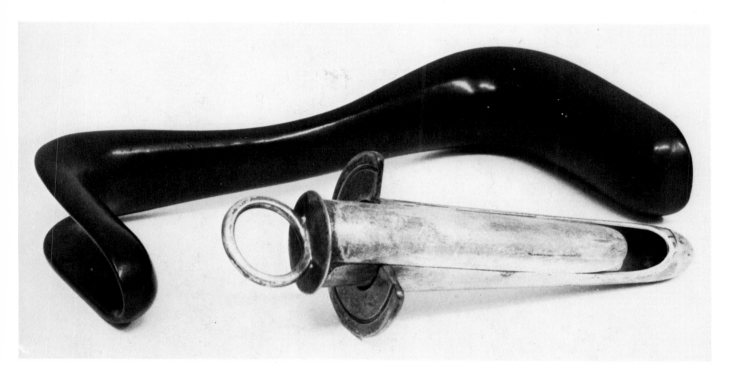

22. *Sim's duck-bill speculum, c. 1850; vaginal speculum in two parts, c. 1860. 17·8 cm, 17·8 cm. (Woolstaplers' Hall Museum, Chipping Camden)*

from an early period, being slightly altered into valves from time to time. Recamier invented a telescopic type of speculum in 1801, afterwards modified by Protheroe Smith in the 1830s.

In 1830 David Davis introduced a four-bladed instrument with a fitting plug; this latter first made of wood and later of vulcanite. A few years later Columbat devised a speculum with five or six blades on a metal collar and in 1837 a most ingenious invention was made by Beaumont, an English surgeon who afterwards worked in Canada. It consisted of four or five blades, each having its own screw and capable of being opened independently.

During the next fifty years many new types came into fashion, notably the tubular glass speculum of Sir William Ferguson in 1855 with a mirrored interior, and the double-ended duck-bill speculum of Marion Sims in 1845. This instrument was apparently improvised by bending a long-handled basting spoon backwards at both ends, but eventually took the form of one jaw of a duck's bill at each end of a central handle, having somewhat the appearance of a shoemaker's last; it was originally made in brass and later in steel (pl. 22).

The main problems with specula had always been a source of light, and pain to the patient. With anaesthesia they came into their

131

own (see Chapter 14). However, the particular problem with vaginal specula was the presumed indecency. The following extract from *Hints to Husbands* shows what respectable opinion was like in 1857:

> 'We allude to the speculum. The adoption of this instrument as we are informed, is now becoming general; and its employment plunges its wretched victim, woman, into the lowest depths of infamy and degradation. We will not pollute these pages by describing its methods of action; suffice it to say, that, to the sense of touch, common to all midwifery practices, is added, in its application, that of sight; exposure the most complete of all which modesty even in the most abject of races, invariably conceals.'

Other gynaecological instruments

A set of uterine instruments chiefly remarkable for their exquisite workmanship, the handles being of porcupine quill and silver, is

23.   *Vaginal speculum of the type described by Scultetus in 1672, but probably earlier. (Musée le Secq des Tournelles, Rouen)*

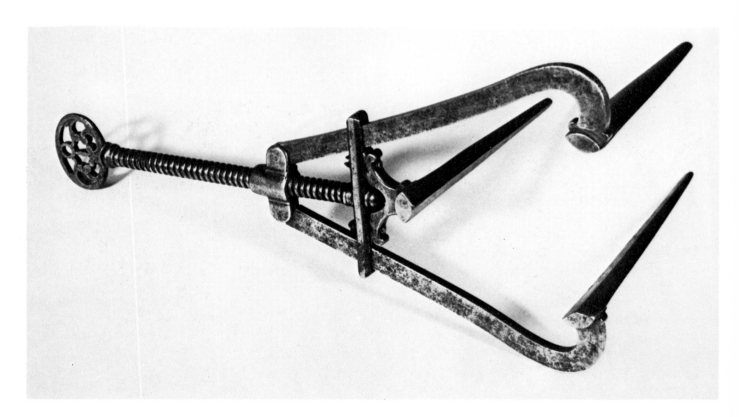

shown in col. pl. IV. This combination of instruments was frequently made in the nineteenth century, a curette with a short lozenge-shaped blade, a swab-holder with ring slide hold, and a caustic holder to take styptic. Women's diseases still being too indelicate to consider, the instance and development of instruments in their cure was not great. Columbat, *c.* 1840, introduced a hysterectomy forceps—four arms each ending in two hooks curving inwards, the arms controlled by a ring slide engaged in all arms together, forcing them inward when depressed.

Guillaume Dupuytren (1777–1835) was the first to amputate the neck of the uterus for cancer. Ephraim McDowell (1771–1830) of Danville, Kentucky, who trained at Edinburgh, was a pioneer of abdominal surgery and the treatment of ovarian cysts. In 1809 he described being sent for to deliver a woman of twins but discovered her not pregnant at all but suffering from a large tumour, found on extraction to weigh 20 lb. The operation was entirely successful.

However, these sallies seem to have exhausted the profession until time beyond the scope of this book.

24. Dilator speculum, c. 1650.
(Germanisches Nationalmuseum, Nuremberg)

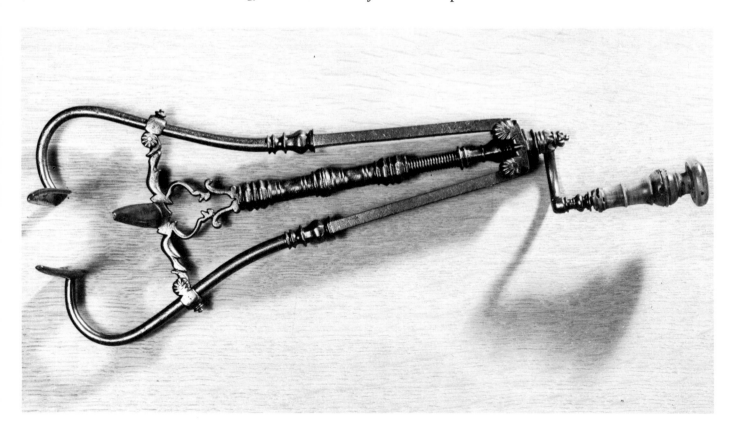

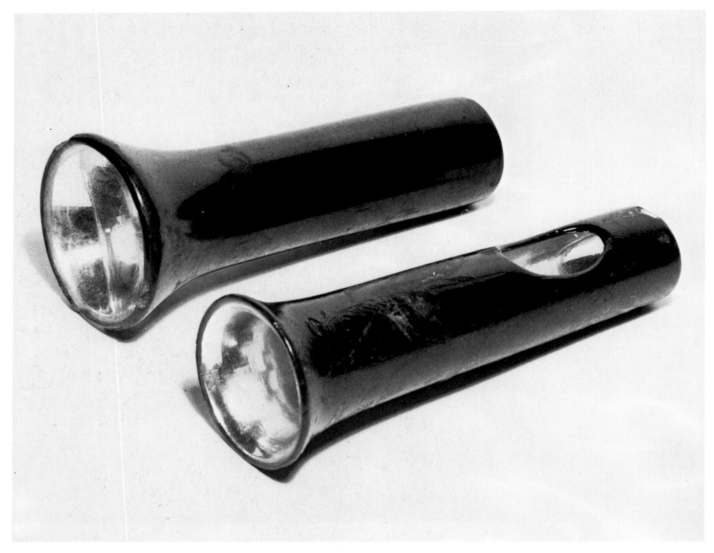

25.   Two examples of Ferguson's glass
speculum, one with fenestration, c. 1855.
17·8 cm.
(Wellcome Collection)

CHAPTER SEVEN

Ophthalmic instruments

*1. Woodcut by George Barlisch, 1583,
showing an early cataract operation.
(British Optical Association Library)*

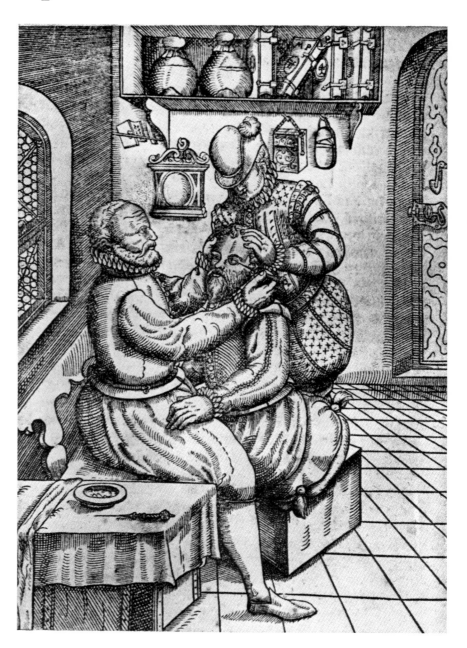

Ophthalmology is one of the oldest specialities. Hammurabi, laying down his code in 2250 B.C., legislated for operations on the eye—10 shekels for a successful operation, or amputation of both hands if it failed. There are descriptions of couching for cataract, i.e. instilling drops to depress the opaque lens, from Roman times, but the study then fell into neglect.

Records do remain of iron splinters in the eye being removed with magnetic iron ore c. 1525. Generally, though, it was cataracts that commanded most attention (pl. 1). J. S. Bach died as a result of his operation and Handel only survived his first one in 1752 to be blinded for the rest of his life. William Cheselden attracted universal attention with a paper he published in 1728 in which he described the case of a boy born blind and only couched at the age of 13. Cheselden was said to have rendered immortal service to ophthalmic surgery by forming an opening to serve as an artificial pupil by slitting the iris. Percivall Pott was another to contribute to the early study of ophthalmics, particularly fistula lachrymalis, for which he advised against probing but used a syringe. The French surgeon Dominique Anel (1679–1730), in the first half of the eighteenth century, invented the first lachrymal probe and introduced a minute syringe to inject fluids into the lachrymal sac without use of knife or cautery (col. pl. IV). These were the positive contributions. Roger Grant (d. 1724) on the other hand, an ex-tinker and Anabaptist preacher, rose to be oculist to Queen Anne and George I without furthering the study at all. The *Spectator* of 1712 referred to him as 'putting out eyes with great success'.

The minute anatomy of the eye, described by Leonardo da Vinci as 'the window of the soul', was only worked out in the late eighteenth and early nineteenth centuries, by which time microscopes were available for study. Old theories of vision were overthrown and it was realised that the eye was a simple optical apparatus with unique properties of focusing objects near and far. Henry H. Southey (1783–1865) the younger brother of the poet and Physician-in-Ordinary to George IV said, with unusual democratic perception, 'In the employment of the iris, the porter and the Peeress are alike.'

Cataract and other knives

Early operations for cataract could seldom have been attended by a special knife designed for the purpose: this would probably have been the smallest scalpel available. Celsus records for us that Heraclides the Tarantine advised cutting very gently with the sharp edge of the scalpel, following adhesions of the lids to the

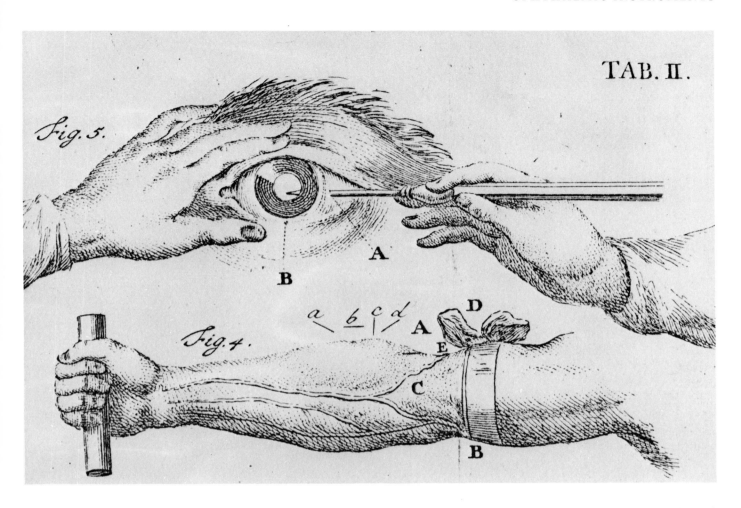

2. *Plate from Samuel Mihles's* Elements of Surgery, *showing couching for cataract, 1764*

white of the eye, to effect separation. During the eighteenth and early nineteenth century, by which time ophthalmics had become a recognised speciality, the technique for removal of the lens in cataract was perfected and entirely replaced the ancient operation for couching or depressing the opaque lens. Samuel Sharp (1700–1778) was the first to cut the cornea with a knife in cataract operations. Heister, meanwhile, had much to say of the itinerant operators who abounded. Chevalier Taylor, for example, couched hundreds in the years 1750–52 but not one in a hundred recovered their sight. The operation, thought Heister, had not been performed when the cataract was 'ripe'—i.e. hard enough. William Cheselden in 1729 had attempted an operation to relieve tension in glaucoma, followed by Joseph Beer in 1798, but success was not achieved until 1857.

137

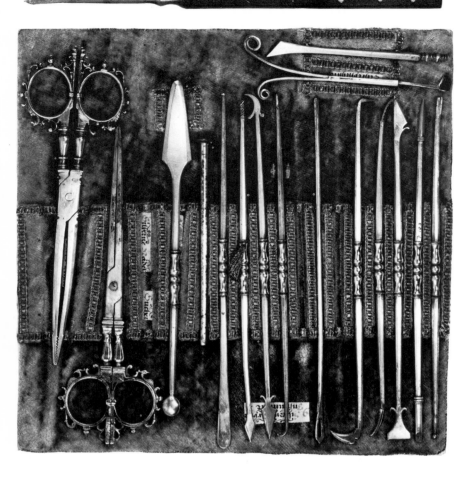

3. *Brambilla's couching needle, c. 1790.
11·5 cm.
(Royal College of Surgeons of England)*

4. *A set of silver-gilt ophthalmic
instruments, c. 1620. Length of case 12·5 cm.
(Kunstgewerbemuseum, West Berlin)*

Samuel Mihles, in his *Elements of Surgery* of 1764, describes
operation for cataract in some detail. The patient is to be placed in a
chair with pillows supporting his back so that his body inclines
forward and his head backwards. The assistant holds back the upper
eyelid and the surgeon the lower, attempting, with his other hand,
to depress the cataract with a needle. His diagram of how this is to be
done is shown on pl. 2. If the cataract rises again, it must be
continually depressed and if it has adhesions they must be broken.
If a right-handed surgeon is to operate on the right eye of the
patient, then he is to do it from behind or place the patient on the
floor with his head on the operator's knees. Afterwards, both eyes
are to be bound and the patient kept upright. He is then to be bled
and purged.

However, the cataract may need to be cut not couched. This was first done in France, he says, by M. Daniel in 1747, but possibly earlier by M. Mery in 1707. The instruments needed, says Mihles, are as follows:

(1) A pointed needle, sharp-edged and semi-lunar to make the first aperture;
(2) A blunt needle, sharp-edged and semi-lunar for enlarging the first aperture;
(3 and 4) Two pairs of crooked, convex scissors;
(5) A small spatula for raising the cornea;
(6) Another small-pointed needle, sharp-edged on both sides for opening the membrane;
(7) Small curette or scoop to extract discharge and fragments
(8) Small pincers for removing portions of membrane.

All these to be ranged in order and given to the assistant who will deliver them in time to the surgeon. Surgeons in France tried to simplify this outlay and two, le Faye and Poyet, invented instruments to that end, but they were found inadequate.

The patient could not expect to escape severe inflammation, even in a successful operation. On average, Mihles felt this might be likely to last six weeks.

Cataract knives, in common with all ophthalmic instruments, are characterised not only by the delicacy of size and weight of the blade, but also by the small and slender handle (pl. 4). Ivory seems almost always the favoured material for the handle, two fine plates riveted on either side of the metal shaft, as often smooth as chequered. The blades are triangular in shape, fine and sharp on two sides, the spine on the hypotenuse just sufficiently strong to prevent flexibility. A variation on this norm, but not one attracting much popularity, was Guerin's spring cataract knife, which he invented in Lyons in 1785 (pl. 6) and it can be seen at the Royal College of Surgeons. The knife is attached to a spring in a brass case. A ring is applied to the eye and a lever is depressed by the thumb; the knife then flies across the lower part of the ring thus making a corneal flap. Secondary cataract knives, often made in the nineteenth century in a variety of shapes, were minute blades, no bigger than a fine needle-eye on a needle-like shaft, as those described above by Mihles.

An instrument for making an artificial pupil was first invented c. 1800 and was much improved by Grossheim who published his treatise *Raphian-kistron* in 1826, and had the piece made by Geiger who in fact gave their name to it.

139

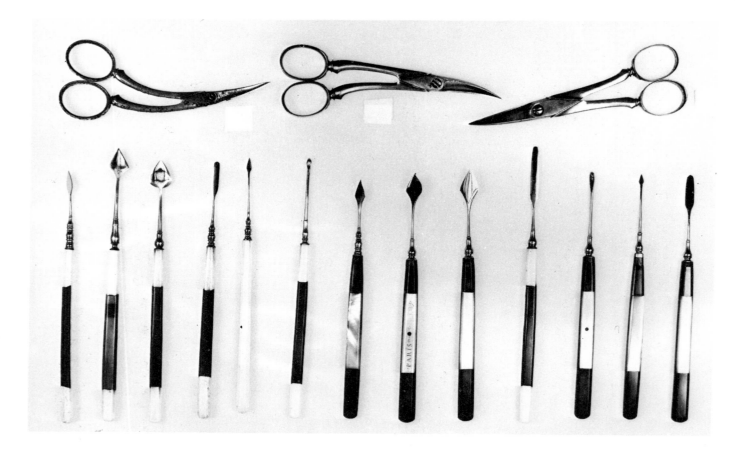

Iris knives were flat, mitre-shaped blades, sharp on both edges and between half an inch and one inch long. The Maw catalogue of 1868 does, though, illustrate one that has a thick central spine. Samuel Sharp's method of cutting the iris was said to need two knives, a spatula and a pointed cutting needle. Bistouries for use in operations for fistula lachrymalis and for separating the false membrane of the iris were as those described below by Mihles or, by the mid-nineteenth century, had a long narrow scoop-shaped blade, sharply pointed at the end and with a very limited cutting edge.

Ophthalmic conditions listed by Mihles, apart from Cataract, are; Ophthalmia or Inflammation; the Contracted Pupil; the Fistula Lachrymalis; and Excoriations of Ulcusculi on the Edges of the Lids. For curing Ophthalmia, he suggests first, repellent applications (his words), then raising blisters, a Seton (see Chapter 3), or formation of matter behind the cornea to be opened by a lancet for discharging, and the eye then bandaged.

5. *Instruments for cataract operation by cutting, c. 1755 (those of J. Daviel, 1693–1762.)*
(Musée d'Histoire de la Médecine, Paris; Cliché Assistance Publique)

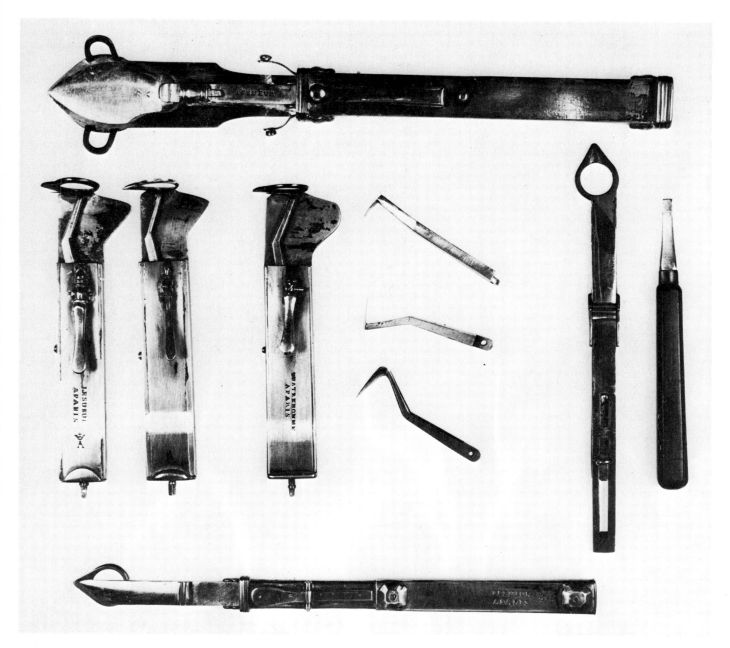

6. *Guerons' spring cataract knife, 1785, and
other cataract-cutting knives of Dumont and
Demours, c. 1770. Right Gueron's knife 11·5 cm.
(Musée d'Histoire de la Médecine, Paris;
Cliché Assistance Publique)*

141

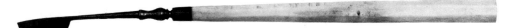

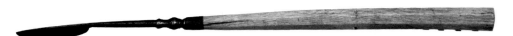

7.   *Cheselden's iris knife, c. 1750. 12·5 cm.*
(Royal College of Surgeons of England)

8.   *Scarpa's bistoury for tumour of the*
eyelids, c. 1805. 12·5 cm.
(Royal College of Surgeons of England)

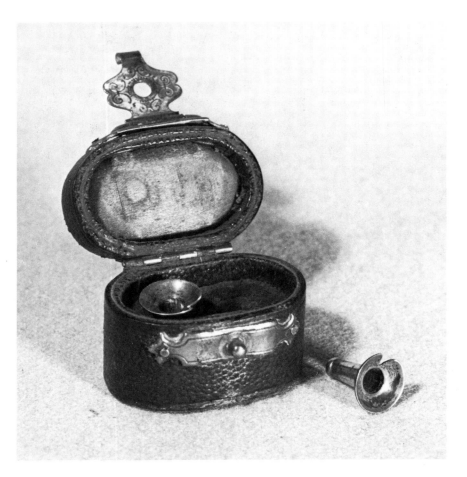

9.   *A very early pair of tubes for the nasal*
ducts, cased, c. 1770. Length of each 2 cm.
(Castle Museum, York)

142

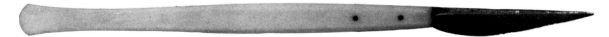

10.   *Frère Côme's cataract knife, c. 1750.*
15 cm.
(Royal College of Surgeons of England)

11.   *Set of ophthalmic instruments, c. 1800.*
(Germanisches Nationalmuseum Nuremberg)

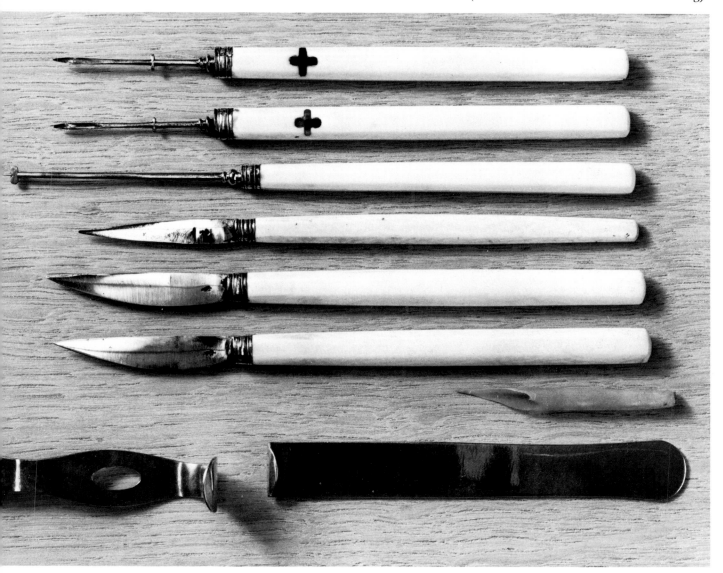

For operating in cases of fistula lachrymalis, slight cases could be cured by Anel's probe (see above) and then syringed. Otherwise, it was necessary to lay open the whole duct with a small crooked bistoury. If this were not successful then one would have to procure a passage through the nasal duct with a silver or whalebone probe, catgut or a plaster bougie, keeping fungus at bay with the application of caustic. Another method used the smallest size of curved trocar (see Chapter 5).

Tumours or cysts on the eyelids might be excised with a small knife.

All these operations were usually impossible on children, says Mihles, because of the difficulty of keeping them still. Many an adult today might feel they would have the same trouble.

12. *Plate from Samuel Mihles's* Elements of Surgery, 1764, *showing ophthalmic and other instruments.*

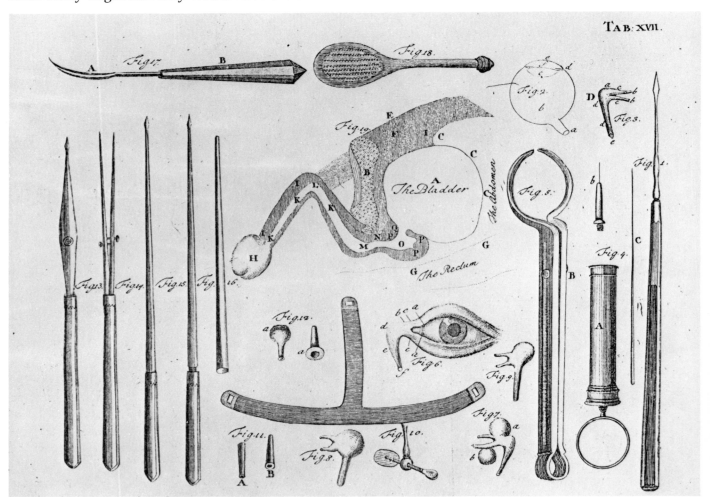

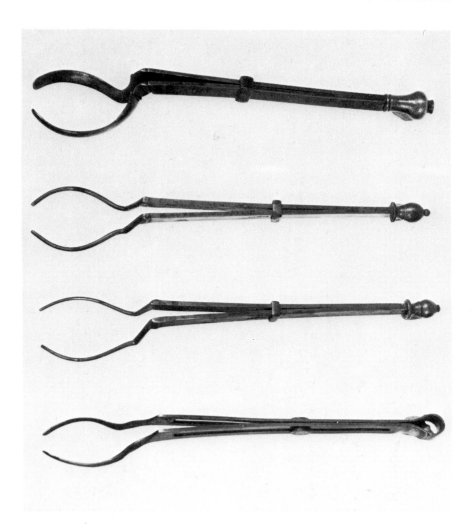

13. *Cheselden/Sharp's eye specula,*
c. 1750. 13 cm.
(Royal College of Surgeons of England)

Ocular forceps

This branch of surgery produced more types of forceps than any other. They are mostly immediately recognisable by the small size of the jaws for use on the eye-ball and for the extraction of foreign bodies, and most have a hinge-hold for instant control. Benjamin Bell introduced an eyelid retractor forceps in 1790 with a spring catch, though an eyelid speculum had been devised by Perret as early as 1772. Both these must have been based on that shown by Samuel Mihles in 1764 (pl. 12). Petit, a little later, had an eyelid retractor with semi-circular blades on the slot-slide principle. There is a rather earlier retractor in the Royal College of Surgeons which

145

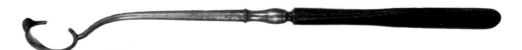

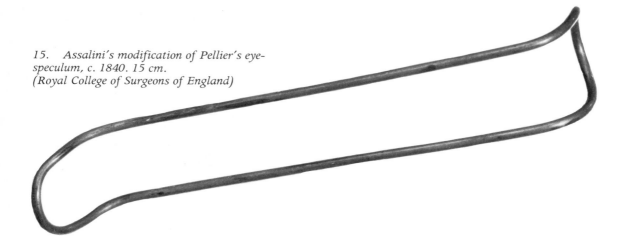

14. *Benjamin Bell's eye speculum, c. 1780.*
12·5 cm.
(Royal College of Surgeons of England)

15. *Assalini's modification of Pellier's eye-*
speculum, c. 1840. 15 cm.
(Royal College of Surgeons of England)

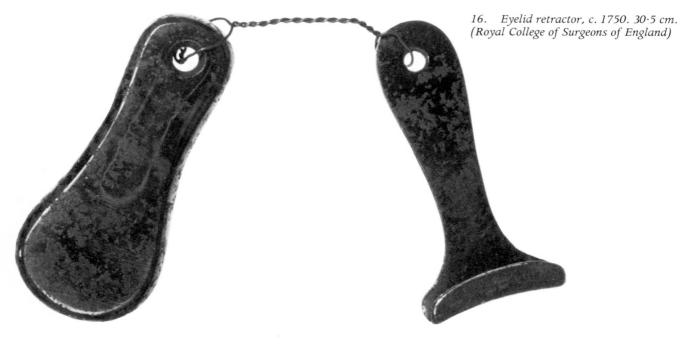

16. *Eyelid retractor, c. 1750. 30·5 cm.*
(Royal College of Surgeons of England)

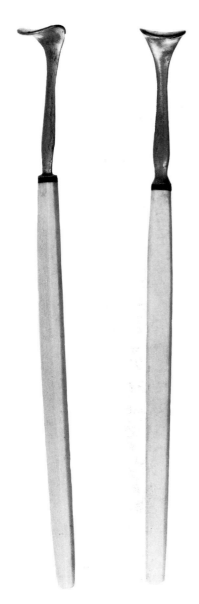

17. *Desmarre's eyelid retractors, c. 1850.*
15 cm.
(Royal College of Surgeons of England)

works with the aid of a weight. Savigny, in 1798, illustrated eyelid forceps with hollow rectangular blades and a ring slide catch. From the same catalogue is 'the forceps of Mr Wathers' with ring-jaws, convex outside, concave inside 'for holding soft, pulpy substances'. Carl von Graefe, the first to produce serious work on surgery of the eyelids, modified this so that the legs were curved and a pin on one ring fitted into the other—a type that is still used today in operations for cataract. Karl Himly (1772–1837) a German professor of ophthalmics was the first to give specialised instruction in the subject. He introduced a fenestrated forceps of circular section for ocular use, and many later trachoma forceps for fixing the eyelid while operating were based on this idea. German surgeons were particularly forward-looking in this branch of surgery, and another ocular forceps, made by Brambilla and Savigny, was that of Baron de Wenzel (1728–1800). Louis Desmarres (1810–82) had a forceps—made by Maw among others—with an oval fenestration in one blade, and a solid oval plate in the other, held by a slot-slide catch. Herman Snellen (1834–1908) modified this to a semi-rectangular shape. The Nyrops catalogue of 1872 shows several of this type as does the Maw catalogue of 1868.

Other eyelid forceps include that by C. M. J. Langenbecke (1776–1851), a German surgeon, which has very curved legs thus allowing other instruments to be used through it when closed. About 1840 an instrument was devised for holding the fold of the eyelid to be excised. It took the form of a self-holding forceps turning at the top on the same axis. All these eyelid retractors were made both for right and left eyes (pl. 17).

Dieffenbach (see Chapter 3) tells us that G. F. L. Stromeir was the first to consider the operation of tenotomy for squint in 1829, and in 1839 Dieffenbach himself performed the first complete and successful operation on a boy of 7. Fixation forceps for this purpose first appeared in the Nyrops catalogue of 1840. They had bifurcated legs and in 1842, a Fricke's catch (see Chapter 3).

H. J. Knapp (1832–1911), later Professor of the University of New York, invented a trachoma forceps the jaws of which are formed by small rollers.

Iridectomy forceps take the form of hooked jaws, which, when closed, lie together as one hook. The best of these was introduced by Franz Reisniger (1781–1853), a German oculist, in 1817. They had minute steel points on an ivory handle, modified later into one with larger hooks.

Another item included in this chapter, but which could equally well fall into Chapter 5, is a pair of minute dilators such as those illustrated by Samuel Mihles in pl. 12. After an operation for fistula lachrymalis it was necessary to keep open the newly made passage to the nose until 'the passage is become callous or cicatrised'. These tubes are carefully angled for each side of the face and measure only 1·9 cm in length. Many and varied have been the suggested purposes for these dilators—from ear drop applicators to nasal membrane protectors while sniffing cocaine. Those found today are usually cased, in pairs, and appear in the nineteenth century catalogues, though the pair from the Castle Museum, York in pl. 9 are of *c.* 1770.

Ophthalmoscopes

The ophthalmoscope, as we know it, was invented in Germany by Herman Helmholtz (1821–99) in 1850 and thus succeeded in making ophthalmics the most exacting science in surgery. It is a device for shining a narrow beam of light through the pupil of the eye so that the retina may be seen. It incorporates a selection of tiny lenses which bring the retina into focus to the eye of the observer, thereby making it possible to work out the degree of long or short-sightedness present. In addition, the ophthalmoscope allows a view of the nervous system and can detect hypertension and diseases affecting the blood vessels. Helmholtz's instrument was inde-pendently devised although William Babbage had constructed a rudimentary version in 1847. Both had a turned wooden handle and brass shaft holding a circular concave mirror with a small central hole. A little later a revolving brass disc containing a variety of inset lenses was added, and these could be adjusted to the hole in the original mirror. Very much larger ones were designed to examine the patient while in bed, and others were mounted in telescopic tubes for easy carrying. By the early 1860s ophthalmoscopes had become more sophisticated and the mirror was made adjustable so that light could be reflected on to the eye; a tube enclosed the eye and was padded at the patient's end for comfort. The Maw catalogue of 1868 shows a simple ophthalmoscope with circular bi-convex lens on an ivory handle.

Optometers

William Porterfield (1683–1760), one of Boerhaave's pupils (see Chapter 1), invented the optometer for measuring sight and, eventually, for fitting spectacles. Thomas Young did much to improve his model but it was not until the mid-nineteenth century

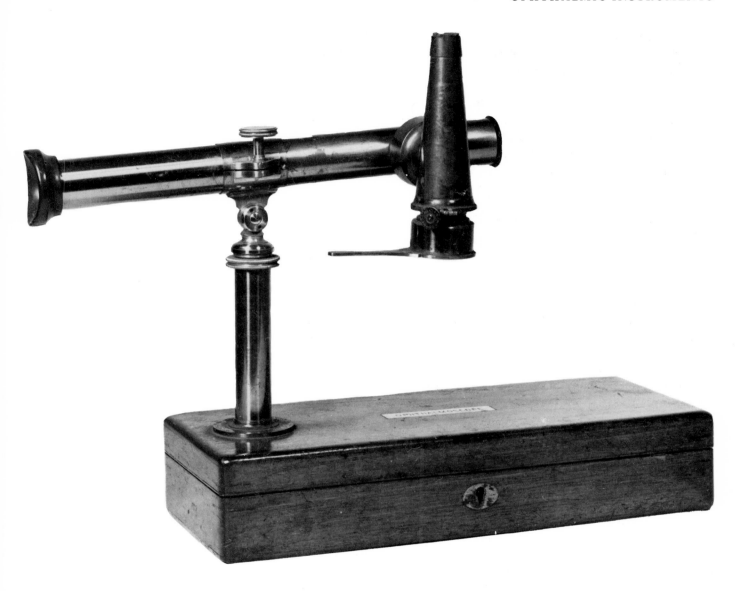

18. *Ophthalmoscope of the type introduced by Beale in 1869 with attached illuminating device, Hawkesley.*
(Wellcome Collection)

that the use of an optometer became at all usual; however, once used they stayed much in vogue. The Wellcome Collection has a 'lens test trial' of 1843, made by Mann of Gloucester. It consists of 40 pairs of lenses in a case, each of which can be slotted into a pair of spectacles on a trial and error basis. There, too, is the Hudson 'Complete Sight Suitor' of 1854, with three ranges of lenses including cataract lenses in cardboard frames from which the customer might select the most suitable. Jaeger introduced his clear type face for sight testing in

149

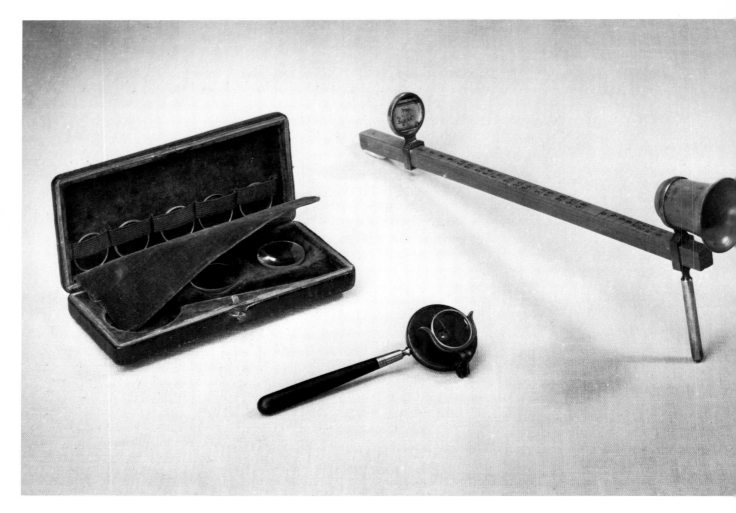

1854 and this was thereafter used on optometers. A curious truncheon-like example in a Pennsylvania Hospital has the script circling the barrel. Most optometers took the form of a rotating selection of lenses which could be slid along a rod a varying distance as required from a sample of written symbols, thus determining the correct power needed. One of the simplest and earliest was that of W. H. Wollaston (1766–1828) and can be seen in pl 19. He was a tireless researcher into optics and invented periscopic spectacles, useful for oblique vision. However, extreme anxiety on behalf of his patients forced him to give up his very lucrative practice. 'Allow me', he said, 'to decline the mental flagellation called anxiety; compared with which the loss of thousands of pounds is as a fleabite.'

19. Boxwood and brass optometer, as designed by W. H. Wollaston, c. 1870; Early ophthalmoscope as devised by R. L. Leebreich (1830–1917) with six supplementary lenses, c. 1865. 9 cm. 30·5 cm. (Simon Kaye Ltd, London)

CHAPTER EIGHT

Miscellaneous instruments

Naval and military items

Surgeons attached to the two services were, in the earliest days, those who won most renown (see Chapter 1). There was an incentive to pay them well and encourage them in their research and endeavours. Nearly all the early surgeons of any achievement served their time in the services. In a Charter of 1462, Edward IV granted them privileges as non-combatant officers, although today's military and naval surgeons often imagine theirs were gained from the Geneva Convention. John of Arderne (1307–90) was at Crecy in 1346, Thomas Moresteyde (1401–50), and Nicholas Covet were at Agincourt in 1415, and Thomas Gale (1507–87), who published the first book on gunshot wounds in 1563, served in Flanders. John Woodall (1556–1643) was surgeon both in the Army and the Navy. He compiled *The Surgeon's Mate* while Surgeon-General to the East India Company, the first book particularly designed to instruct ships' surgeons. It examined scurvy for the first time and he is credited with advising the use of lime juice, though it was not until 1779 that the Admiralty enjoined its use and scurvy disappeared almost overnight. Woodall's book became an unofficial textbook that every naval surgeon had to have, and included passages on gangrene, plague, and gunshot wounds. He invented a form of trephine still in use today (see Chapter 2) and was the first to advocate amputation of the leg at the ankle, thought to be a hazardous undertaking.

The Roundheads and Cavaliers each had their own surgeons. James Cooke (1614–88) was a Puritan who achieved fame by editing *Select Observations on English Bodies* by Dr J. Hall, the son-in-law of Shakespeare, and by writing himself *The Marrow of Surgery*— but he was not as great a surgeon as the Cavaliers had, Richard Wiseman. Richard Wiseman (1622–76) enjoyed a life of high adventure; in and out of prison and exile, he eventually became Serjeant Surgeon to the King on the Restoration. He made notes on every case he treated and wrote, not for students, but for educated and experienced surgeons. He advocated immediate amputation for gunshot wounds 200 years before Larrey (see Chapter 3) in his book *Treatise of Wounds*.

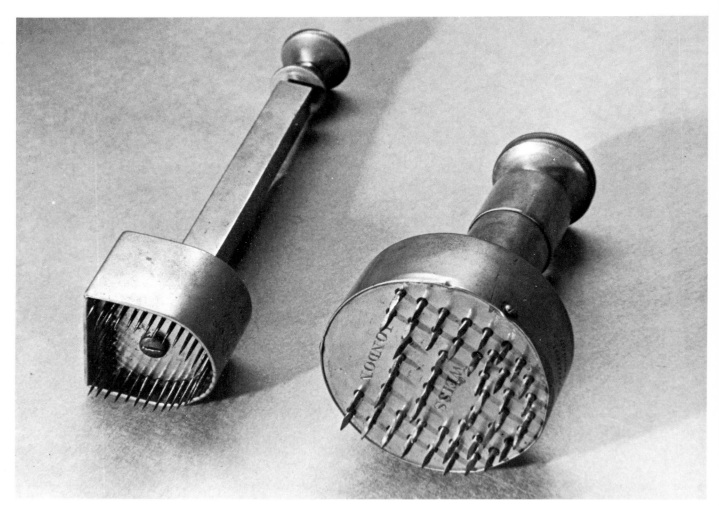

Naturally, certain instruments have particular application to warfare. Thomas Moresteyde (1401–50) in his *Fair Book of Surgery* gives a detailed description of an instrument to remove an arrow from the head: 'the wych instrument was mad in the maner of a tonges and was Rownde and holowysche.' Others such as bullet extractors and post-mortem pieces are described below. It is doubtful if any set of instruments described as 'field-surgeon's kit' can be treated as such, if it does not include at least one of these.

Another instrument peculiar to the Army is a branding device for deserters (pl. 1). When a deserter was caught, the whole regiment would be drawn up to see his punishment. The left arm was raised and to a roll of drums, a bunch of needles in the shape of the letter 'D' was thrust into the armpit; it was then the duty of the drummer-boy

1. *Instrument for branding deserters from the army. Invented by Weiss in 1850. 14 cm. (R.A.M.C. Museum, Aldershot)*

2. *Contents of naval surgeon's case: spring-socket knife with three blades, Maw, c. 1860; dental forceps, c. 1830; catheters, forceps, saw, etc., mostly Weiss, c. 1800. (Commanding Officer, H.M.S. Victory, Portsmouth)*

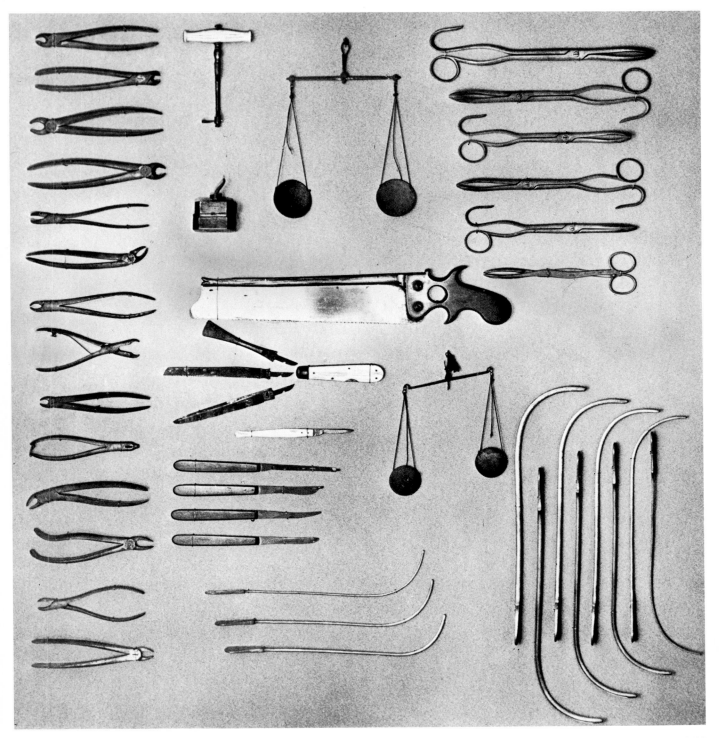

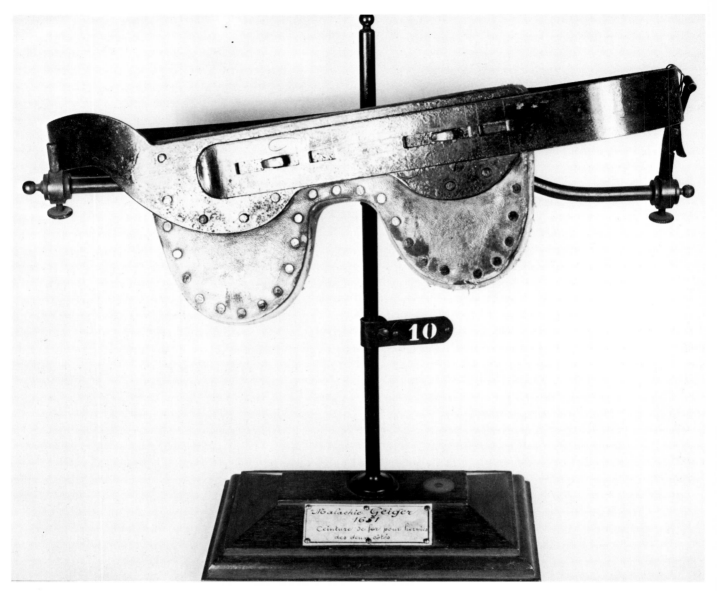

to rub a mixture of lampblack and gunpowder into the wound, thus branding the offender for life. In 1850 Weiss invented an instrument for the purpose—a heavy brass truncheon from which shot, on the release of a spring, the series of spikes that effected the 'D'. One of these may be seen at the Museum of the R.A.M.C. at Aldershot. The practice was abolished in 1871.

Naval surgeons were undoubtedly those who endured the worst conditions in the execution of their duty. During the Armada wars

3.   Hernia truss as introduced by Geiger in 1651.
(Musée d'Histoire de la Médecine, Paris; Cliché Assistance Publique)

154

it was accepted that the wounded would be laid upon the ballast while the ship was in action and naturally wait for reaching land to receive attention. Even 100 years later and well into the mid-nineteenth century, surgeons complained of lack of room both for their equipment and for performing operations. Medicine chests served as both operating table and a sleeping place, and the allotted space was often below the water line, always dark and candlelit, and had no ventilation; added to which the ship was rocked and shaken by the recoil of the cannon overhead. Edward Ives's advice of 1755 to have six knives at the ready rather than the regulation two, as there was no time to sharpen them in action, says much.

In Tudor days apprentices often ran away to sea and posed as surgeons to the authorities whose only concern was to assure the crew there was a surgeon on board. Later, completely ignorant men were press-ganged as surgeons. In addition to their ordinary duties, they were required to be in attendance at all punishments, when flogging and keel-hauling were commonplace. The provincial Barber–Surgeons' companies, such as those of Bristol and Newcastle, and not only the company in London had authority over the ships' surgeons and had to examine their medicine chests. These chests were a constant source of contention. At first the surgeons had to provide instruments and drug chests at their own cost. From the time of Charles I an allowance was given for this purpose but it was never enough and some young surgeons were known to sell their instruments to recoup their expenses. In the St Vincent reforms of 1799, all naval surgeons were required to carry a set of pocket instruments with them at all times, either on or off duty; this was only abolished during the 1930s. Another recommendation of c. 1805 was that 10 per cent of the whole ship's crew should be trained in First Aid but it seems doubtful if this was ever implemented.

The isolation of the sea surgeon meant that he placed much reliance on the books available. In addition to those mentioned above, books specifically for the sea included *Marine Practise of Surgery* by William Northcote (1770), and Turnbull's *The Naval Surgeon* of 1806.

Apart from injuries sustained in action the most common condition on board ship was hernia and other forms of rupture (pl. 3). The enormous physical strain of lifting and hauling, working the windlass, etc. combined with chronic constipation due to the diet, made hernia an occupational hazard for the seaman. The first order to supply free trusses to naval vessels was in 1744, and in 1753 the Sick and Hurt Board said the expenditure of £303 on trusses over the past three years must be regarded as normal. These free trusses were made of straw and were fairly rudimentary, but it is interesting to note that there were 35 patents for trusses applied for between 1617 and 1852. For bandages on board, the surgeon often relied on outworn and fragmented ensigns; a lucky break was provided by the surplices confiscated from the City churches by the Roundheads in the seventeenth century. Improvisation at sea was inevitable, and Hugh Ryder recorded in 1685 an operation he performed using the chisel and mallet of the ship's carpenter.

Bullet extractors

Attempts to extract bullets from the body date from *c.* 1250 when the introduction of firearms into warfare presented a new challenge to the surgeon. At first, treatment was primitive and

4. *Brass and steel screw bullet extractors, c. 1520. 30 cm.*
(Germanisches Nationalmuseum Nuremberg)

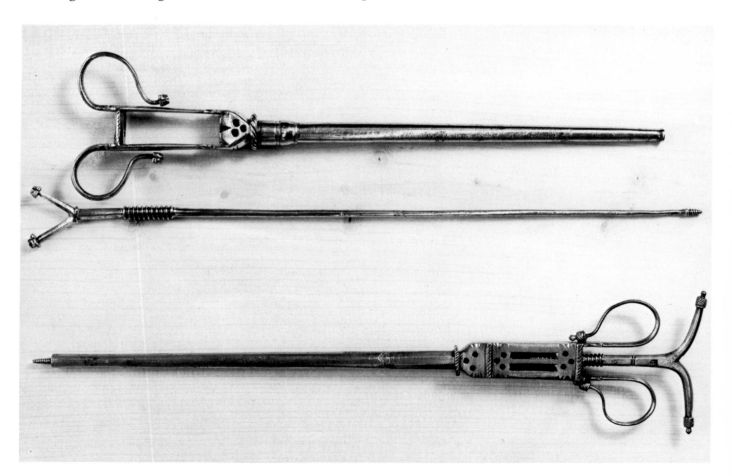

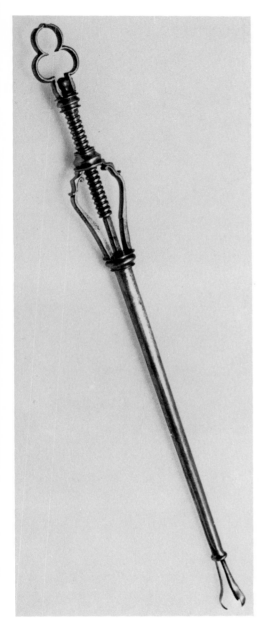

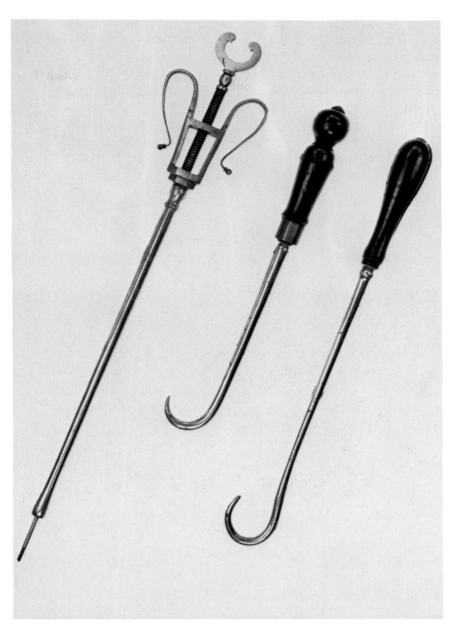

5   *Seventeenth-century bullet forceps.*
(Museum Boerhaave, Leiden)

6.   *Screw bullet extractor and scoops,*
Prujean Collection, c. 1653. 20·5 cm.
(Royal College of Physicians of England)

ineffective except in cases where the bullet was lodged near the surface. No special instrument appears to have been known until the screw extractor of *c.* 1535. This consisted of a hollow rod encasing a long screw which was pushed into the wound, the screw engaged in the lead-bullet and was then withdrawn (pl. 4). An example of this type is illustrated in *The Surgeon's Mate* by John

157

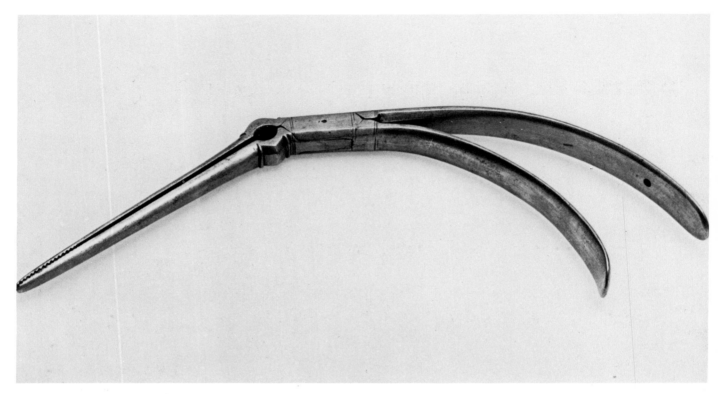

7.   'Crane's beak' forceps used as bullet
extractors, c. 1700. 20·5 cm.
(Museum Boerhaave, Leiden)

8.   Bullet extractor, c. 1700.
(Musée le Secq des Tournelles, Rouen)

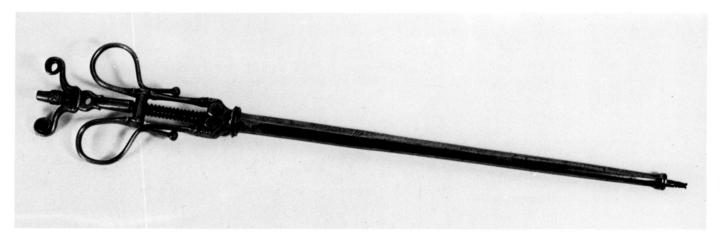

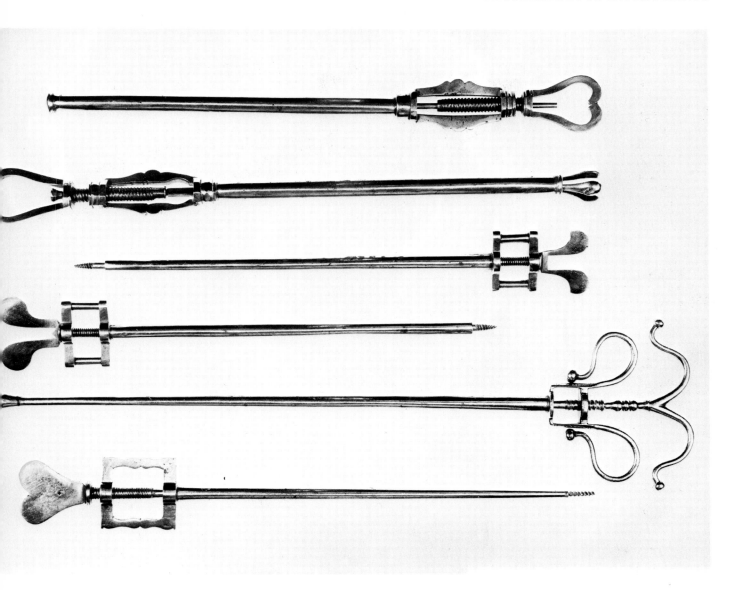

9.   Seventeenth- and eighteenth-century bullet
extractors. Second from the top is the type
introduced by Diderot, c. 1790. 20·5 cm.
(Musée d'Histoire de la Médecine, Paris;
Cliché Assistance Publique)

Woodall (see p. 151). With modifications, this type of extractor was
used down to the nineteenth century. Alongside it came the bullet
forceps with curved points, the insides of which were heavily serrated
for a firm grip. In 1552 a variation in the form of an ornate three-legged
forceps was introduced from Naples by Alphonso Ferri (1515–95) and
became known as an Alphonsine. However, it was not much liked
and the previous type of forceps was preferred with the addition of
rings which encircled the blades and fixed them once the bullet was
found. Scultetus in 1674 found it necessary to warn of the need to

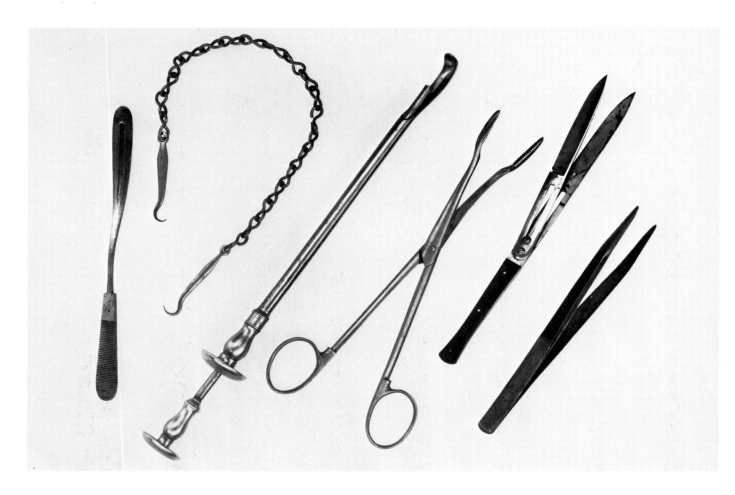

keep the forceps closed while probing the bullet and on no account to open them until it was located. Nevertheless, during the eighteenth century, bullet forceps were often found to have such an injurious distending effect that forceps in two parts, similar to midwifery forceps, and with a midwifery hinge, were devised and introduced by Savigny early in the nineteenth century. Another type that came from the Continent at the turn of the century, the Diderot type as illustrated in his *Encyclopaedie*, consisted of an ornamental handle, usually elaborate, with a screw which worked three or more retractable inward-facing hooks at the end of a tube which engaged the bullet on the turn of the screw. Weiss made one with a lever which raised the bullet from its bed and a spring which secured it for extraction. Different again is the one by Aitken of York in pl. 10 believed to have been used in the Crimea.

10. Contents of a Field-Surgeon's case, containing director and file, Valentin knife, cross-legged forceps, chain hooks, tweezers, and bullet extractor, c. 1850, Aitken, York. Director 15 cm.
(Simon Kaye Ltd, London)

160

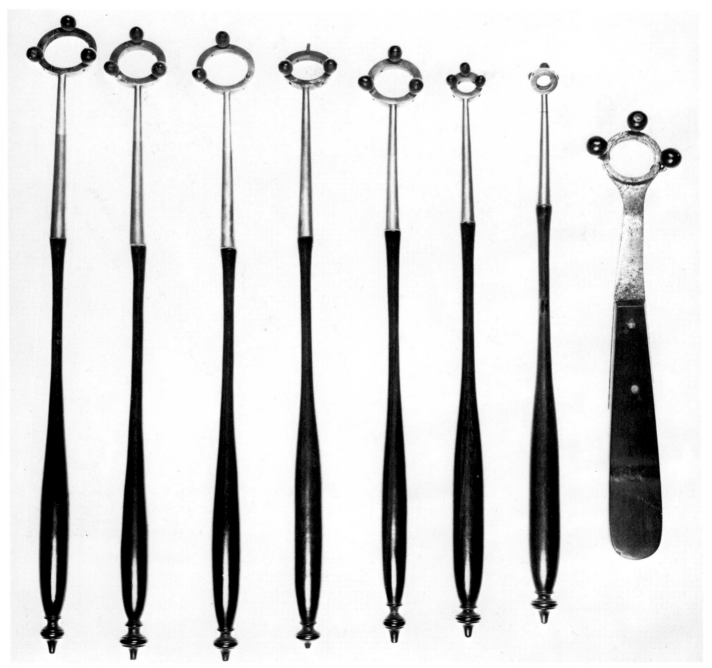

11. A set of early nineteenth-century portes-moxas—holders for the Japanese burning herb, moxa, which was burned and applied to the skin as a counter-irritant; a form of treatment widely used in France. Longest instrument 20·5 cm.
(Musée d'Histoire de la Médecine, Paris; Cliché Assistance Publique)

12. *Instruments used by Dr Antonmarchi at the autopsy of Napoleon on the 6 May 1821. (Musée d'Histoire de la Médecine, Paris; Cliché Assistance Publique)*

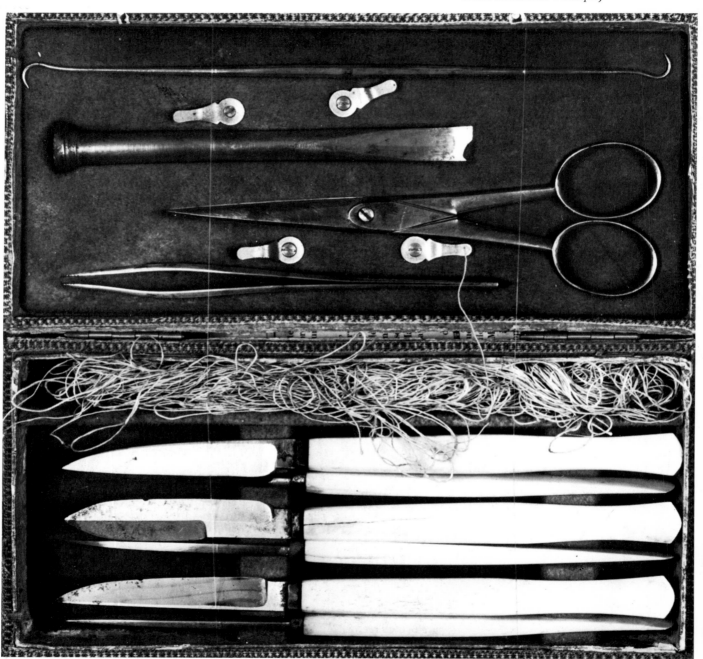

162

Post-mortem items

The lack of corpses allowed for anatomical demonstration meant that post-mortem examination was an opportunity often seized. James Yonge's writings suggest the practice was well established in his day (1670) and Robert Wright, demonstrator in anatomy at Surgeons' Hall between 1643 and 1646, took care 'lest he be criticized' to 'straightaway open the body' and show the inevitability of death.

Corpses felled on the battlefield could seldom be retrieved before *rigor mortis* had set in, and various instruments for use in straightening the corpse for burial were necessary to the field surgeon. The science of diagnosis was not well developed until the second half of the nineteenth century and the practice of examining the bodies to determine the cause of death in unexplained circumstances did not become generally accepted until then. The least number of instruments a field surgeon would need would be a steel mallet and chisel (pl. 13), and possibly a spine-wrench.

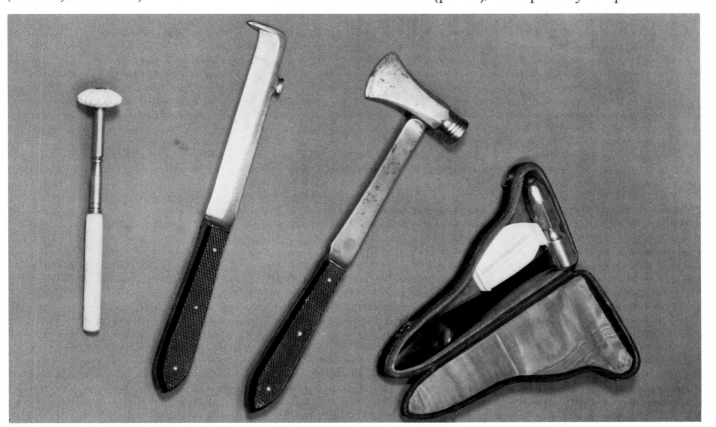

13. *An ivory and brass reflexmeter, c. 1870, 15 cm; A post-mortem mallet and chisel, c. 1840; Dr Bennett's percussor and graduated pleximeter, cased, c. 1870. (Simon Kaye Ltd, London)*

Nineteenth-century cases of instruments for the purpose would include much more. An early nineteenth-century set by Coxeter is in the Wellcome Museum and a fine set at the National Army Museum *c*. 1858 by Ferris of Bristol contains the following:

    a pair of bowel scissors, with guarded blades;
    a tenon saw with hinged handle;
    a cartilage knife;
    4 scalpels of varying sizes;
    a pair of tweezers;
    a chisel;
    a set of chain hooks;
    a spine wrench.

Spaces are provided for a pair of sharp-pointed scissors and a hammer, though the instruments themselves are missing (pl. 14).

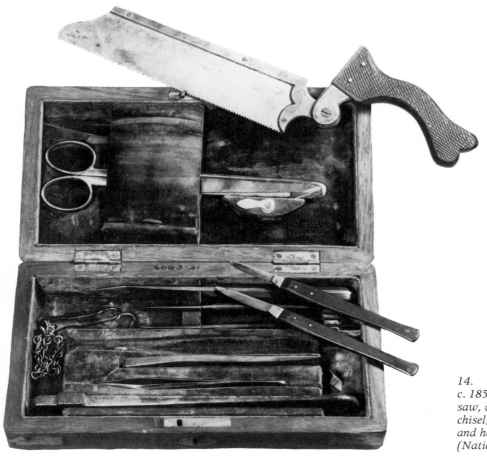

14.   *Cased set of post-mortem instruments, c. 1850, Ferris, containing: bowel scissors, saw, cartilage knife, 4 scalpels, tweezers, chisel, chain hooks, spine wrench (scissors and hammer missing). 30·5 by 25·5 cm. (National Army Museum, London)*

Stethoscopes

The Breton doctor René Laennec of Quimper (1781–1826) first invented the stethoscope in 1816. Finding that a percussor alone was inadequate to diagnose the chest condition of the stout, and being, it is said, embarrassed at putting his ear to the bosom of his female patients, he first used rolled up paper secured with string, to listen, as it were, at second remove. Far from being less efficient, he found the method amplified the sound and was an improvement. He published his treatise on the stethoscope—literally Greek for 'I look into the chest'—in 1819, but the first English translation did not appear until 1825 so there are unlikely to have been many here before that date. His paper entitled 'On Mediate Auscultation—a classification of all cardiac and respiratory sounds—with signification, condition, doctrines and interpretations' was much acclaimed.

The first monaural stethoscopes were of turned wood, either cedar, boxwood, or ebony, approximately 30 cm long and 3 cm in diameter though they became much more slender in time (pl. 16). Some had the cylinder dividing in the middle and screwing together for easy carrying. As time went on, the ear and chest pieces became more elaborate with ivory mounts or the entire instrument was embellished with painting. A few may be found in metal, notably pewter, or rubber. The Wellcome Collection has a syringe-shaped one and some most elegant turned wood examples have been found.

15. Original Laennec stethoscope, 1819. 30·5 cm.
(Musée d'Histoire des Sciences, Geneva)

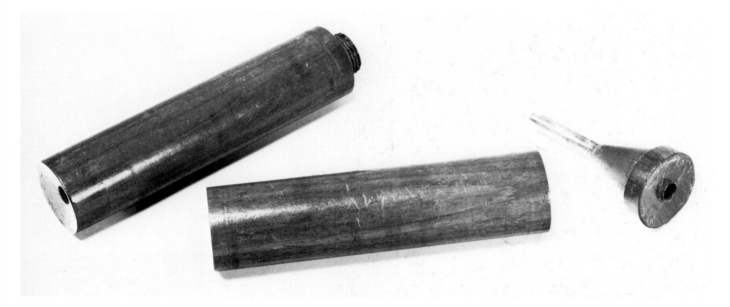

165

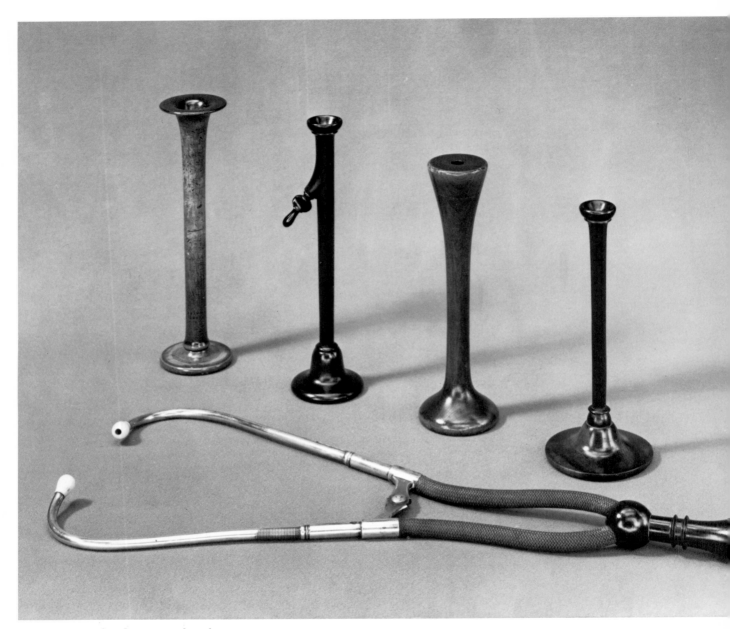

16.   *A group of early monaural stethoscopes.
From left: fruitwood, Grumbridge, c. 1840,
18 cm; ebony, with second outlet to which
tube could be attached for a student, c. 1870;
as Sir James Paget's, Bigg, c. 1830; ebony
and tulipwood, c. 1850; early binaural
stethoscope, c. 1860.
(Simon Kaye Ltd, London)*

One of the original Laennec types with a funnel section at the top is at the Royal College of Surgeons. Another, from Geneva, is shown in pl. 15.

The monaural stethoscope was modified into the binaural type around 1850 by G. P. Caniman of New York who patented his invention in 1855. The first ones were of steel with ivory ear pieces and ebony chest pieces of two sizes were provided. The flexible tubes were either cord or silk bound becoming uncovered gutta-percha and afterwards plain rubber. Of those now found with rubber tubes it is difficult to pretend that many still have the original rubber (pl. 16).

The monaural type, however, died a slow death and even in 1868 the Maw catalogue showed several, some with a graduated or revolving ear piece. Monaural stethoscopes are, of course, still commonly used today in maternity hospitals. It is therefore an over-simplification, as with many other instruments, to suggest that the earlier type must have been made prior to 1855 and the affectation of using a longer and longer stethoscope was high fashion for some time.

Galvanisers

Electricity was first used for medical purposes in Germany in 1743. It was generally thought to have a therapeutic effect on the physiological processes of the body. Several surgeons, including John Hunter, worked on this theory and found it an important factor in the functions of the body. It was thought to cure, among other things, consumption, palsy, dropsy, dysentery, stone, venereal disease, cancer, blindness, and worms. By 1800 to 1830 many large and cumbersome machines, mostly involving rotating glass vessels with friction procured by a leather flap, transferred electricity to a Leyden jar with curved brass rods to transmit it to the patient. Clarke invented an electromagnetic machine c. 1832 that was the forerunner of the medical galvanic machine. From about 1840 onwards, many varieties of these were used and may be found today, though seldom complete. In pl. 17 can be seen a pair of galvanic tractors patented by Benjamin Douglas Perkins in 1798. These, he said, drawn across the body would ease a variety of aches, pains, and diseases. The tractors are made of a careful combination of various metals. W. H. Halse produced many galvanisers in the years 1855–80. Well made of rosewood with brass fittings, they look a little like a cross between a miniature steam engine and a clock, measuring approximately 20 by 10 cm and about 13 cm high.

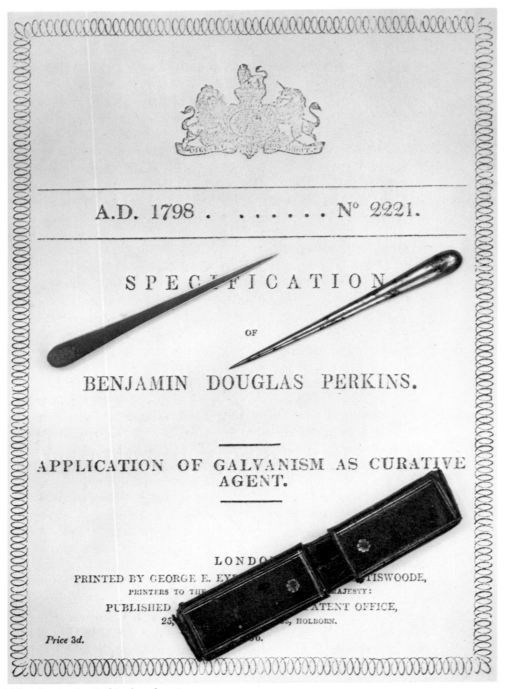

17. *Benjamin Perkins's galvanic tractors*
with case and patent, 1798. 7·6 cm.
(Simon Kaye Ltd, London)

Syringes

Syringes for many purposes were used early. The Romans had a nasal syringe—the outer case of metal with a disc plunger—and made frequent mention of clysters. John of Arderne (c. 1350) recorded that he had a syringe for enema but did not describe it. He recommended an enema to be administered three times a year. Early English syringes are heavy and cumbersome, often made in pewter or silver. They were developed in the seventeenth century and were probably multi-purpose. They have an extended head and a barrel from 10 to 20 cm long that possibly suggests a vaginal or rectal intention. Smaller ones of silver or bone were made, however, as John Moyle in 1693 recommends syringeing of the ears with wine or sack; 'but if there be a noise in the Ears like the singing of Grasshoppers, then that is Wind and Water, from coldness and moisture of the Brain'. The French Surgeon, Dominique Anel (1679–1740), in the first half of the eighteenth century, invented a small suction syringe to take the place of the 'soldier-suckers'—bands of men and women employed on the battlefield to suck the wounds of the soldiers, obviously removing much of the dirt and infection and resulting in quicker healing. This became the forerunner of the modern aspirator. Another of Anel's small syringes was for use in the lachrymal duct (see Chapter 7).

A beautiful silver syringe appeared recently, about 8 cm long and 4 cm in diameter of the barrel. Dated c. 1780 it unscrews to remove head and plunger and is indeed a precision-made instrument. Ivory and bone were used for syringes for aural and nasal use, mainly in the late eighteenth and early nineteenth century, the plunger being made of wood with either linen or tow binding to provide suction. From 1800 onwards tiny hypodermic syringes were made for minute injections often of preserving fluids both for embalming and dissecting uses. These were usually made in steel, brass, or a combination of both, with perhaps a ring thumbpiece of ivory, and might have either curved or straight needles. Side ring attachments did not appear before c. 1800.

Another type of small syringe made in the mid-nineteenth century was for the application of lotions or other medicaments on-to or into the body. It was of silver or silver-plate with a screw adjustment, each turn of which released one drop.

John Weiss took out a patent for a syringe in 1824 and Frederick Weiss for another in 1851, but it is difficult to learn the form they took. John Read (1760–1847), patentee of the stomach pump, gave his name to an enema-syringe of brass with ivory attachments.

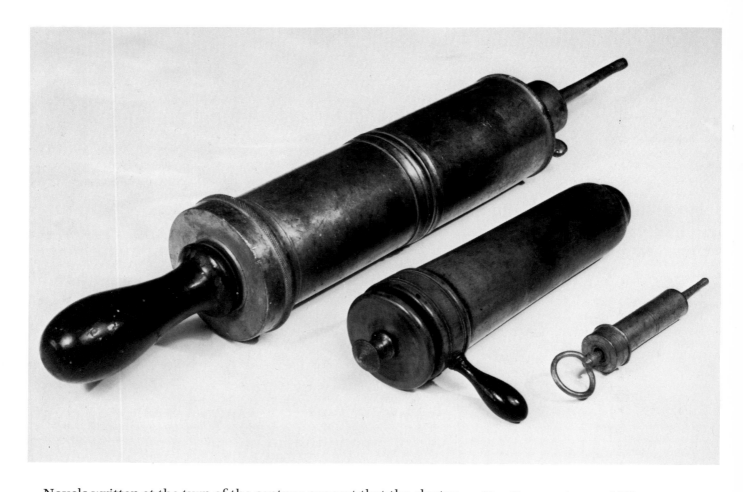

18. *Enema syringes, c. 1800.*
(Musée d'Histoire des Sciences, Geneva)

Novels written at the turn of the century suggest that the clyster or enema was already taking a place in the lives of the healthy as well as the sick, and indeed the wide and ingenious variety of apparatus from that time on bears testimony to it. Those fanatics of colonic irrigation, the Victorians, could have chosen from 39 varieties offered by the Maw's catalogue of 1868, and for their delight they were made of every material, some wildly decorated but all discreetly fitting into anonymous cases. The smaller ones were from 18 cm long and were made of brass or pewter, or even glass, with a rubber or twine bound plunger; some would have been attached to a bladder full of liquid. A silk covered rubber tube ended in either an ivory plug for rectal irrigation or a long brass-mounted rubber tube for the vagina—the latter gaining ground from the 1860s onwards as a contraceptive measure.

A larger variety, sometimes of quite breathtaking size, was the

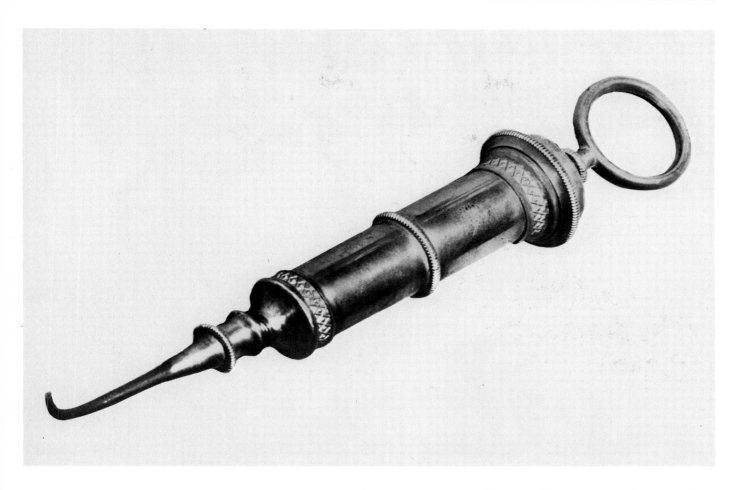

*19.   Large brass syringe, c. 1820.
(College of Physicians, Philadelphia)*

plunger and reservoir type. The vessel containing the irrigation liquid stood independently and was worked by a brass pump from the top, a brass mounted tube with attachments led from it. Thomas Machell patented an enema of this kind in 1818 and the Pharmaceutical Society owns a wide selection, the cylinders of porcelain and engraved silver-plate as well as glass and japanned metal all stand at least 25 cm high (pl. 22). One was introduced by Maw in 1830 and was known as 'Maw's Domestic Medicine Machine'. A very rare form of enema introduced in the first half of the nineteenth century was telescopic, made in several sections of strong metal as it was designed to be sat on and collapsed as it became effective. Hutchinson brought in another self-administered variety *c.* 1840 with a telescopic barrel and nozzle at right angles to the handle.

An apparatus of similar purpose to a syringe might be mentioned

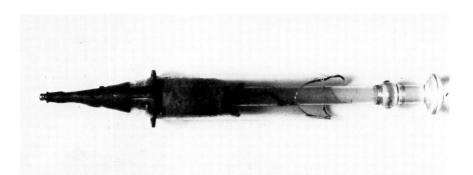

20. The hypodermic syringe used by Alexander Wood for the first subcutaneous injection of morphia, c. 1853. 10 cm. (Royal College of Surgeons of Edinburgh)

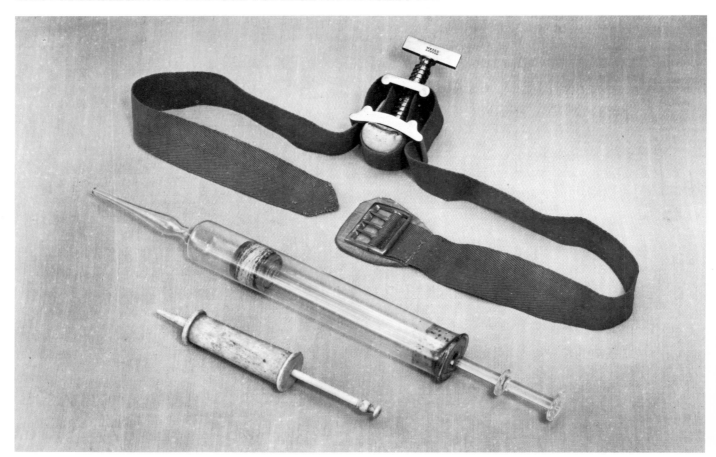

21. Screw tourniquet of the Petit type, c. 1820, Weiss; Glass syringe, tow plunger, c. 1860, 23 cm; Early bone syringe, c. 1680. (Simon Kaye Ltd, London)

172

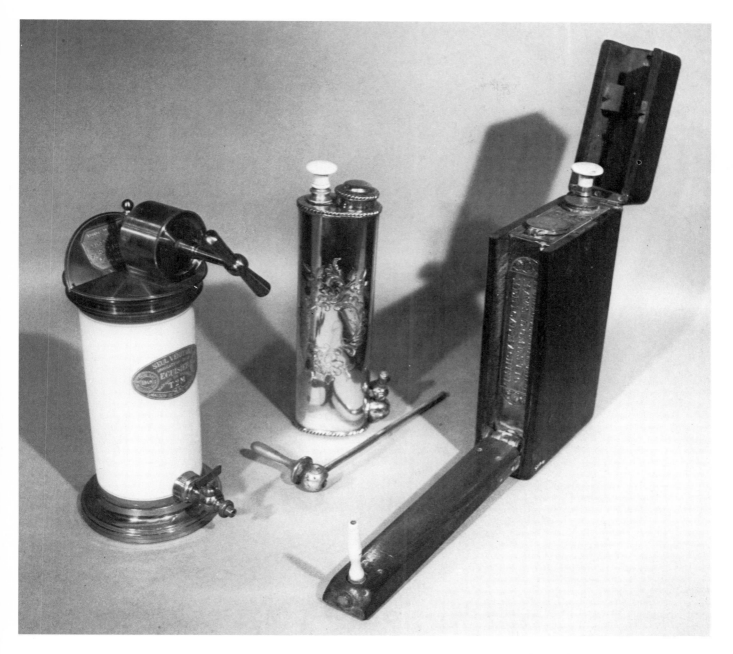

22. *French porcelain enema, c. 1860.*
30·5 cm; French silver-plated enema, c. 1870;
Wooden-cased enema shutting into book-
form, Maw, c. 1870.
(Pharmaceutical Society of Great Britain
Museum)

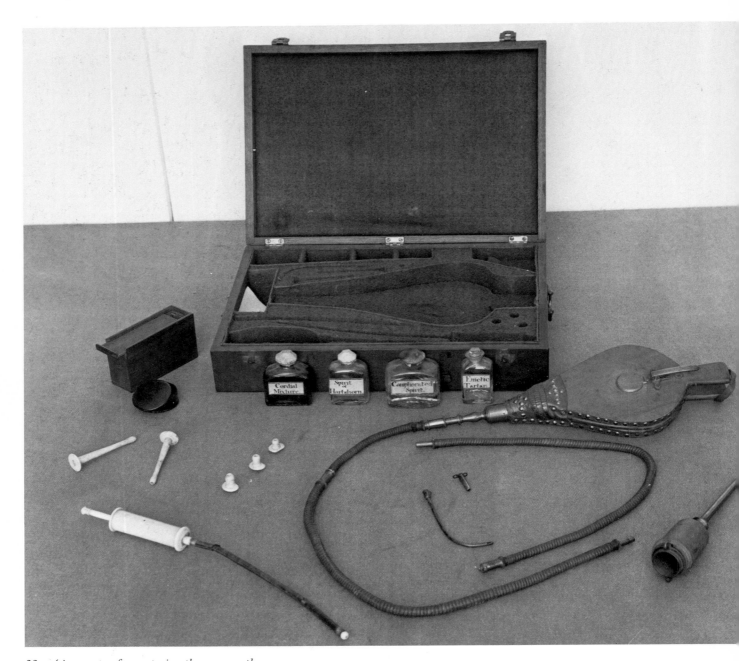

23. 'Apparatus for restoring the apparently
drowned' kept by Bedford canal for that
purpose from c. 1800. As recommended by the
Royal Humane Society. Length in case
45·7 cm.
(Bedford Museum)

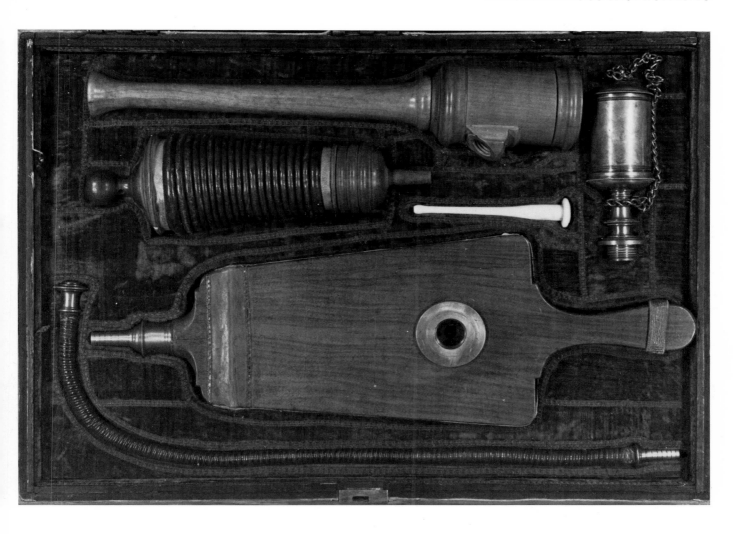

24. Tobacco enema, 1785.
(Institute of Medical History, Vienna)

here. This was an instrument made about 1776 onwards by, at least, Evans, and recommended by the Royal Humane Society (founded 1774) for the revival of 'temporary lapse of animation' (pl. 23). It took the form of a pair of wood and leather bellows with brass mounted tube attached, ending in a circular ivory mouthpiece. By the application of the bellows the lungs might be induced to work. However, should this be to no avail, another tube could be attached, this ending in a long brass finial for rectal insertion and tobacco smoke was then pumped into the wretched inert patient. The latter use was first introduced by John Woodall in the seventeenth century, though he advocated it principally as a laxative. One of these early types, from Denmark is in pl. 25.

175

25. *Tobacco enema, 1661. Length 45·5 cm.*
(Museum of Historical Medicine,
Copenhagen)

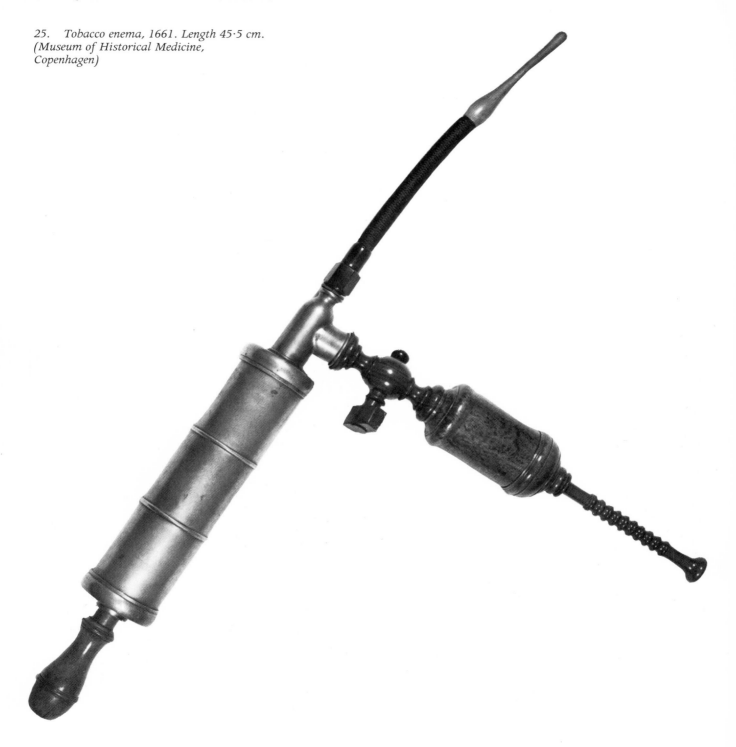

Vaccinators

In the East, attempts to combat smallpox had been tried from earliest times; children were wrapped in the clothes of smallpox victims and Chinese doctors ground the scabs of sufferers to a powder and blew it into the nostrils through a tube. The first attempt to control smallpox was introduced to Europe from Turkey, and to England by Lady Mary Wortley Montague, wife of the British Ambassador to Constantinople, about 1720. The Turks were administering inoculations of actual smallpox, but this was naturally dangerous and might actually have spread the disease. They tried it out on the female slaves who only lost a little in price because of pockmarks. Lady Mary had all her children done and they escaped infection, which recommended the idea to the Princess

26. Early eighteenth-century case of circumcision instruments. (Musée d'Histoire de la Médecine, Paris; Cliché Assistance Publique)

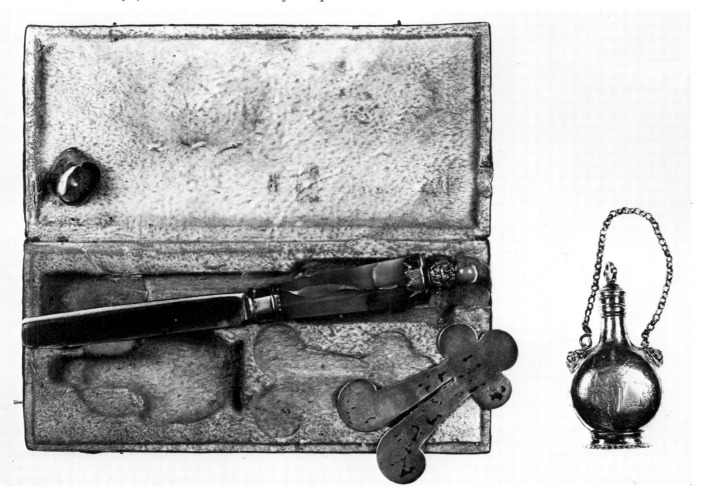

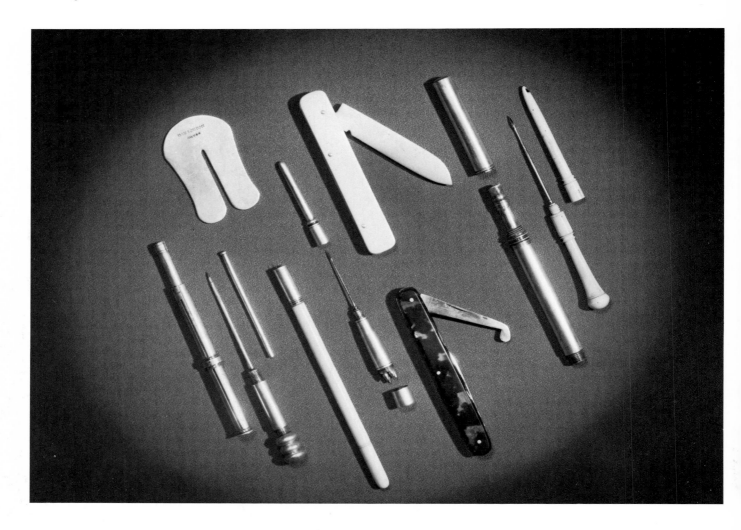

of Wales. The Royal princes were done in 1772 (though in those unliberated days the Royal princesses were done first to test the efficacy) thus giving the practice the social seal, but it was not appealing to the fastidious. It was not infrequently ineffective; the diarist William Hickey was vaccinated in 1756 at the age of seven. Having been dosed at the home of the operator for two weeks previously, as was the custom, he recalls '. . . an incision made in each arm as if the operator intended to cut me up, the wound being at least two inches in length and nearly to the bone in depth, the scars of which remain very visible to the present day. Yet all this butchery (which was the mode then universally pursued) was of no avail, for owing to the matter being too old, or from some other

27. *From right: trocar and cannula, ivory case, c. 1855, 10 cm; caustic-holder, silver and gold, 1836, (possibly) Theophilus Merry; ivory vaccinator, c. 1790; gum lancet, tortoise-shell guard, c. 1860; Southey 4-point trocar and cannula, silver, c. 1840; vaccinator, ivory handle, c. 1840; circumcision guard, silver, c. 1850, Maw; combined lance and caustic-holder, 1842. (Simon Kaye Ltd, London)*

unknown cause, I did not take the infection!' Edward Jenner (1749–1823), an apprentice of John Hunter, is generally credited with the introduction of vaccination by cowpox and published his report in 1798. By 1801 the sailors of the British Fleet were all vaccinated and the practice was here to stay.

The type of operation endured by Hickey was clearly performed by a lancet or small scalpel, but the post-Jenner instruments were usually ivory bladed, folding into a guard like a lancet or like the one in pl. 27. Ivory was the preferred material as the lymph could be preserved on it for a few days. A vaccinating scarificator was made by Millikin early in the nineteenth century, followed by Spratley's vaccinator, a minute steel blade on the end of a long shaft which could be screwed into the handle when not in use. By mid-century Weir introduced his vaccinator—an ivory shaft from which slid, at one end, a 1·5 cm long steel blade, and from the other, four small pins on an ivory mount. This would be the same principle as that of the vaccinator in pl. 27. Another type was an arrow-head lancet with a grooved blade to hold the vaccine and c. 1865 Cooper-Rose devised a vaccinating curette.

Tourniquets

Arresting bleeding from open wounds was, in early times, chiefly attempted by the application of some absorbent substance covered by a bandage. This was followed by boiling oil or pitch, or a cauterising iron. Not until Paré used a ligature did the idea of a tourniquet first begin to take shape (pl. 28). The first shape it took was in 1674 when Morell used a field garotte to stop the haemorrhage of a soldier; this was a simple cord with a wooden rod pushed beneath it and twisted to tighten it. In 1678 a naval surgeon again used a garotte successfully in amputation, but this time first put a hard lined pad over the vessel concerned. A device was then developed that used a rack through which the strap was passed with a handle to turn and tighten it.

It was not until 1718 that Jean-Louis Petit (1674–1760) invented a screw compressor which limited the pressure to the artery, and he gave his instrument the name of tourniquet. The other advantages of this were that it could be held without assistance and the pressure relaxed or released at will. This type of tourniquet was copied with variations (such as the Garot type in pl. 29) but superseded all others. Rudimentary tourniquets on board ship were described in 1782 as being of stiff leather with a linen compress and a wooden cylinder to twist the tape for tightening; many lives must have been

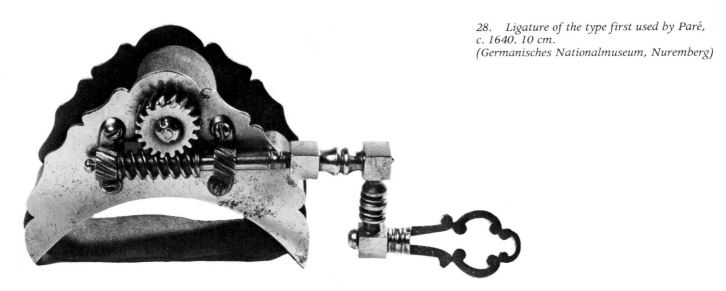

28. *Ligature of the type first used by Paré,*
c. 1640. 10 cm.
(Germanisches Nationalmuseum, Nuremberg)

29. *Garot tourniquet, c. 1750.*
(Royal College of Surgeons of Edinburgh)

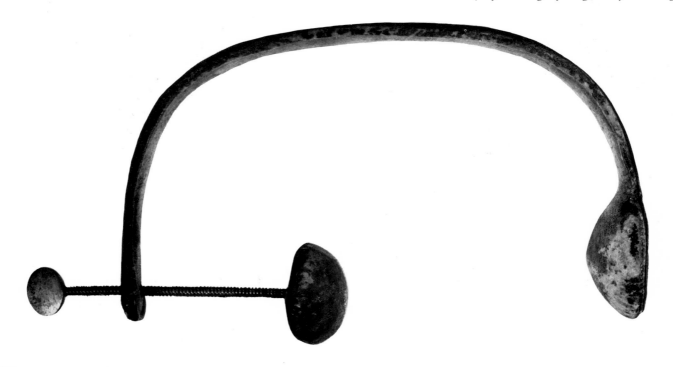

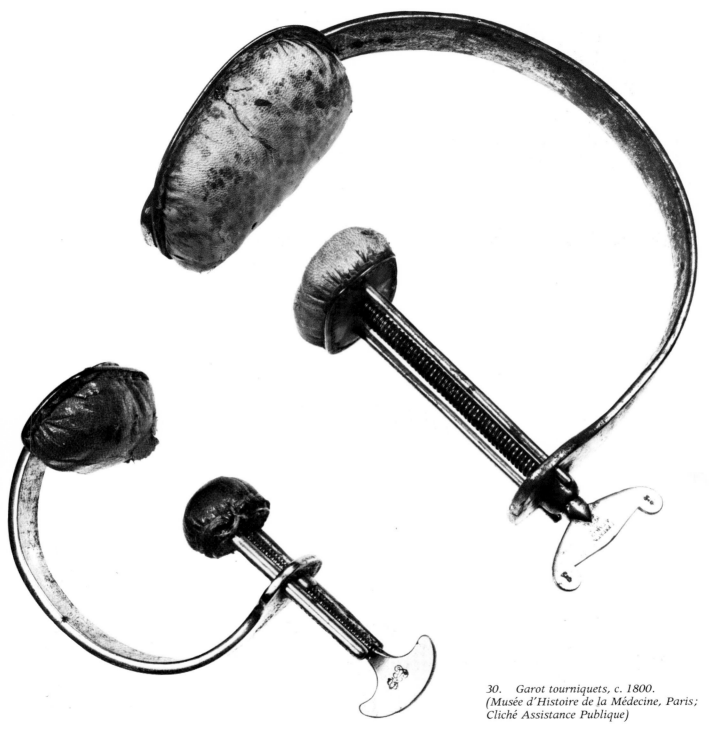

30.   Garot tourniquets, c. 1800.
(Musée d'Histoire de la Médecine, Paris;
Cliché Assistance Publique)

saved by it when over a hundred men might be queueing for the services of the surgeon at a time. Early in the nineteenth century a tourniquet with a cog and the wheel mechanism was tried and found wanting. The original tourniquets were of wood but later brass was used with a strong linen strap, the compressor often being covered in fine kid (pl. 31).

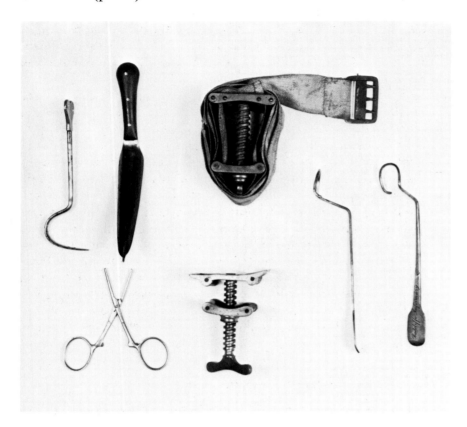

31. Two Petit-type tourniquets. Extreme left, an aneurysm needle and right, two perineal sutures, c. 1830. (Pitt-Rivers Museum, Oxford)

Thermometers

The Greeks knew that air expanded if heated, but Galileo was the first to put a scale by the tube. Attempts to measure body temperature were first made *c.* 1600 in Padua, using the thermoscope of Galileo, but this was slow and inaccurate. Santorio's thermometer of 1611 took the form of a glass bulb held in the patient's mouth from which a long serpentine tube led to a bowl of water. The higher his temperature, the lower the water level in the tube dropped. William Cockburn who wrote *A Continuation of the*

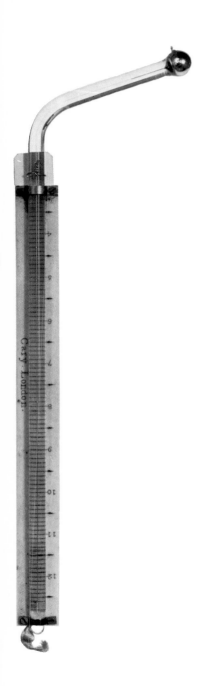

Account of the Distempers . . . Incident to Seafaring People in 1697, based much of his observation on pulse and temperature though no facts were so far established in this regard. We are told he used 'a clumsy and fragile oil thermometer'.

The thermometer, as such, was invented by Gabriel Fahrenheit in 1720. George Martine (1702–41), one of the Boerhaave brigade (see Chapter 1), was a pioneer in its use and his thermometer was in general use until the invention of the short clinical thermometer. James Currie (1756–1805) of Liverpool introduced a thermometer with curved ends that could be read while standing behind the patient (pl. 32), but the Hunter-type of *c.* 1800 was more popular. This was approximately 18 cm long with a large bulb and was fitted into a turned wood case. Most had either a paper scale or the scale engraved on to the ivory or wooden outer case. Professor Phillips of Oxford invented a self-registering thermometer that used a minute air-bubble to break the thread of mercury; one of these, made by Casella of London, was exhibited at the Great Exhibition of 1851. However, it was only in 1868 that the work of Karl August Wunderlich (1815–77) showed how important the thermometer was in diagnosis and the practice of compiling temperature charts grew from that time. Thermometers, though, were still massive and took five or more minutes to register accurately. Sir Clifford Allbutt (1836–1925) of Leeds introduced one in 1866 in which a contraction broke the mercury thread, allowing the maximum temperature to be read. Harvey and Reynolds were the original makers of this thermometer and it developed into the short, modern, clinical thermometer we know today.

Cauteries and caustic-holders

Two early Arabian surgeons of the tenth century established the use of the red-hot cautery as being a cure-all for a wide range of afflictions—epilepsy, headache, toothache, piles, pleurisy, dropsy, melancholia, and many another might be cured by this means. Most of the cauteries were of iron but a few seem to have been gold and came in an amazing variety of sizes and geometric patterns. In medieval Italy they were used as cutting instruments. William Clowes, surgeon to Queen Elizabeth, was very fond of using a cautery; 'The yron', he said, 'is most excellent but that it is offensive to the eye and bringeth the patient to great sorrowe and dread of the burning and the smart.' It is obvious that it was widely used and most surgeons would have had a cautery in their collection (pl. 33). There are several in the seventeenth-century Prujean

32. Early clinical thermometer to be read from behind patient, c. 1800. 17·8 cm. (Royal College of Surgeons of England)

183

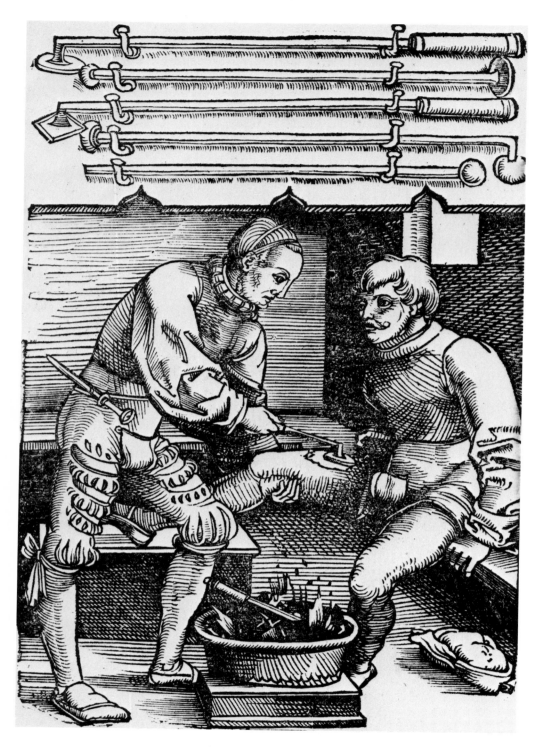

33.   The use of the cautery;
woodcut from Albucasis,
Chirurgicorum omnium, 1532.
(Wellcome Museum Library)

Collection ranging in size from a small bead to a lozenge 2·5 cm across (pl. 34). A case of instruments *c.* 1715 at the R.A.M.C. Museum includes one with a forward-curving shaft and a head the shape and size of half a large pea. Percivall Pott completely abandoned the cautery and such was his example that it virtually passed out of use. The fall in its popularity brought about the development in the use of the cauterising styptic and holders for it. In the latter part of the eighteenth century and the beginning of the nineteenth, these were usually silver, approximately 10 cm long, and the thickness of a pencil with a screw cap. A firm band of silver held the styptic in the hollow tube, and the more sophisticated ones had a button and slide to raise it as it wore down. A fine one dated 1836 by Theophilus Merry has five bands of decorative rope-work in gold and is illustrated in pl. 27. In time, however, it was found that the caustic burned through the solder of the tube and about the middle of the nineteenth century one finds holders engraved 'Seamless', clearly a welcome advance. However, use of the iron cautery had not entirely died out for the Maw catalogue of 1868 shows four types, each priced 9*s*.

34.   Cauteries, c. 1653. Prujean Collection.
25·4 cm.
(Royal College of Physicians of England)

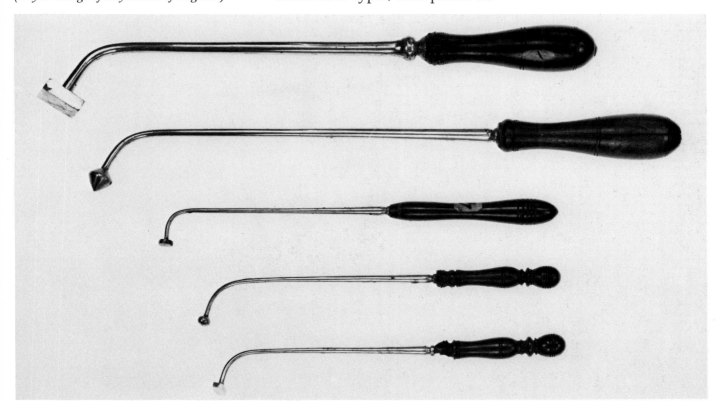

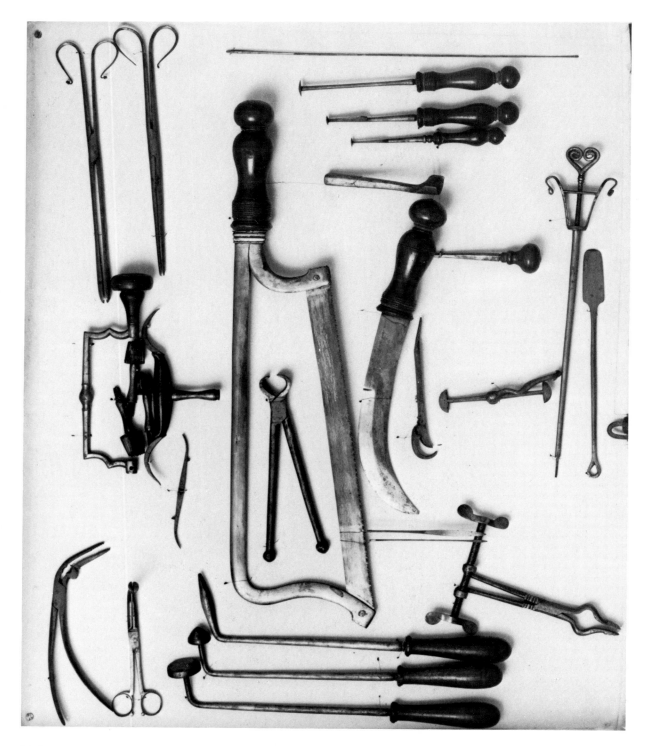

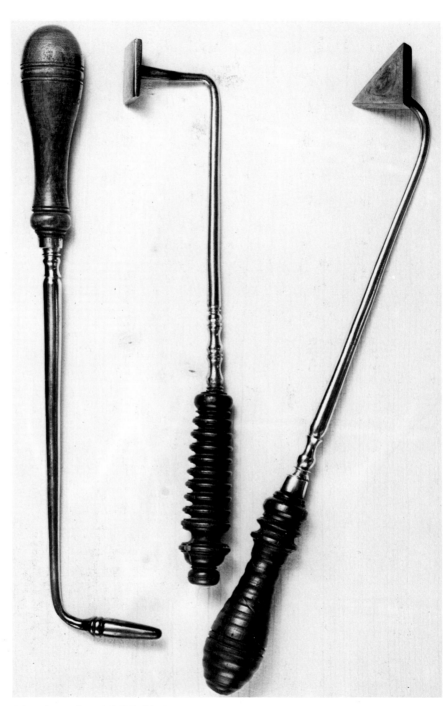

35. *Set of surgical instruments, 1703.*
(Society of Antiquarians, Newcastle upon
Tyne)

36. *Cauteries, c. 1750. 30·4 cm.*
(Germanisches Nationalmuseum, Nuremberg)

37.   Cautery, c. 1750. 25·5 cm.
(Museum Boerhaave, Leiden)

38.   Cauteries, c. 1780.
(College of Physicians of Philadelphia)

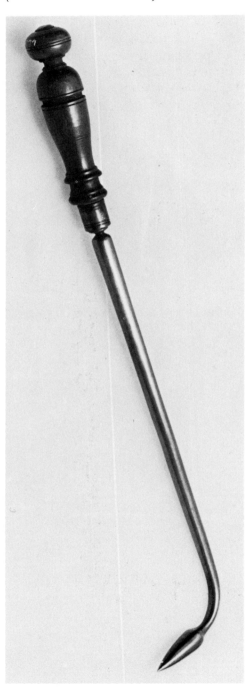

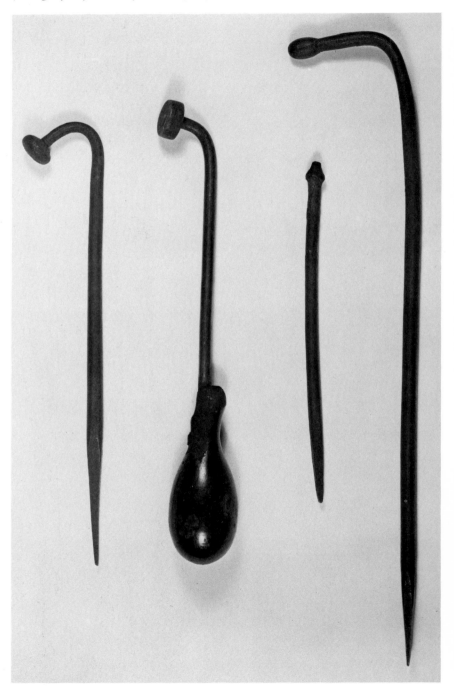

Anaesthesia masks and inhalers

Mandragora and other anaesthetic drugs were much used in medieval surgery but they are seldom referred to since. Mild doses of laudanum or brandy were all the luckless patient might expect until the advent of ether and chloroform, though a compressor might occasionally have been applied to stultify the senses before amputation. Benjamin Bell, in his *System of Surgery* mentions 'The ingenious proposition by Mr Moore of London for diminishing and preventing pain in several operations of surgery. It is done by compressing the nerves of the limb.' A Moore's compressor is shown in pl. 39. Even after the introduction of anaesthesia one

39.   *Moore's nerve compressor, c. 1780.*
(Royal College of Surgeons of Edinburgh)

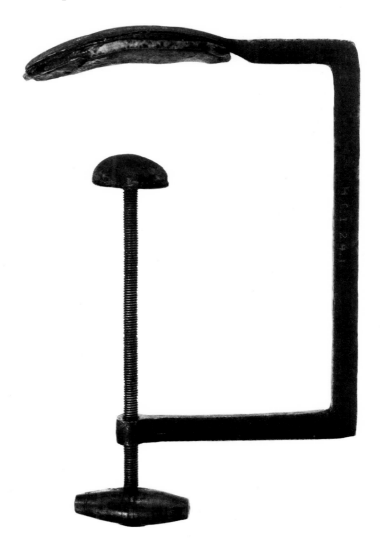

189

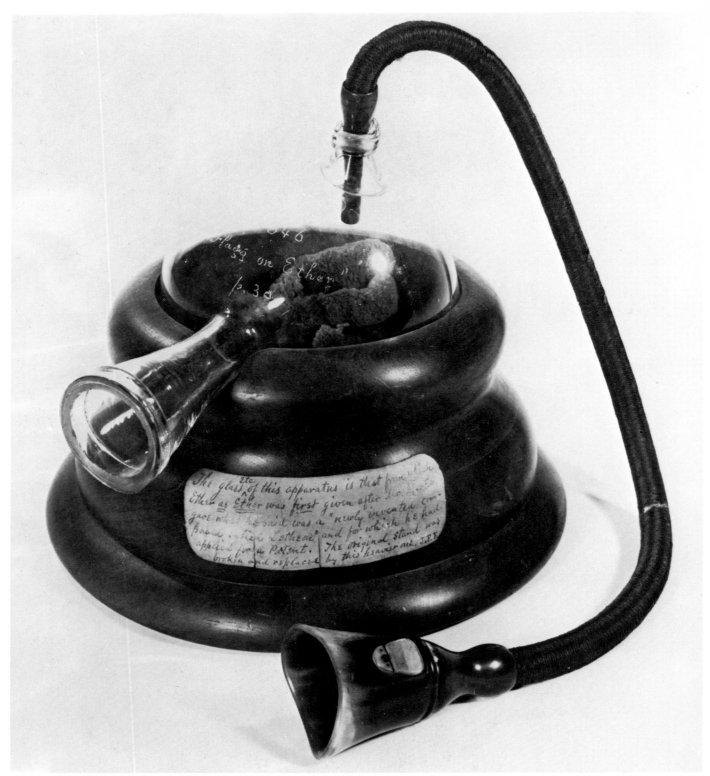

might not count on it. The notorious Dr John Hall deliberately restricted its use in the Crimea. '. . . the smart of the Knife is a powerful stimulant,' he said 'and it is better to hear a man bawl lustily, than to see him sink silently into his grave.'

The earliest form of inhaler, in use from late 1846, was an oval silver-plated box with a concave and perforated mouthpiece presented to the patient. The body of the box held a sponge soaked in ether or chloroform and a plate behind the perforation prevented the liquid being drawn into the mouth. For use with this was a metal nose-clip consisting of a doubled piece of metal with flaring ends that fitted over the nostrils.

An ether inhaler was made by Attlee & Co. in 1847 and an example can be seen in the Wellcome Collection. It is made of brass with a screw adjuster and a perforated mouthpiece.

Mouth gags were used in the administration of chloroform from 1862, and in dentistry. These took the form of forceps with a rack between the handles and S-shaped blades. A mask designed by Thomas Skinner of Liverpool at the same time was more sophisticated than the earlier type and was a folding metal frame about 10·5 by 7·5 cm, intended to be covered by gauze on to which the chloroform was dropped. Dr John Murray, in 1868, modified this so that the framework enclosed the nose as well as the mouth, making the nose clip obsolete. Dr John Snow was the first professional anaesthetist and did much to make the practice acceptable (see Chapter 1).

Blood transfusion apparatus

That man of many hats, Sir Christopher Wren, experimented with blood transfusion and was wont to say, 'It will probably end in extraordinary success.' In 1667 Drs Lower and King transfused sheep's blood into a Bachelor of Divinity at Cambridge. Samuel Pepys, who met him, wrote, 'I was pleased to see the person who had his blood taken out. He speaks well . . . he had by 20s for his suffering it.' And suffer he did, idiotic to the end of his days. Jean Baptiste Denys (1625–1704) was the first to make a real study of the subject, but the Australian Aborigines are said to have practised it for thousands of years. Denys first experimented with animals to humans—compatibility not being understood—but when a patient died there was considerable scandal.

A gap of over 100 years elapsed before James Blundell of Guy's Hospital performed the first human-to-human transfusion in 1818. He used a brass syringe with a valved thumbpiece. A glass funnel was attached at right angles to the barrel, which could contain 2 oz; it had a silver pipe for insertion into the vein and was made for him by Philp and Whicker. Blundell's experiments were mostly on patients whose condition made their lives past hope anyway, but in 1829 he made the first successful transfusion to a woman in childbed. The method he used this time is illustrated in the Maw Catalogue of 1830 in a drawing believed to be by J. M. W. Turner. (J. H. Maw was a very close friend of Turner, David Cox and J. F. Lewis, all of whom provided him with sketches from time to time.) It is unlikely that much of the early apparatus will be found still complete, but in 1863 J. H. Aveling introduced a portable transfusion case, much used in the Franco–Prussian War, and this

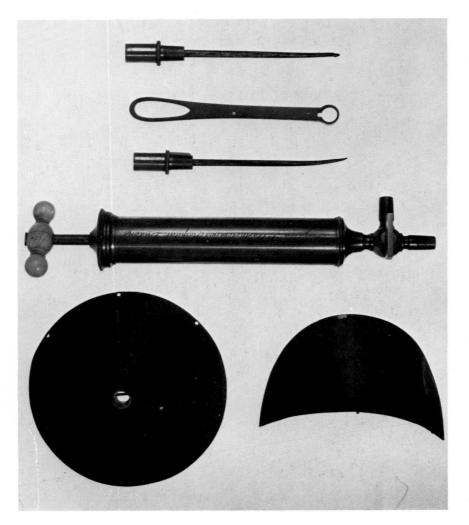

41. *Blood transfusion apparatus of 1830.*
(Royal College of Surgeons of England)

42. *Aveling blood transfusion apparatus,*
c. 1865.
(Wellcome Collection)

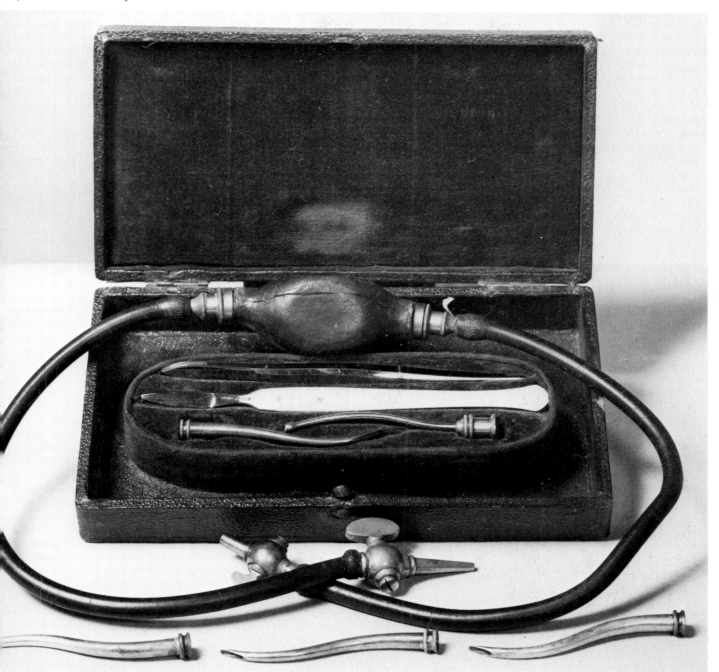

would make for a more reasonable search (pl. 42). It took the form of a rubber tube to form a connection between the vein of the donor and the recipient, with a bulb in the middle to act as an auxiliary heart.

Percussion hammers and pleximeters

Nineteenth-century percussion hammers took many forms but were more or less standardised by Henry Vernon of the Great Northern Hospital in 1858. He introduced a flexible whalebone handle with a 1 oz metal head enclosed in a rubber ring. Pleximeters for use with these and other hammers were usually of ivory, a 5·8 cm long oval with upright sides, or occasionally were made of metal with hinged sides. These were much criticised as they did not produce a suitable sound. A combined hammer and pleximeter was designed by Gibson in 1850. A well-carved ivory hammer is shown in pl. 13. The handle unscrews to reveal a shaft for drawing across the sole of the foot to test the Babinsky reflex.

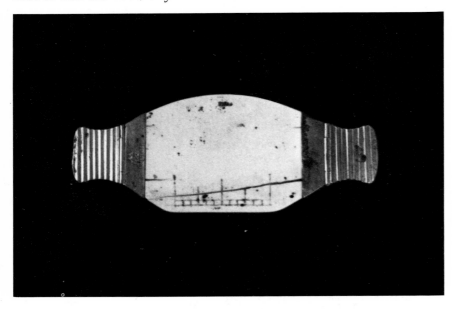

43. Pleximeter, c. 1850. 7·5 cm. (Museum of Historical Medicine, Copenhagen)

Orthopaedic instruments

The prevalence of rickets among the poor and the deformities it caused, were chiefly responsible for the birth of orthopaedic surgery as we know it today. It is hardly surprising, therefore, that the Liverpool slums were the setting for the first serious work on the

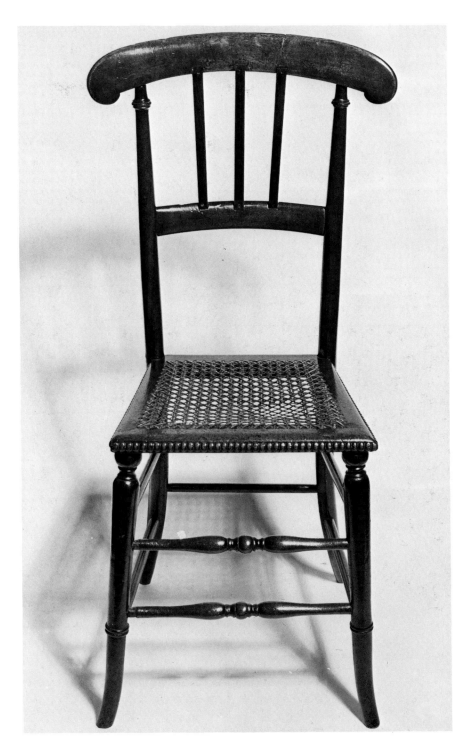

44. Corrective chair for spinal disorders, designed by Sir Astley Cooper, c. 1800. (Strangers' Hall Museum, Norwich)

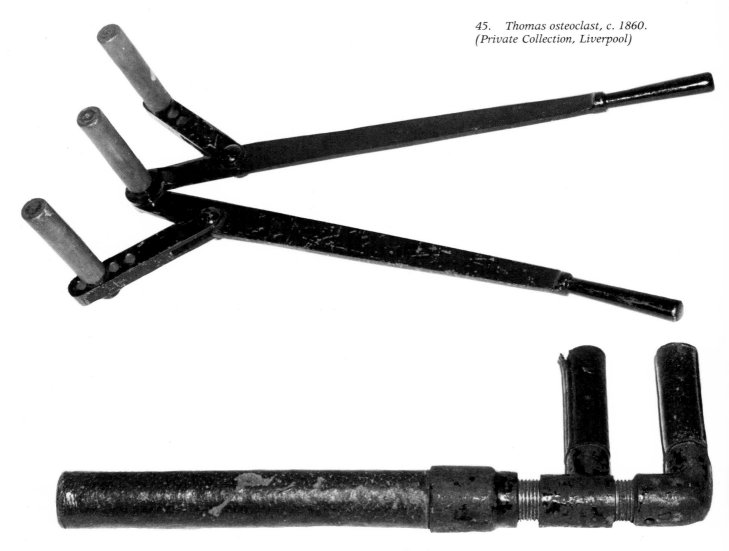

45. *Thomas osteoclast, c. 1860.*
(Private Collection, Liverpool)

46. *Thomas wrench, c. 1865.*
(Private Collection, Liverpool)

speciality, and gave Liverpool pre-eminence in the subject both at home and abroad. Hugh Owen Thomas was the leader in this field and the inventor of many of the early instruments. Pl. 46 is the Thomas wrench, used to untwist club feet. This was introduced *c.* 1865 and it was later used for other deformities, particularly those of the wrist and ankle. As well as a variety of ingenious splints, Thomas invented the osteoclast, a sadistic instrument for breaking the deformed bones of children between its three legs (pl. 45). However cruel this may seem it was a great advance on the previous method of cutting through to the bone and breaking it with a mallet and chisel similar to those in pl. 13.

196

CHAPTER NINE

Dental instruments

Anyone fearing the extraction of a tooth today may draw comfort from the thought of what it was like in the eleventh century. On no account could the tooth be broken as it was realised that bits of the root remaining in the gum would cause yet more trouble in the future. The gum, therefore, was cut down with a sharp scalpel and the tooth then rocked and shaken to loosen it. The patient's head was held firmly between the operator's knees, and all efforts were made to extract the tooth in a straight direction. Repellent mouthwashes were afterwards prescribed, and often the wound was cauterised with a red-hot iron.

Extraction and rudimentary scaling were, for many centuries, the only form of dental treatment available other than crude potions for toothache. In the early days the Barber–Surgeons were concerned in these activities, to be overtaken later by the Fairground toothdrawers and blacksmiths.

Separation of dental science from general medicine started noticeably in the sixteenth century and became accentuated in the next, showing the very poor standard of treatment available. It was still generally believed that worms in the teeth were the cause of dental pain; some even maintained that on scraping a decayed cavity they had seen them issue forth and that, putting them in water, had actually seen them move about. It is possible that on splitting open a decayed tooth, the nerve could have looked like a worm. The fact that pain in the ear sometimes caused toothache gave rise to the belief that the two were connected, and many treatments for toothache were directed to be given through the outer ear. Some remedies suggested were bleeding of the arm, followed the next day by a strong aperient; cupping in the spinal region and behind the ear; or the burning of the nerve with a cautery or strong acid in the hope that the tooth would gradually fall to pieces.

The first book on dentistry in the English language was by Charles Allen, *The Operator for the Teeth*, published in 1685, but generally jealousy and fear of the scant knowledge being used in competition, accounted for the very slow dissemination of learning among dental practitioners, and there was an entire lack of adequate teaching. However, in the early eighteenth century small progress

197

was made and greater care was taken of the teeth by the individual, with more common use of toothbrushes (see Chapter 15) and personal scaling sets, By 1757 a book had appeared advocating extraction of teeth to reduce unsightly appearance caused by overcrowding, and even suggested removal of corresponding teeth on the opposite side of the jaw to afford symmetry. William Rae, who practised in Adam Street, Adelphi, *c.* 1775, was the first to give lectures in dentistry.

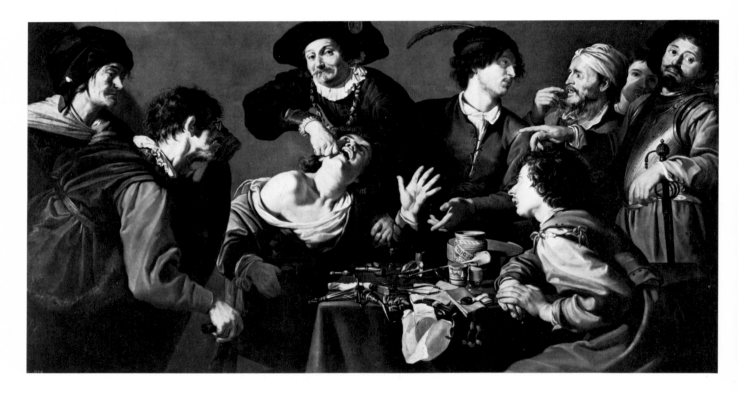

Despite these small advances, dental treatment was practised by charlatans well into the nineteenth century, often a sideline occupation of blacksmiths or of mountebanks, who drew teeth as entertainment at Fairs—the cries of the sufferer being drowned by raucous music from an assistant. As can be imagined, advertising of these events was lurid in the extreme. There was still no recognised training, nor qualification for practice. Knowledge had to be self-acquired, or instruction sought from an established practitioner. In 1820, L. S. Parmley who suggested that an anatomist, a surgeon, and a good mechanic would be a desirable combination for a successful dentist, offered instruction in the art for 100–200 guineas. Another

1. Theodor Rombouts (1597–1637), The Dentist, *Flemish School. (Museo del Prado, Madrid)*

offered a day's instruction in gold-filling for £50. The terms of apprenticeship that existed were harsh, and the boy was enjoined to strict secrecy about what he learnt. For the 5–7 years' service he was not allowed to marry, play at cards or dice, or to visit taverns or playhouses, but had to work faithfully at the tasks set, only acquiring such surgical knowledge as might drift his way from the poor who came to be treated early in the morning. Sometimes the premium for all this might be as much as £500.

Since there is no record of the numbers of those in practice at one time, or any kind of journal devoted to dentistry, it is hard to form a complete picture. Those few who practised with any skill or success were probably qualified surgeons, but the vast majority were obviously uneducated and disreputable. It was said: 'The adage that any fool will do for a parson may be applied with still greater force and truth to the profession of a dentist'! In 1841 an appeal was made to recognise dentistry as a legitimate branch of medicine, but not until 1856 was the first Dental Society in England formed by Samuel Cartwright and its transactions published in the *British Journal of Dental Science*. A little later, Cartwright also helped form the Odontological Society of Great Britain.

It can be seen that little progress was made until the nineteenth century. In addition to the scarcity of knowledge, poor equipment had contributed to the low standard of treatment, and by the mid-century finer instruments made the evolution of treatment more rapid. The foot drill made cutting and shaping the cavity of a tooth more accurate, and anaesthesia for tooth pulling, brought into general use only at the end of the century, made for a more humane relationship between dentist and patient. With these advances, schools of dentistry were set up, as it was now thought to be a lucrative calling. Restraint had to be exercised to see that training was under medical control and many dental schools have grown as part of an existing medical school. The first one was attached to University College in London, and in 1858 the Royal Dental Hospital was founded. By 1880 a four-year course of professional study was established, ending in a Diploma from the Royal College of Surgeons.

Extractors

The Greeks were probably the first to use extraction as a form of dental treatment, but the first illustration of extraction instruments did not appear until the works of Albucasis (1050–1122). These, however, are crudely drawn and unreliable; the first acceptable source of illustration is Walter Ryff (*c.* 1500–1562) Officer of Health in Nuremberg, who wrote *Major Surgery* in 1545. The instruments used are grouped as pelicans, elevators, screws, keys, and forceps.

Pelicans were named after the bird from their resemblance to the shape of the beak (pl. 2). The earliest reference to a pelican was by Guy de Chauliac (1298–1368) in 1363, and an early drawing was made by Arcoli in 1542, showing a straight shaft, wheel-shaped bolster, and a single claw attached to the shaft by a rivet. Before then, teeth were sometimes extracted by coopers' forceps used to force the last hoops on the barrels. Gabriele Ferrara published a book on surgery in Milan in 1627 that gives a good idea of dental instruments in seventeenth-century Italy. The pelicans are ornate and heavily-built with a convex, serrated bolster and a deep, smooth cleft; sometimes they are double-clawed for use on alternate jaws. By 1719, Heister introduced an ivory knob-handled pelican on which the claw could be adjusted up and down the shaft by a screw operated by the handle; the shanks of the claw were either straight or curved. Throughout the eighteenth century those with broad bodies and single claws were favoured. Perret's catalogue of 1772 shows ebony handles and a much simpler screw mechanism, and Savigny's catalogue of 1798 has long octagonal ebony handles with a well-made firm steel bolster, broad and rounded. Double-ended pelicans were first illustrated by Francisco Martinez (d. 1585) in 1557 with two bolsters and two claws. John Woodall, in 1617, showed one with concave bolsters. Within twenty years there were

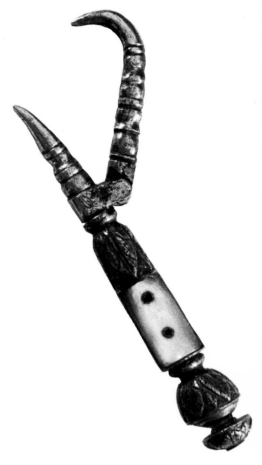

2.   Pelican, c. 1580. 12·5 cm.
(*Musée le Secq des Tournelles, Rouen*)

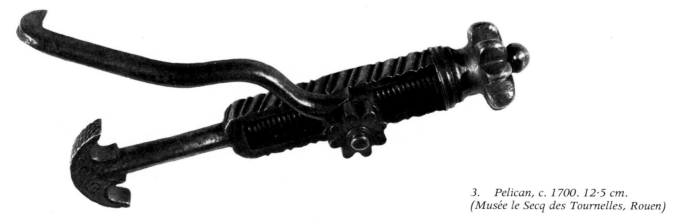

3.   Pelican, c. 1700. 12·5 cm.
(*Musée le Secq des Tournelles, Rouen*)

200

illustrations of pelicans published in several different countries, so it may therefore be concluded that they were in general use by the middle of the sixteenth century. Early in the eighteenth century, shafts had become more slender and convex, and serrated bolsters became standard. By 1810, forceps-type pelicans were introduced into use—they had appeared in the seventeenth century but had found no favour. Benjamin Bell said of pelicans in 1786 that they did not possess any advantage over toothkeys and could not be used when it was necessary to turn the tooth towards the inside of the mouth.

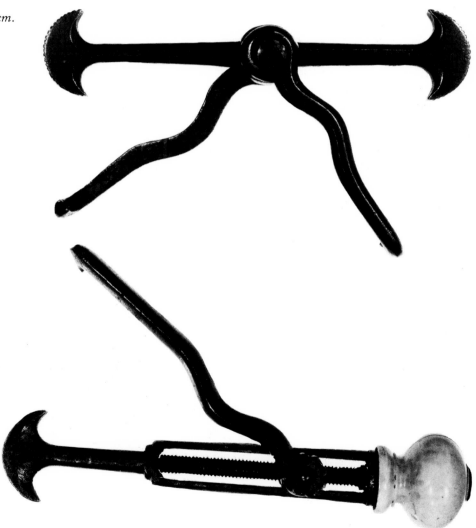

4. *Mid-eighteenth-century pelican. 11·5 cm. (Royal College of Surgeons of Edinburgh)*

5. *Mid-eighteenth-century pelican. The handle controls an endless screw to accommodate any size tooth. 12·5 cm. (Royal College of Surgeons of Edinburgh)*

201

Elevators were principally used for incisors and canine teeth but were suitable for roots and stumps as well (pl. 8). One of the most popular forms was known as the 'goat's-foot', owing to the cleft and angle of the head which resembled a goat's-foot. Scultetus showed early versions with ornate handles and double-cleft head, one side of which is serrated, but there were many variations—curved shafts and diverse heads which could be spatula-shaped, hook-ended, arrowheaded or a simple point; Gariot introduced an elevator in 1805 known as the 'carp's tongue' owing to its shape. Gums were separated from the stump by a single-bladed scarificator, and the tooth was raised by pressure from the elevator against the base of the root. By the end of the eighteenth century, handles were sometimes placed at right angles as on a toothkey.

Thomas Bell was chiefly responsible for making the elevator popular and devised one in 1829 with a long handle, short curved blade, and a lance-shaped point which was said to be good for the extraction of lower third molars. A very complicated form was patented by W. Fitkin in 1861 but there is no evidence of its popularity.

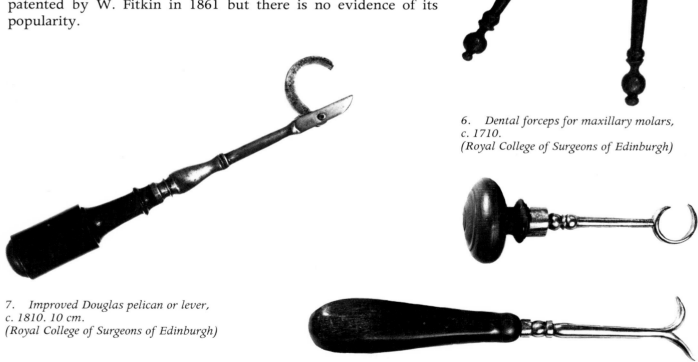

6.   *Dental forceps for maxillary molars, c. 1710.*
(Royal College of Surgeons of Edinburgh)

7.   *Improved Douglas pelican or lever, c. 1810. 10 cm.*
(Royal College of Surgeons of Edinburgh)

8.   *A goat's-foot elevator and an elevator for roots, c. 1780. 10 cm.*
(Germanisches Nationalmuseum, Nuremberg)

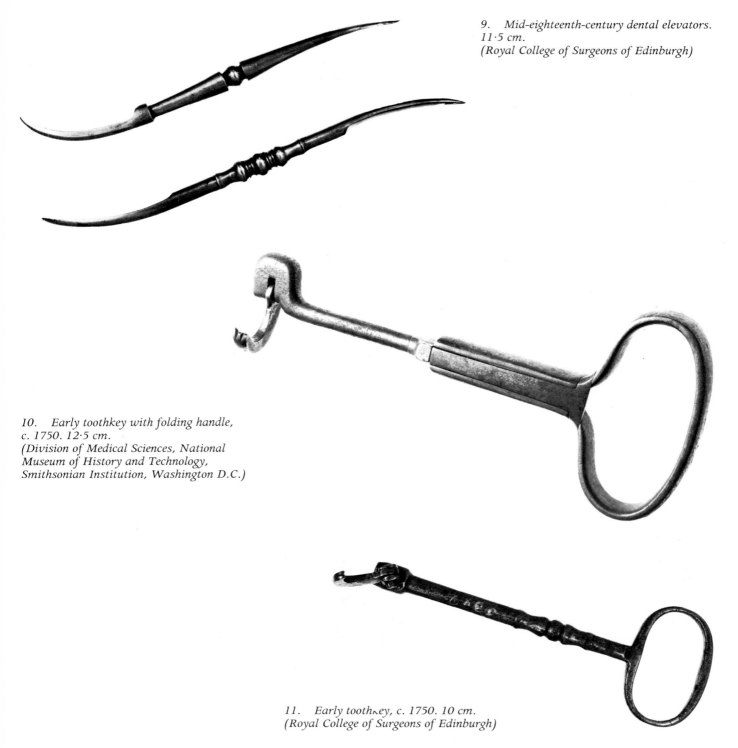

9.   Mid-eighteenth-century dental elevators.
11·5 cm.
(Royal College of Surgeons of Edinburgh)

10.   Early toothkey with folding handle,
c. 1750. 12·5 cm.
(Division of Medical Sciences, National
Museum of History and Technology,
Smithsonian Institution, Washington D.C.)

11.   Early toothkey, c. 1750. 10 cm.
(Royal College of Surgeons of Edinburgh)

203

Toothkeys were first mentioned in 1742 and looked exactly like a key of the period with a large ring handle and straight shaft—the French called them the 'clef Anglais' (pl. 12). Earlier keys had a claw with two points but later examples had levelled off by the end of the eighteenth century and had a grooved inner surface. A key illustrated in the *British Magazine* in 1762 shows that the handle can be removed and used as an elevator. Perret in 1772 favoured a key with a single cleft and the inner surface well serrated. A rare find is a double-ended key. By 1770 a slight bend had occurred in the shaft and later, a double bend to prevent strain on adjacent teeth. Savigny's catalogue of 1798 stated that the principal defect of keys had been the depth of bolster which had raised teeth in too wide an arc; they were now introducing a narrower bolster so that teeth might be raised almost perpendicularly. Fox, in 1806, had keys made to be used in different positions—with a double bend in the shaft and an auxiliary bolster that could be placed against an adjacent tooth, which was very useful in cases of abscess. In 1810, Charles Laforgue (1763–1823) introduced a key with a deep curve in the shaft and a concave bolster and Knaur, in 1796, made a key with a movable bolster—undoubtedly the same ideas were occurring to different people simultaneously. In 1816 came the smooth, egg-shaped bolster to prevent injury to gums, but by 1834 efforts to alleviate pressure on adjacent teeth were condemned. F. S. Prideaux, in 1843, devised a claw with a cutting edge that operated in this way—the handle of the key was turned in the reverse direction so that the claw cut deeply round and a little under the tooth; it was then turned in the ordinary way so that the tooth was extracted more completely. Many and various were the ingenious devices on the toothkey theme, but it is doubtful if many of the more diverse were produced beyond the prototype. Several instruments were introduced similar to the key but with strength like that of a forceps. Most have twin handles united by a pin and terminate in a claw on one shaft and a bolster on the other. Some of this type can be seen at the Royal College of Surgeons.

Screws probably came into use in the early nineteenth century and were first illustrated in 1803 in the works of Serre and Laforgue. They were used in the extraction of roots of incisors and canines where no part remained which could be grasped. They consist of a handle and shaft similar to a key with a screw end which was turned and engaged in the root which was then scooped out by the other end of the instrument. The 'Compound Screw-Forceps' patented in 1848 was a pliers-like instrument for splitting roots and in 1851,

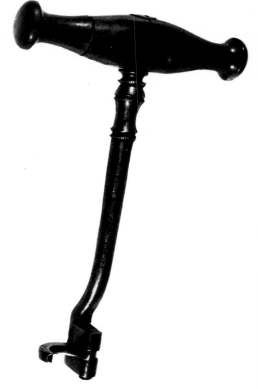

12. *Toothkey (known on the Continent as Clef Anglaise), c. 1770. 10·2 cm. (Musée le Secq des Tournelles, Rouen)*

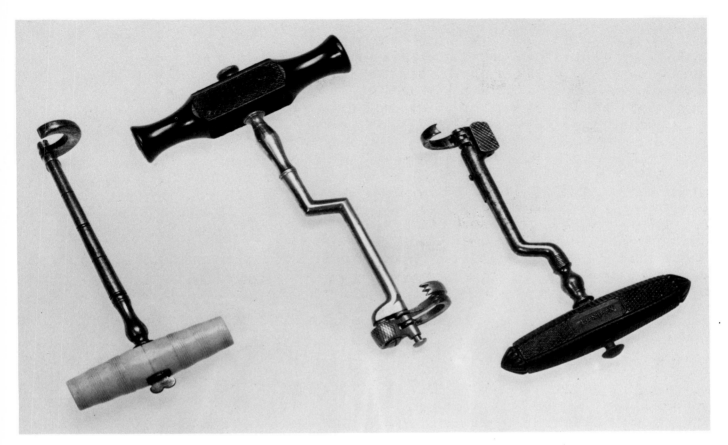

13. *Toothkeys: early straight shaft, ivory handle c. 1760; double-type (as introduced by Fox), c. 1820; standard type c. 1825, Weiss. 10 cm.*
(Simon Kaye Ltd, London)

Wadsworth introduced a screw-lever—a double instrument—the one part a fork-ended elevator and the other a bulbous-handed shaft with a detachable screw end.

Forceps. Early forceps of damascened iron with notched beaks were as much for shaking the teeth as for extracting them, and seem ill-designed for the job. John of Gaddesden (1280–1361), in the early fourteenth century, recommended a sharp-pointed lever rather than forceps and Ryff, in 1545, illustrated several. They had curled handles and short, curved beaks, although Martinez, in 1557, showed very angular pliers-like forceps. Several pairs were necessary to the operator. Paré advised 'now one, now another as the greatness and site shall seem to require'. They were only used after the tooth had been freed from the gum by a scarificator. Woodall listed three to be included in a surgical chest. Dionis in 1708 described three types—tooth-forceps of pincer-like form with crooked and cleft blades; a tooth-root drawer with sharp, pointed

205

blades; and crow's bill forceps with an aperture between the blades but touching at the points. Scultetus illustrates forceps with a screw between the handles to regulate pressure and this was reintroduced at intervals during the late eighteenth and early nineteenth centuries. Savigny, in 1798, showed forceps for children's teeth. By the early nineteenth-century forceps were very heavy with a firm grasp, the inward-curving handles had a serrated grip and strong beaks. No attempt was made to fit forceps into the necks of individual teeth until 1826 when this defect was remedied by Cyrus Fay and beaks became sufficiently curved to clear the tooth they were extracting. James Snell, in 1831, advocated one handle being curved round in a hook to accommodate the operator's little finger, which prevented slipping in warm weather. The Weiss catalogue of 1843 shows nineteen different stump forceps, and in the same year J. Chitty Clendon published an illustrated book showing the shape of teeth and the different forceps needed, all made by Evrard. Forceps with inter-changeable beaks appeared *circa* 1850 but enjoyed short popularity. Weiss made a complete set of forceps with gilded handles as an example of their workmanship for the Great Exhibition of 1851 (pl. 15).

Instruments for Perpendicular Extraction of Teeth were mostly on the ratchet elevator principle. There were several objections to this method as it took a long time, adjacent teeth might be injured, and

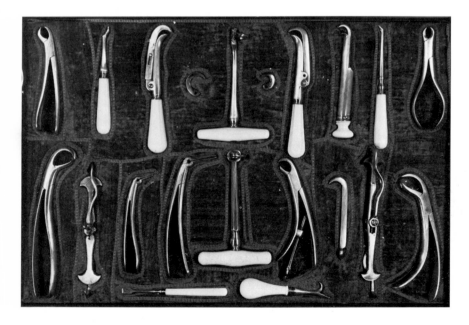

14. *Case of dental instruments, ivory handles, c. 1785.*
(Institute of Medical History, Vienna)

sometimes there were no adjacent teeth on which counter pressure could be put. These instruments date from the latter half of the eighteenth century and are all immensely complicated engineering pieces. Some may be seen at the Royal College of Surgeons.

Compound or Multi-purpose Instruments are very occasionally found, such as that in the Wellcome Collection of which one end is a key and the other a lever. Another, described by Heister in 1719, can be a pelican or an elevator, but the most interesting is at the Royal College of Surgeons. It comes from Virginia, was possibly owned by the Surgeon of the *Mayflower*, and is a combined pelican, elevator and forceps.

15. Set of dental instruments, ivory and gold handles, made by Weiss for the Great Exhibition of 1851. (John Weiss & Son Ltd)

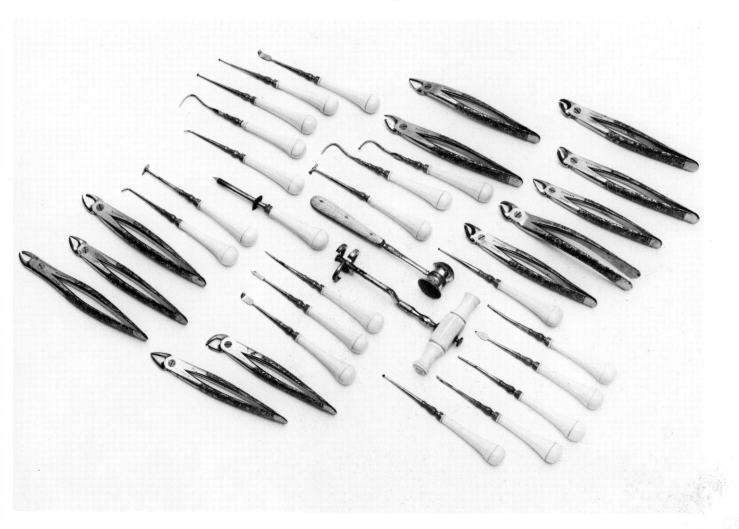

Scaling instruments

Small cased sets of scalers were made for personal use from the seventeenth century. These included anything from five to twelve different headed instruments which were interchangeable on one, usually ornate, handle. The set of *c.* 1750 (col. pl V) has a chased silver handle and fits into a sharkskin case with a mirror in the lid for home dentistry. Each head only measures 3·8 cm and the handle is the same size.

Others made use of ivory, mother of pearl, and tortoise-shell, and on the whole became larger with time. Victorian scalers of about 1840 measuring 14 cm including the by now fixed handle, were for the dentist and no longer for the patient to use himself. Napoleon's dental set, now at the R.A.M.C. Museum, was obviously meant for the dentist. It contains, in addition to the scalers, 4 toothkeys, and some forceps and probes.

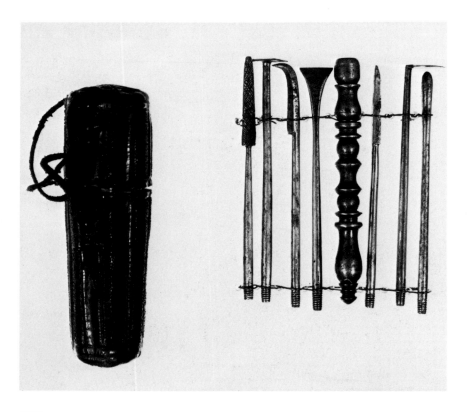

16. *Set of dental scaling instruments and cylindrical case, c. 1650. Case 6 by 3 cm. (Royal College of Surgeons of Edinburgh)*

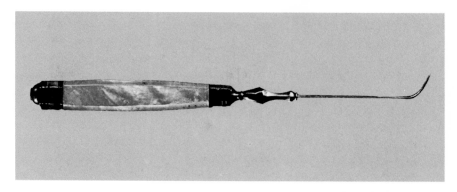

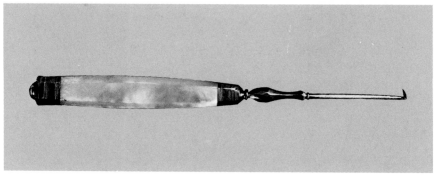

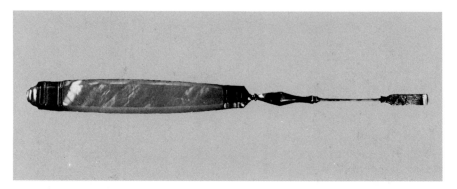

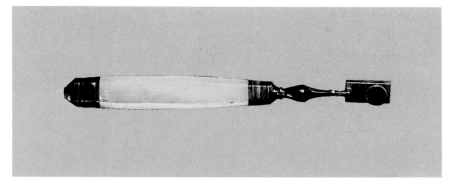

17–20. Four dental scaling instruments, mother-of-pearl handles, c. 1800. 10 cm. (Stedelijk Museum, Amsterdam)

Dental mirrors

For use with these scalers, and possibly with toothpicks, tiny mirrors with a magnifying glass were made. Their small size, the oval frames were only about 4 cm long, inspired delicate workmanship and they are one of the prettiest finds for the collector. From plain silver frames in the late eighteenth century they progressed to a useful hinged handle, though the one illustrated in col. pl. V of chased silver-gilt with an engraved mother-of-pearl handle, must be one of the most exquisite made. Richard Corson suggests that these were in fact the true quizzing-glass (see Chapter 11) and could be used at the Assembly to see what was happening behind one—but that is not the view of this writer.

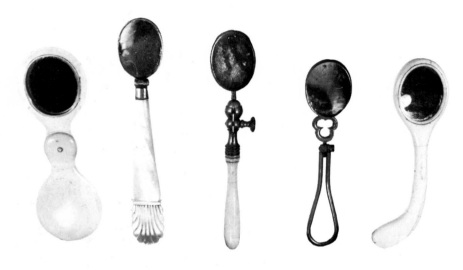

21. A group of dental mirrors, c. 1790–1830. 6·5 cm. (Royal College of Surgeons of Edinburgh)

Excavators and files

It is impossible to be very specific about the precise purpose of some of the earlier dental pieces, but it is known that teeth were filed down. In the Tudor period uneven teeth, 'so particularly disfiguring to women', were sometimes filed down to make them even. It was recommended that the filing take place over several days in order not to loosen the teeth too much—which speaks for the coarseness of the file. Excavations of decayed cavities were carried out as early as the first half of the eighteenth century, and then filled with lead, tin, or gold. Some dentists apparently would colour the lead or tin with yellow, and then charge the patient for

Colour plate
Two dental scaling sets: one with silver handles, c. 1750, the other with ivory handles, c. 1800. Four dental mirrors top right, silver, 1824, John Collings and 1820, John Crawley; centre, silver hinged mother-of-pearl handle, c. 1815; bottom, silver-gilt, mother-of-pearl handle, 1843, Thomas Diller. (Simon Kay Ltd, London)

PLATE V

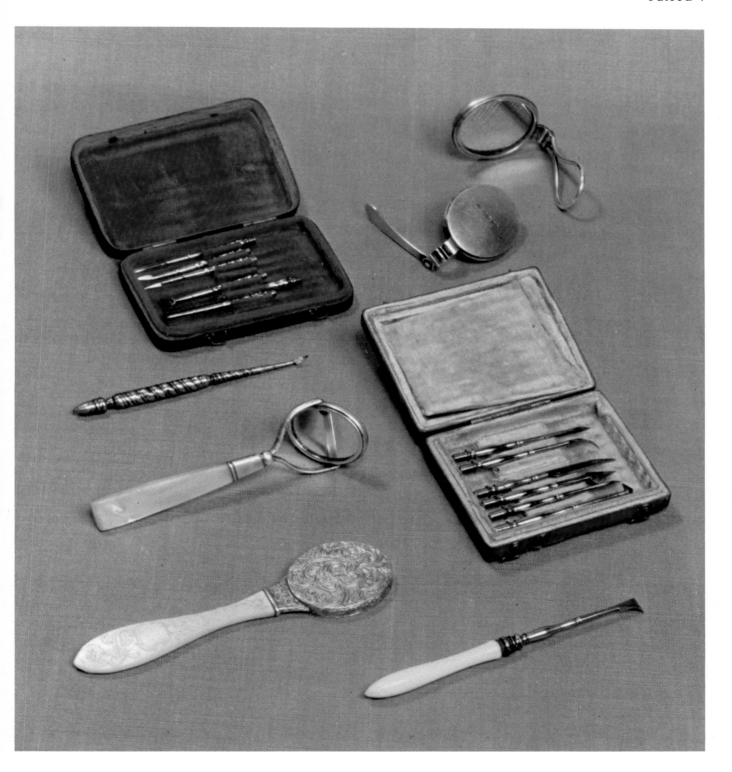

PLATE VI

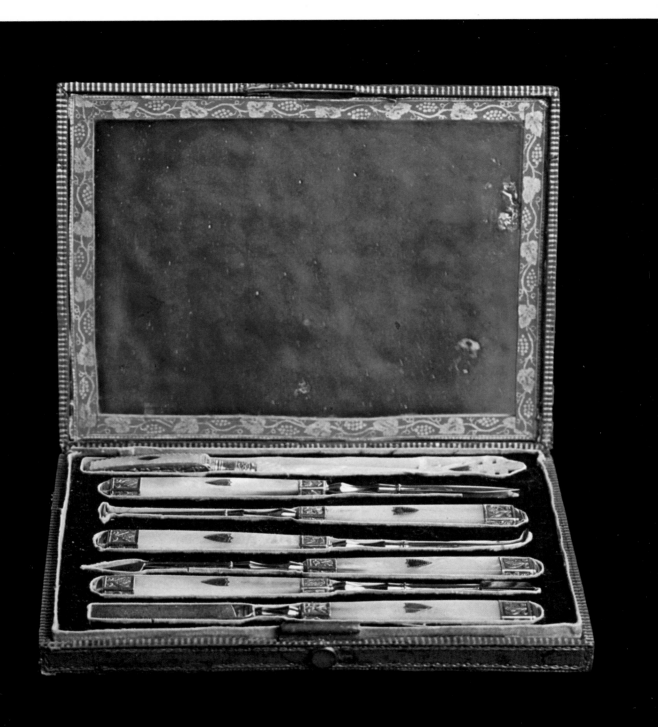

gold. Rudimentary probes, files, and excavators are to be found, though they are often indistinguishable from some of the pieces of a scaler set.

A type of dental drill operated by bow-string appeared in the early eighteenth century, and in 1790 John Greenwood of Boston (George Washington's dentist) adapted the spinning-wheel to rotate the drill. However, most dentists of the time used a joiner-type drill with a handle until, in 1829, James Nasmyth invented a method of making rotary power turn corners by using a coiled steel spiral in a sleeve. A beautifully made set of instruments by J. & J. Arnold & Son c. 1840 contains a drill to be hand-operated on a ratchet principle. Charles Merry of America patented a hand-operated drill with a flexible cable in 1858, and in 1864 George Harrington in England invented the first motor-driven drill which was a hand-held clockwork device (pl. 22).

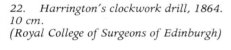

22. Harrington's clockwork drill, 1864. 10 cm.
(Royal College of Surgeons of Edinburgh)

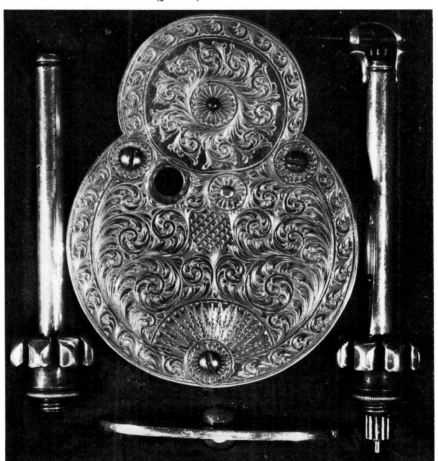

Colour plate
Set of French mother-of-pearl and silver-gilt dental scalers with toothbrush, c. 1800. 10 cm.
(Nicole Kramer, Village Suisse, Paris)

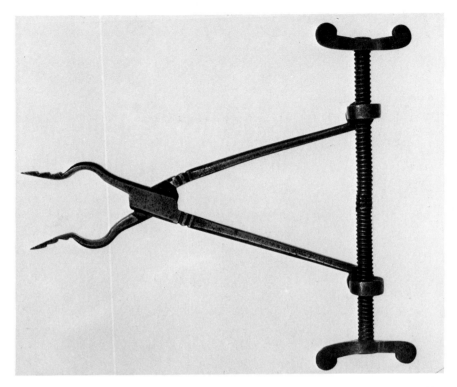

23.   *Paré's mouth gag, c. 1570.*
(Royal College of Surgeons of England)

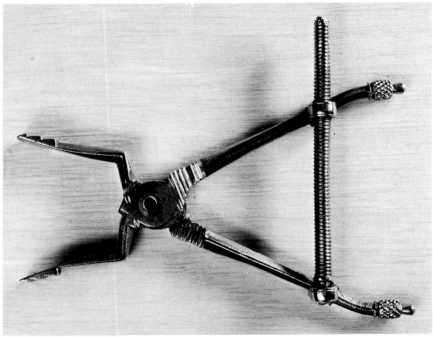

24.   *Mouth gag used by dentists and for*
epileptics, etc., c. 1680.
(Germanisches Nationalmuseum, Nuremberg)

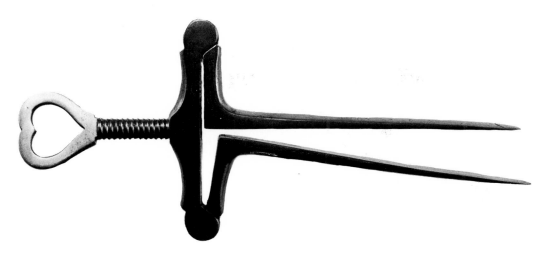

25.   Dental mouth gag with screw, c. 1780.
(Stedelijk Museum, Amsterdam)

The spherical rose-head file was not introduced until the mid-nineteenth century, and groaning patients had to wait until 1872 when the invention of the dental engine produced a grinding tool for simpler and better fillings. Without doubt it remains to this day the most unpopular piece of dental equipment. It is not within the confines of this book to trace the history of the materials used for fillings, but better materials required more accurate excavation, and heads for hand drills became more elaborate and diverse throughout the nineteenth century.

Notes on artificial teeth appear in Chapter 11.

213

CHAPTER TEN

Veterinary instruments

The veterinary art and science is of great antiquity. The laws of Hammurabi, 2100 B.C., mention a 'doctor of oxen and asses'. Treatises on the subject were written by Simon of Athens, Xenophon, and Aristotle. One of the most detailed was by the Roman, Apsyrtus, chief army veterinary surgeon to Constantine the Great. Apart from the importance of the horse in warfare, the Romans were great farmers and set up a remarkable tradition of medical knowledge applicable to all domestic animals.

In this country, by the fourteenth century, we find practitioners of the art known as Marshalls and by 1356 the Master-Marshalls had formed a trade guild. Later, however, the practice fell into the hands of the farrier, the 'beast-leech', who handed down his recipes from generation to generation, and by the end of the eighteenth century veterinary surgery was in disrepute. Through the efforts of the Odiham Agricultural Society and others interested in the welfare of horses and cattle, a Veterinary College was set up in London in 1791. A French veterinary surgeon, Charles Vial de St Bel (1750–93), was appointed the first professor. In 1823, William Dick (1794–1866) established a similar college in Edinburgh, and by 1844 these two schools had granted certificates of competency to about a thousand practising veterinary surgeons. In that year a Royal Charter was granted incorporating the Schools into the Royal College of Veterinary Surgeons, and declaring the practice to be a profession. But Joseph Gamgee, who entered the College c. 1822, wrote later '. . . the greatest disaster of my life has been the erroneous teaching of my professional school'.

The course of study for a Diploma was fixed to cover two sessions after a period of apprenticeship, though this was extended later. The examinations were practical and did not include a written paper until 1892.

The instruments used by these early veterinary surgeons would appear to have been mostly individually designed and made to order by the local blacksmith, a practice that pertained well into the present century, making recognition difficult, and dating of each item seldom possible. A few surgical instrument makers, however, did produce veterinary pieces, notably Arnold and Weiss. In his catalogue of 1830 John Weiss quotes many testimonials to his instruments from the Royal Mews and the Royal Horse Infirmary, Woolwich, of which the following is a mere sample:

Savile Row, May 14th,1824
I think so highly of Mr Weiss's talents as a surgical instrument maker that I now employ him for making and repairing the greater part of the instruments I require for the use of the Royal Military Asylum, Chelsea, the Lock Hospital, and my private patients. I therefore feel myself justified in recommending him to the favourable notice of the Director-General of the Army Medical Board.

P. Macgregor.

The development of root crops, selective breeding, and other changes in eighteenth-century agriculture, enabling farmers to keep stock alive more easily during the winter, encouraged greater skill among veterinary surgeons. Again during the later nineteenth century changes in husbandry and scientific advances led to radical changes in techniques. Some were discredited, others rendered obsolete, and some neglected. Many of the instruments found today are in fact the farrier's or the farmer's own tools, rather than those of the veterinary surgeon.

Success, however, remained problematic and one feels the following story of an old Yorkshire vet says much for what kept one animal alive and killed another. He was widely renowned for his quite phenomenal success; before every operation he insisted on being left quite alone in the farm kitchen for a while, though no one ever discovered what he did there. On his death-bed his son begged for his secret. Making sure no one was listening, the old man whispered, 'I boils me tools.' A most succinct definition of antisepsis.

Some of the earliest sets of tools to be seen in this country are now thought not to have the veterinary association they once held. A sixteenth-century hunting trousse in the White Tower of the Tower of London, dated 1581, another from the Londesborough collection, and the very handsome set from the former Russian Museum at Tsarskoe-Selo, have been repeatedly described as *trousses de vétérinaire*. Exquisitely engraved and richly handled, these sets consist of, on average:

1 large cleaver;
1 small cleaver;
1 small frame saw;
1 bodkin;

1 file and chisel combined;
1 mallet;
1 pair of small shears;
1 small paring knife;
an instrument with a swivelling arc-shaped blade (pls. 1 & 2).

Howard Blackmore firmly states that their purpose was the chase, though one feels that where the use of such a set was available and the care of animals was necessary, they might well have been dual purpose.

In 1668 appeared 'Markham's *Masterpiece*, containing all knowledge belonging to the Smith, Farrier, or Horse-healer. Touching the curing of all Diseases in Horses.'

A type of conundrum, the 'Cutt or Figure' is explained as follows:

'The Figure one a Compleat Horseman shews
That rides, keeps, cures and all Perfection Knows

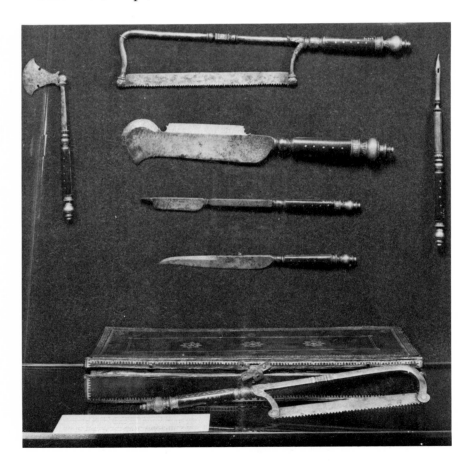

1. *Hunting trousse, 1570, from Heydon Hall, Norfolk.*
(Wellcome Collection)

The two diet; the three letting Blood
Rest Balm of Balms, for inward Griefs most good;
The four wounds, Galls and Sores doth firmly cure,
The five helps Nature's Marks; Six doth procure
Helps for the Sinew's Griefs, as Slip or Strain
Knock or Convulsion, all are helped again
The seven Wholesome Drink; the eight doth take
Blood from the Mouth, which Sudden Death doth Slake,
The nine Slows the Horse-Caudle, or the Mash
Good as the Best, yet some fools count it Trash.
The ten shows Fury in untamed Things,
The only Fountain whence Diseases Springs.'

The book shows a page of fifteen instruments—'The Farriers instruments expounded, with their names and properties' (pl. 3).

'The Fig. I sheweth the Hammer, Which driveth in the Nail.
Fig. II Pincers, which breaketh off, cleaneth and draweth the Nail.
III the Buarteris is that which pareth and openeth the Foot.
IV the Rasp or Rape, which maketh smooth the Hoof.
V the Cutting-knife, which taketh away the Superflous Hoof.
VI the Fleam with which he letteth Blood in the Neck or in the Gross places where the Vein is great.
VII the Farrier's Lancet which openeth Small veins and Threads where the stroke may not be used.
VIII the Incision-Knife to open Impostumes, and to cut away Superfluous Flesh.
IX the Crouet to take up Veins.
X the drawing, cauterising Iron to open and separate the Flesh either found or Imposthumated.
XI the round button cauterising Iron to bore holes in the Skin and Swelled Places.
XII the Mellets to Cleanse Wounds.
XIII the Barnacles to pinch a Horse by the Nose or Ears to make him endure pain patiently.
XIV the Needle to Stitch up his Wounds.
XV the Probe to search the Depth of wounds.

and there you have a full Explanation of all the needful Instruments belonging to the skillfull Farrier.'

Number VIII is a most elaborately designed scalpel with a curved and pointed blade folding like a penknife into a double-sided guard,

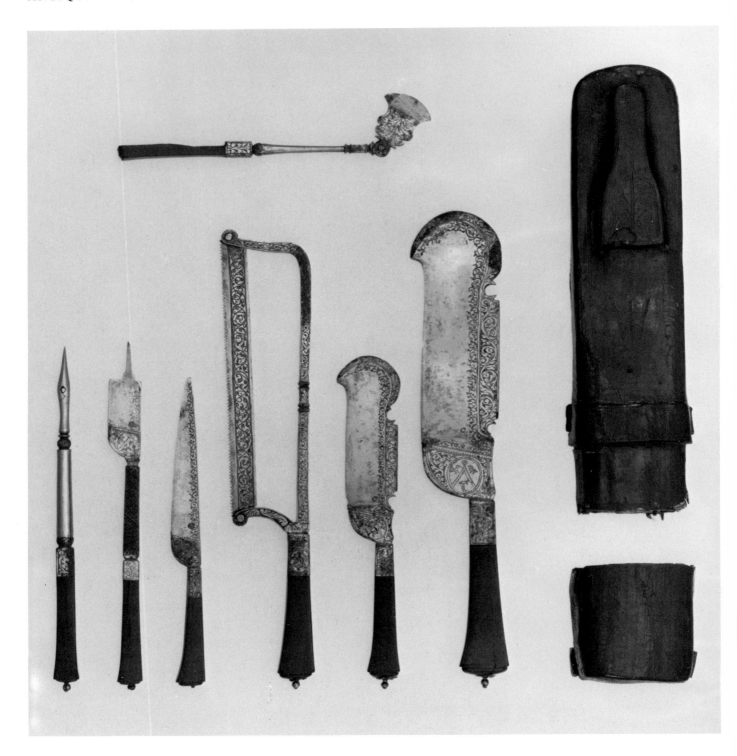

2. Hunting trousse with case, dated 1581. (The Armouries, H.M. Tower of London) (Crown copyright; reproduced with permission of the Controller of H.M. Stationery Office)

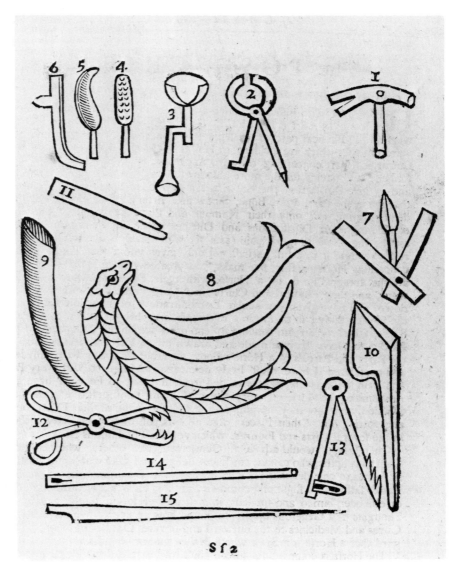

3. 'The Farriers instruments expounded' from Markham's Masterpiece, *1668 (see text, p. 217). (Royal College of Veterinary Surgeons Library)*

which is chased into the shape of a fish with head, tail, and scales. The rest of the instruments are straightforward but very rudimentary.

As in human surgery, blood letting was the universal panacea, doing as much for a frisky horse as a recently confined cow. As can be seen from Markham's instructions above, a veterinary fleam was used for the purpose, with a lancet and spring-fleam or scarificator. The fleam (flem, fleame, flue or flew) was a two- or three-bladed instrument usually folding into a brass or horn case. Each blade was

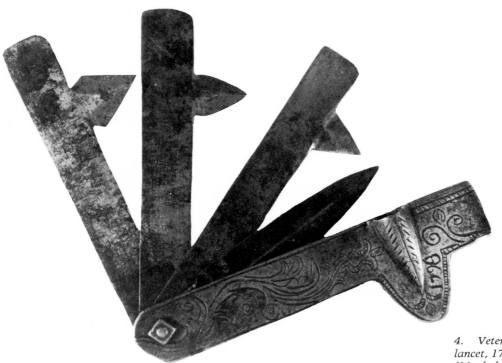

4. *Veterinary fleam in ornate case with lancet, 1798. 10 cm.*
(Musée le Secq des Tournelles, Rouen)

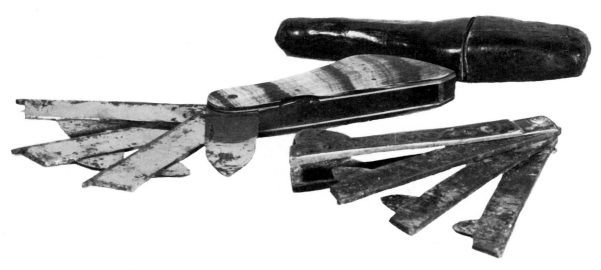

5. *Two veterinary fleams. The upper has three blades and a lancet with horn guard and case, c. 1820. The lower has an engraved brass guard, c. 1840. 10 cm.*
(Castle Museum, York)

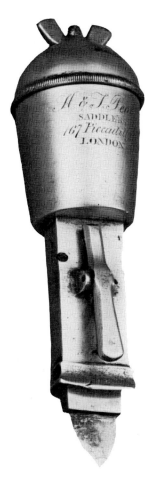

triangular in shape and they were graduated in size, their use corresponding to the size of the animal to be bled (pl. 5). Used with the fleam was the fleaming stick or bloodstick, a heavy truncheon-like piece of wood, usually boxwood, with a leaded head. The scarificator, or spring-fleam in pls. 6 and 7 is a coarse version of the schnappers mentioned in Chapter 2, and was probably used as much in veterinary dentistry as for blood letting. For the more delicate types of venesection small lancets were used, with slightly stouter blades than those for humans, but of the same over-all design. One was found recently, from the second half of the nineteenth century with an enamelled handle depicting a racehorse.

6. *Veterinary spring-fleam, Savigny, c. 1825 (inscribed H. and T. Peat, Saddlers, 167 Piccadilly). 12·5 cm. (Simon Kaye Ltd, London)*

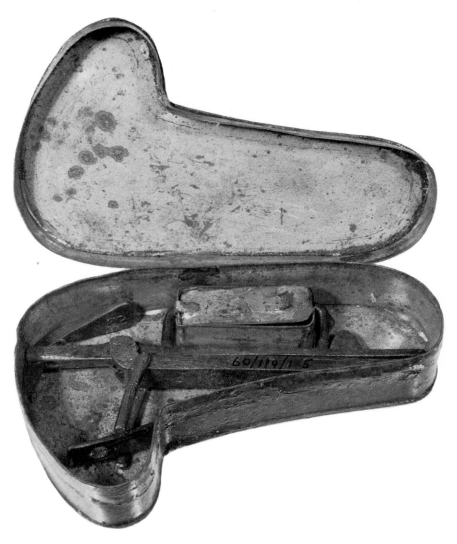

7. *Late eighteenth-century veterinary spring-fleam in case. 10 cm. (Museum of English Rural Life, Reading)*

ANTIQUE MEDICAL INSTRUMENTS

Many and varied were the devices used to induce medicine down an animal's throat. The earliest was probably the drenching horn— a simple cow's horn, occasionally having a metal mount at the wider end and opened at the tip, which would be pushed as far as possible down the throat and the draught poured into the horn (pl. 9). These are often found pierced at the wider end to take a leather thong. They were partly superseded by the drenching bottle, a tall wooden barrel with side nozzle. One such, in the Curtis Museum, is inscribed with instructions, one of which is, 'should the animal begin to cough, lower the head instantly or the medicine in the mouth may run into the windpipe and dangerous results ensue.' For medicine in pill form the balling gun was necessary (pl. 10). In effect it was a type of blowpipe consisting of a beechwood case with an oak inner rod acting as a plunger and shooting the pill far down

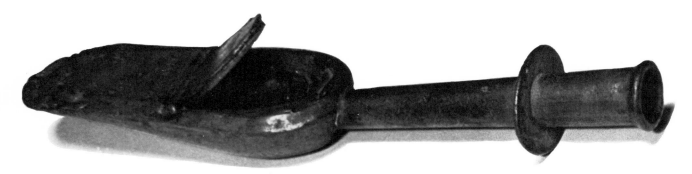

8.   A very interesting veterinary version of the Gibson spoon, pewter, c. 1840. 17 cm. (Wye College, Kent)

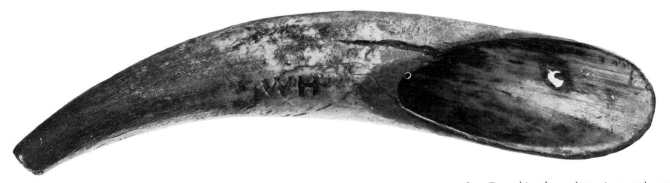

9.   Drenching horn, late nineteenth century. 20·5 cm. (Museum of English Rural Life, Reading)

the animal's throat. Against this, an instrument with an almost opposite purpose, was the chokepipe, a long curved pipe with a hose end, used to cure wind.

Dental instruments followed the development and design of those in Chapter 9, though naturally of a coarser, larger type. Toothkeys abounded and there is a tooth file and rasp in the Wye College collection, a spade-shaped instrument on a long shaft with wooden handle (pl. 11).

Searing and cauterising irons (pl. 12) were used for wounds long after the haemostatic clamp was innovated and can be differentiated from a branding iron, as the latter usually had one shaft with a variety of interchangeable heads of fairly obvious design.

10. Two balling guns. The upper operated by lever, c. 1870; the lower on a piston principle, brass bound wood, c. 1860. 51 cm.
(Castle Museum, York)

11. Horse tooth file, c. 1865. 58·4 cm.
(Wye College, Kent)

An instrument peculiar to veterinary surgery is the Seton's needle. This was a fine piece of metal about 6·5 cm long with a ring handle and a narrow eye which was used to insert strips of fabric through skin lesions to produce suppuration. Setons soaked in the blood of animals dead from blackleg were commonly inserted in the dewlaps of young cattle as a crude form of vaccination. The principle was the same as the setaceum forceps mentioned in Chapter 3.

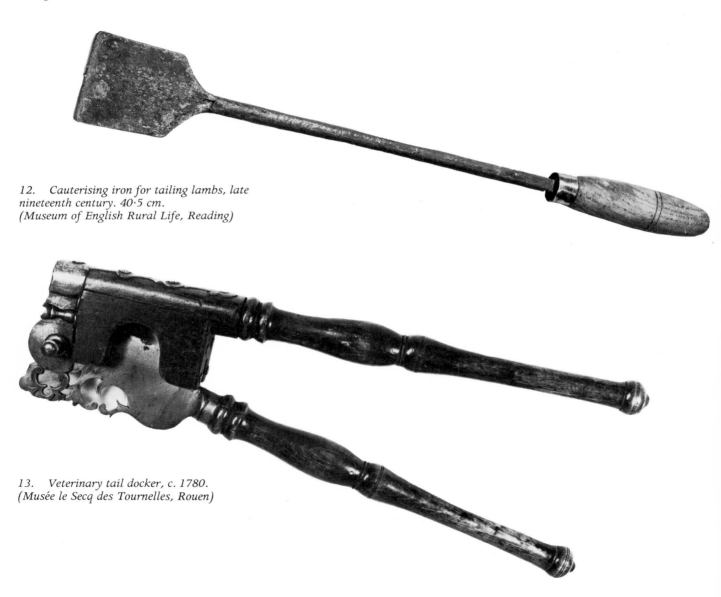

12.   *Cauterising iron for tailing lambs, late nineteenth century. 40·5 cm.*
(Museum of English Rural Life, Reading)

13.   *Veterinary tail docker, c. 1780.*
(Musée le Secq des Tournelles, Rouen)

Small trephines were used, not for trepanning, but for opening the nasal sinuses prior to irrigation, and there are trocars, syringes, and vast enemas found, and forceps of fairly obvious use, but very uncertain age.

It is obvious that much effort had to be put into the task of holding the animal still during treatment, and there are a variety of gags (pls. 14 and 15) and muzzles for the purpose. At the Curtis Museum there is a calf muzzle with a spiked leather hood for the nose, but spiked leather collars and wooden pillories were used too.

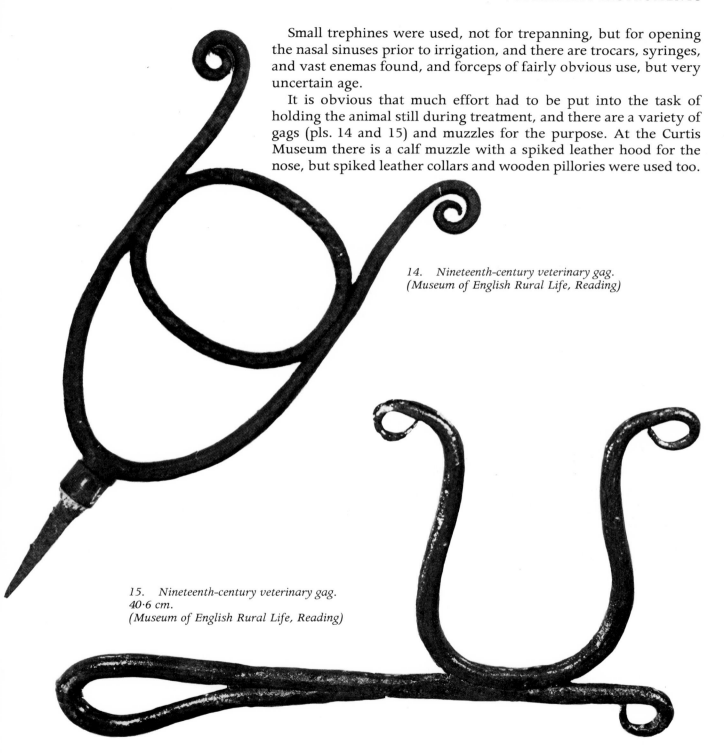

14.   *Nineteenth-century veterinary gag.*
(Museum of English Rural Life, Reading)

15.   *Nineteenth-century veterinary gag.*
40·6 cm.
(Museum of English Rural Life, Reading)

225

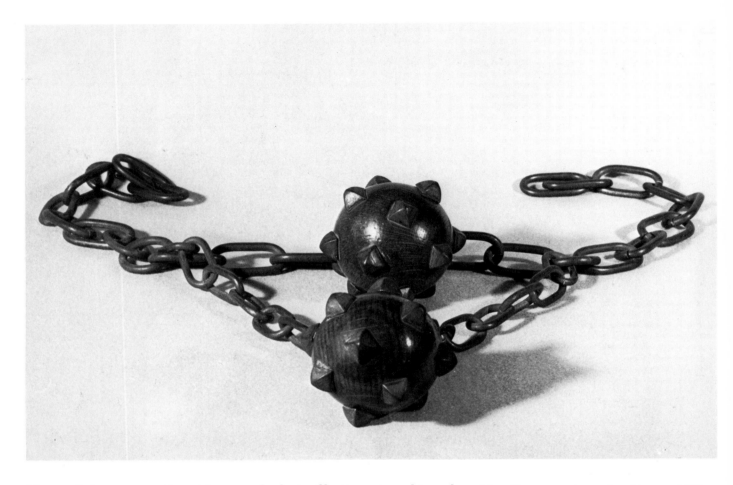

The twitch was another idea, crude but effective; two hinged wooden poles, deeply turned, had a leather strap at the unhinged end. These thongs were wrapped round the tongue and twisted tight. Many types of rigid bull leaders were made, designed to fit on to the nose ring and keep the animal at bay. Docking irons for horses, but more frequently for lambs and puppies, look like wide-bladed shears with the pivot at the top of the blade, and often with a metal catch to hold the handles together. They can be confused with a clam or clamp, which was used in castration and hernia repair. This was applied to the appropriate part and progressively tightened until the isolated tissue sloughed away.

A large number of veterinary instruments are in the Museum of Rural Life at Reading where they are attractively displayed, but totally without description or date. One was told, 'who is to say?' This remains one of the most undocumented subjects ever.

16. 'Ram-scarer', wood and iron, c. 1870. (Castle Museum, York)

PLATE VII

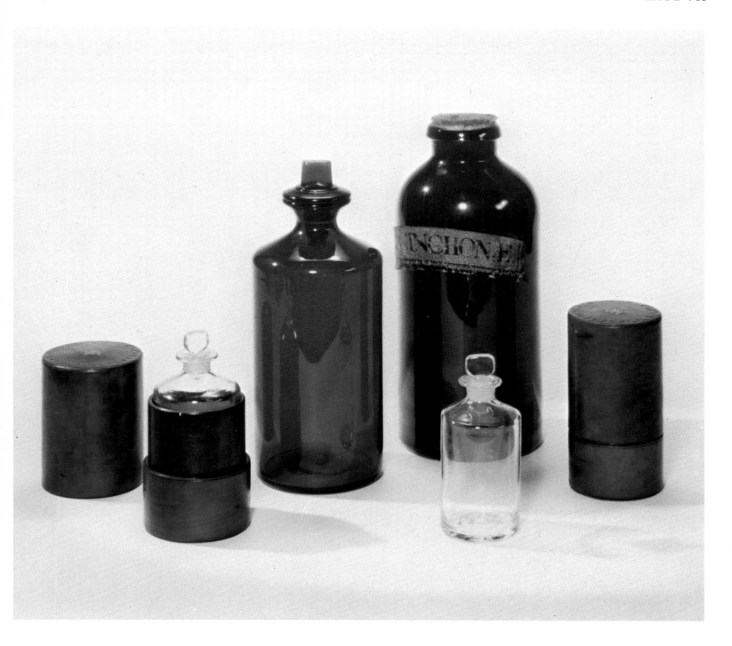

*A pair of leather-cased travelling medicine
bottles, c. 1845; Bristol glass medicine bottle,
c. 1820; large purple glass medicine bottle,
c. 1820. Height of first 12.5cm.
(Simon Kaye Ltd, London)*

PLATE VIII

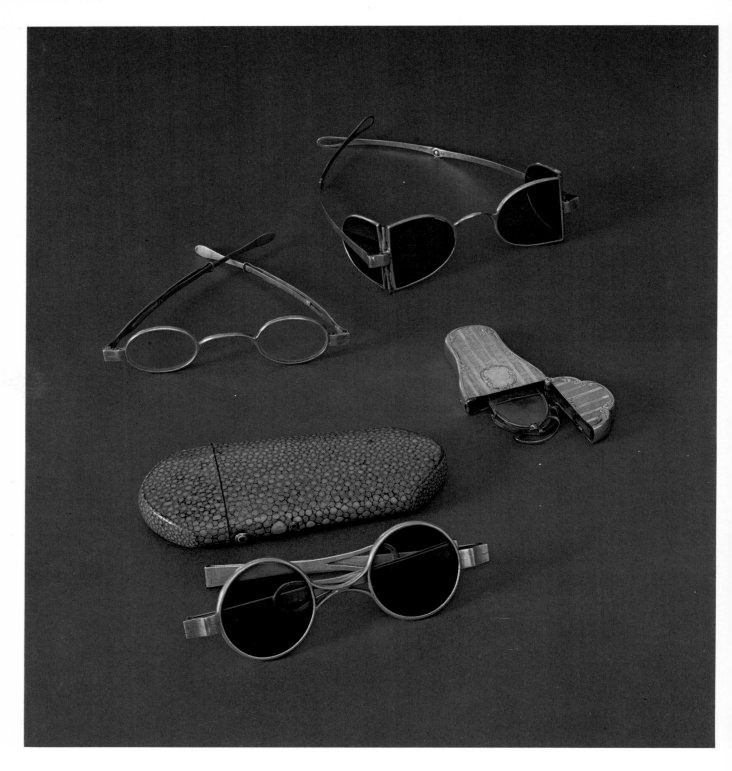

CHAPTER ELEVEN

Functional aids

Ear trumpets

Methods of amplifying sound by holding a trumpet-shaped object to the ear were known and used from the earliest times. First to be used were cow horns, particularly the long, curved type that would curl round to the front of the hearer and not necessitate turning the head. In the sixteenth and seventeenth centuries these were sometimes silver-mounted or had the addition of an ivory ear-piece; they can be differentiated from silver-mounted drinking horns by the narrower tip and the shape of the finial.

Despite Samuel Mihles's assertion in 1764 that deafness could be cured by syringeing with warm milk and water followed by plentiful bleeding, the most elegant silver ear trumpets were made in the eighteenth century and inspired a variety of design and ingenuity. Edward Wakelin made three for Richard Bull in the 1770s; it is not recorded why one was not sufficient. Decoration followed silver designs of the period, bead-edge and bright-cutting, reed-edge and half-fluting, until in the early nineteenth century every kind of voluptuous enrichment was employed.

A telescopic trumpet for carrying in the pocket made of Old Sheffield Plate with silver mounts by W. B. Pine, dated 1820, is in the Sheffield City Museum (pl. 2). Phipps and Robinson made a similar one in silver in 1814 with a ring at the narrow end, presumably to take a ribbon suspended round the neck.

A magnificent example in silver was made by Rawlings and Sumner in 1835 (pl. 3) and is in three parts, each screwing neatly into the other to make a trumpet 42 cm long, and fairly smothered in engraving of flowers, foliage, birds, and a dragon. On the outer end two Chinamen of unidentified purpose sit either side of an Italianate rural scene,. while on the inner lip are the arms of Milton and Golbourne. The original owner must have been exceedingly deaf to need the considerable amplification afforded by this piece.

In the years 1865 and 1866 a series of delightful silver-plated ear trumpets was produced by the firm of F. C. Rein & Son, Aurists and Acoustic Instrument Makers, who inscribed the base of all their pieces with their name and the words 'Patentees and Sole Inventors and Makers, 108 Strand, London.' These, for the most part are small

Colour plate
Early nineteenth-century spectacles: from top to bottom, silver sliding-action frames, 1830; travelling spectacles, c. 1820; pince-nez in silver case, 1849, Nathanial Mills: green lenses in shagreen case, 1822, Gilkerson and McAll; Diameter of lenses 6·5 cm. (Simon Kaye Ltd, London)

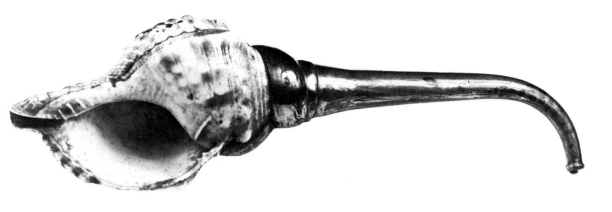

1. *Ear trumpet with shell, Itard (1773–1838), c. 1820.*
(Musée d'Histoire de la Medécine, Paris; Cliché Assistance Publique)

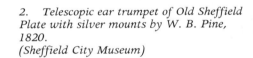

2. *Telescopic ear trumpet of Old Sheffield Plate with silver mounts by W. B. Pine, 1820.*
(Sheffield City Museum)

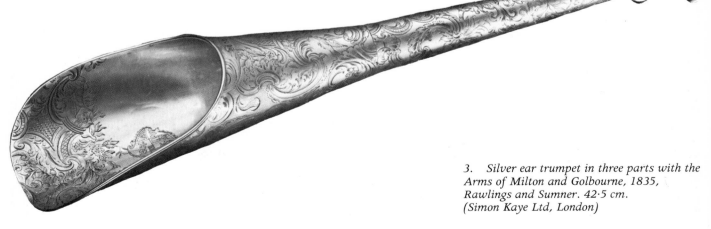

3. *Silver ear trumpet in three parts with the Arms of Milton and Golbourne, 1835, Rawlings and Sumner. 42·5 cm.*
(Simon Kaye Ltd, London)

228

trumpets, completely covered in typical Victorian engraving and having an ivory earpiece. Among the many shapes and designs put out by this firm are variations on a 'double trumpet'. The tube leading from the ear doubles back in a U-turn with a circular aperture; fixed over this opening is a large hood that is then facing to the front of the user and is covered by a scrolled grille. The hood therefore acts as a collective sounding board for conversation and throws the sound back into the tube leading to the user's ear, a principle which works very well. One of this type turned up recently in a London saleroom and, unrecognised, was catalogued as a 'balsam inhaler'. A collection of Rein trumpets is in pl. 4.

4. A group of plated Rein ear trumpets, c. 1865. Length of first 7·5 cm. (Simon Kaye Ltd, London)

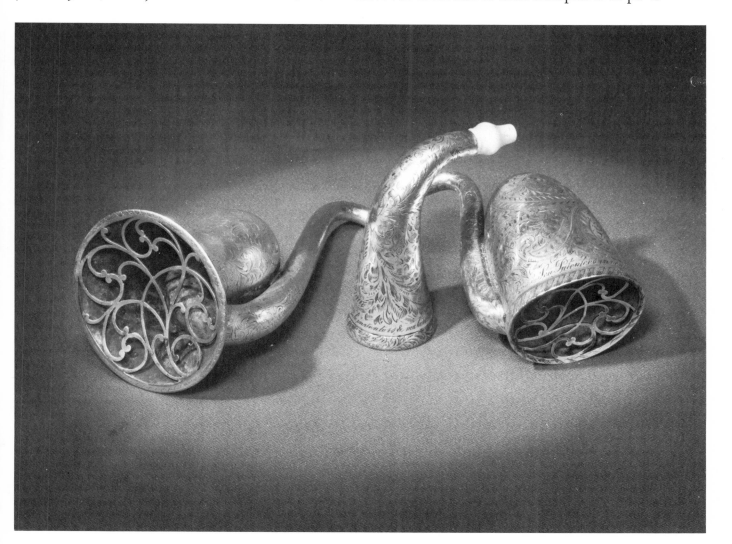

For the humble deaf there were more modest affairs in bronzed tin made by S. Maw & Son, though these too came in every shape and size, collapsible and not, and could be either silver- or gilt-plated. Some were of the 'double trumpet' variety described above, some were plain cones, others looked exactly like a shallow-bowled wine funnel. One trumpet in the catalogue of 1868 is 'adapted for churches'—possibly indicating that if one didn't care for the sermon one could remove the trumpet.

In the latter part of the century, tortoise-shell was much employed for ear trumpets, occasionally silver-mounted but more often plain with a wide flare at the lip.

Another form of hearing aid in the mid-nineteenth century was the conversation tube—a length of silk-covered rubber tubing between 88 and 176 cm long with a small, usually ivory, speaking trumpet at one end, and an ivory earpiece at the other (pl. 7). One, with large ivory mounts and described as 'very powerful', cost one guinea. Finally, there were ear cornets, a pair of tiny cones, plugged into the ears and connected over the head by a band of flexible metal. The cones were either bronzed, plated, covered in silk for the ladies, or were gutta-percha for the *hoi polloi*.

Probably unique is the forerunner of modern hearing aids used by the Duke of Wellington in the latter part of his life, which can be seen at the R.A.M.C. Museum at Aldershot. This has an earpiece 2·5 cm long which is attached to a brass shell-shaped coil with a bell opening. The whole piece has a diameter of not more than 7·5 cm (pl.8).

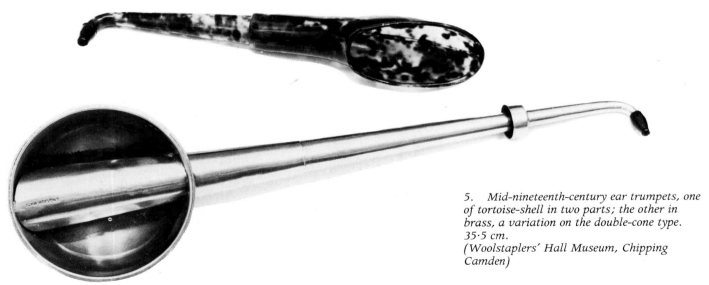

5.   *Mid-nineteenth-century ear trumpets, one of tortoise-shell in two parts; the other in brass, a variation on the double-cone type. 35·5 cm.*
(Woolstaplers' Hall Museum, Chipping Camden)

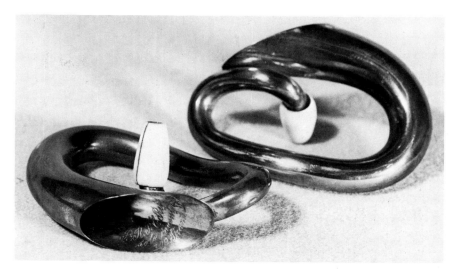

6.   *A pair of copper ear trumpets with ivory ear-pieces, Rein, c. 1865. 6·5 cm.*
(Castle Museum, York)

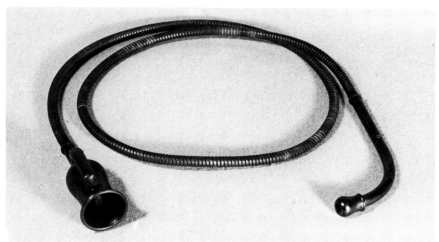

7.   *Conversation tube, c. 1850.*
(Castle Museum, York)

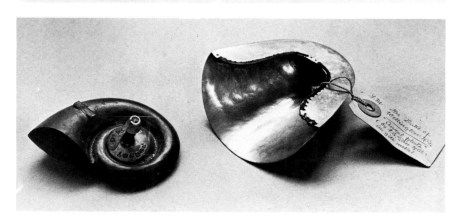

8.   *Hearing aid and case of the first Duke of Wellington, Rein, c. 1850.*
(R.A.M.C. Museum, Aldershot)

Spectacles

Before spectacles were invented, the ill-sighted hired a scholar to read to them, looked through a globe of water or resorted to one of the many quack remedies. One such remedy started 'catch a fox alive' and ended, after something approaching a cross-country obstacle race, 'spit thrice'—which must have been one of the most efficacious spurs the inventors of spectacles could have had. The English philosopher Roger Bacon, writing in 1268, suggested looking through crystal or glass for magnifying purposes. However, the obscurity of the original inventor is the probable effect of medieval church teaching that afflictions should be borne in patience, thus setting up great opposition to their alleviation. Spectacles were most probably invented by Armati of Florence, who died in 1317, and Fra Giodano di Rivalto, writing in 1305, said 'It is not yet 20 years since the art of making spectacles, one of the most useful arts on earth, was discovered.' Excavations at Troy and

9.   *St Peter with an eye-glass, c. 1470; a picture behind the High Altar of the Church of St Jacob, Rothenberg, Bavaria. (British Optical Association Library)*

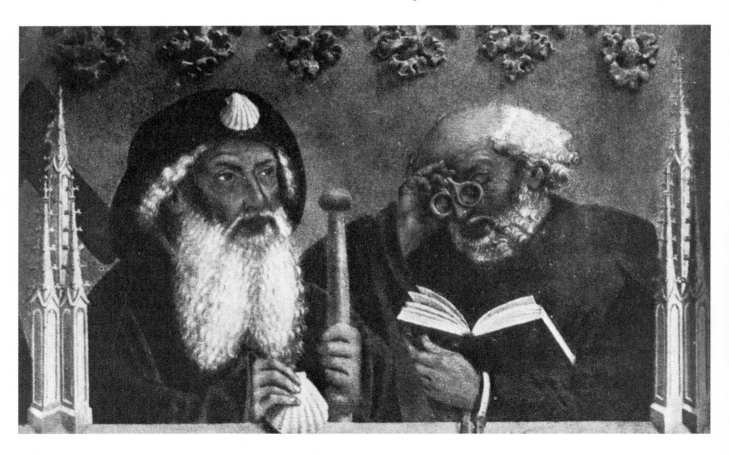

Tyre revealed leather-framed lenses but these are thought to have been mere trinkets as there is a hole pierced through the centre. The thirteenth-century invention is more likely to have been based on Arab sources.

These earliest glasses were probably a single lens in a frame with a handle and in time two handles, one for each glass, would have been joined. Despite church opposition a fifteenth-century altarpiece at Rothenburg in Bavaria shows an ageing St Peter with the keys in one hand and just such a pair of spectacles in the other (pl. 9). Variations on the type of frame were developed but it was a long time before flexibility allowed glasses to rest on the nose without help. In the late fifteenth century they were occasionally held on by an extension over the forehead. Early frames were made of brass or iron and then of horn, bone, gold, silver and even of leather. The first lenses were only for long-sightedness and were ground from berillus or beryl, a smoke coloured glass. From beryl came the French *bericle* and later *besicles*, meaning spectacles. The word 'lenses' comes from the Italian word for lentils, and for three centuries they were called glass lentils. Eye-glasses, being precious, required cases, and these were often the most intricate and beautiful works of art, made of wood, metal, or ivory or, for the *hoi polloi*, leather, horn or parchment. Sometimes, since spectacles were only

10. Sixteenth-century leaf-spring pince-nez, horn rims.
(Ramstein Collection, Basle)

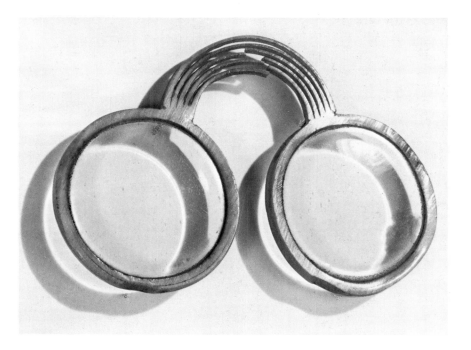

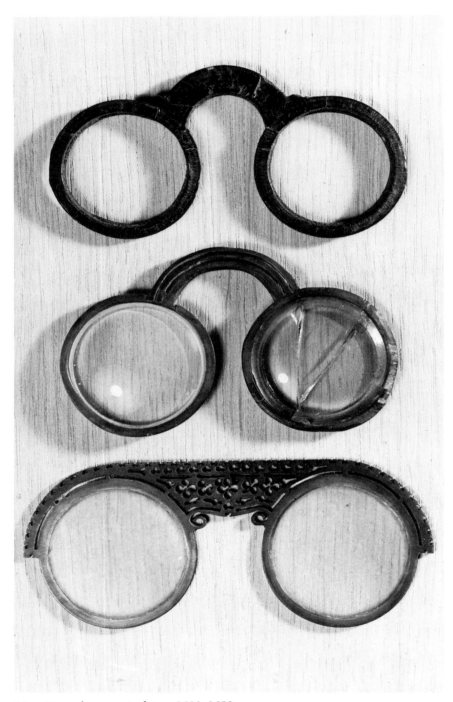

11. *Nuremberg spectacles, c. 1600–1650.*
(Germanisches Nationalmuseum, Nuremberg)

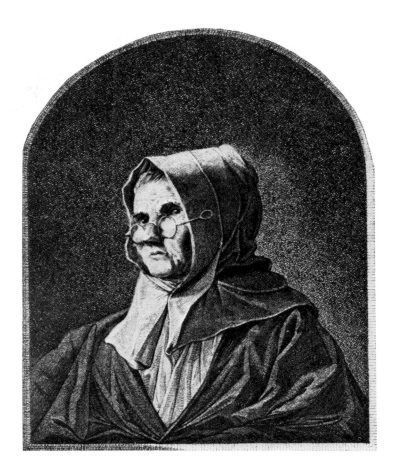

12.   *Dutch engraving by J. Bemme showing temple spectacles, c. 1760 worn outside the head-dress.*
(British Optical Association Library)

used for reading, the case was contrived in the cover of a book. With the invention of the printing press in 1476 more and more people wished to read, resulting in large scale production for the spectacle-maker. Prices fell and spectacles were sold by pedlars; glasses were available to almost all. The first known spectacle-maker was one in Nuremberg in 1478 and by 1567 that city had entirely regularised the craft (pl. 11).

The sixteenth century saw the introduction of concave lenses for the short-sighted, and the innovation of oval lenses meant that one might look over them for distance vision. Frames were becoming slightly more flexible; some were strapped round the head with leather, others had cord around each ear, and others still were attached to a hat. A book entitled *A Briefe Treatise touching the Preservation of the Eiesight*, published in 1586, mentions the usefulness of tinted glasses, and by 1591 lenses of amber, soaked in linseed oil, were used as a protection against the sun.

235

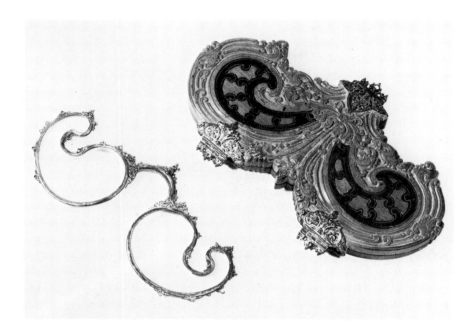

13. Italian silver nose spectacles with carved wooden case, c. 1770. (British Optical Association Museum)

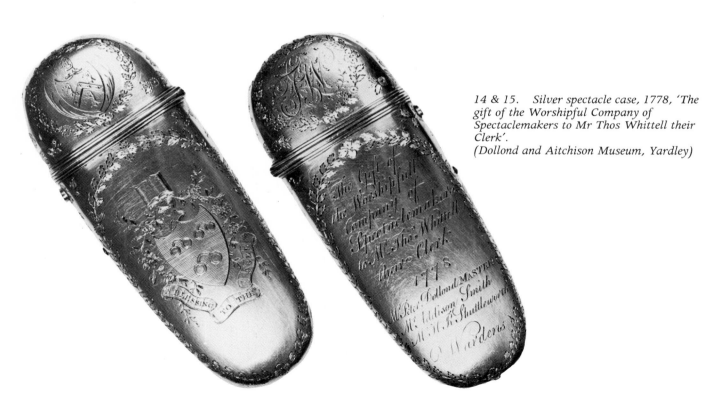

14 & 15. Silver spectacle case, 1778, 'The gift of the Worshipful Company of Spectaclemakers to Mr Thos Whittell their Clerk'. (Dollond and Aitchison Museum, Yardley)

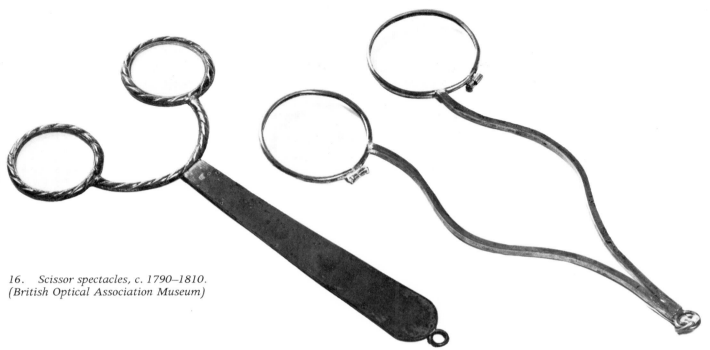

16. Scissor spectacles, c. 1790–1810. (British Optical Association Museum)

In 1629 the Worshipful Company of Spectacle Makers was established, with the strictest regulations. William Spencer, in 1668 was castigated and then sued at Common Law for employing his son who was neither an apprentice nor had served his seven years in the trade. In 1669, a haberdasher's shop was found with spectacles not made by members of the guild and 'was thereon destroyed'. One feels this speaks more of closed-shop tactics than a desire to maintain standards.

The seventeenth century saw a return to the single eye-glass, mostly for the rich who did not wish to be associated with double ones now that they had become available to all. As far as fashion was concerned, this remained so until early in the present century. All was managed much on a hit or miss basis and customers chose glasses as one might a hat, the lens-maker having scratched on to them the age for which he thought they might be suitable. The 'common' double spectacles were now made in light steel frames, though still available in silver and brass, and had a semi-circular spring across the nose-piece, allowing them for the first time to grip the bridge of the nose. The form of mid-seventeenth-century spectacles is not clear as the books of the London Spectacle Makers' Company were burned in the Great Fire, but by the end of the century we read of black frames for sale at 5*d* the pair and ordinary white ones for 7*d*. Samuel Pepys, whose bad eyesight regrettably caused him eventually to stop writing his diary, nevertheless in 1666, 'did this evening buy me a pair of green spectacles to see whether they will help my eyes or no'. The British Optical Association has a pair with supplementary green lenses made to fold across the untinted ones when necessary (pl. 17).

At this period two books appeared to advance the optical science—Isaac Newton's *Opticks* of 1704 and an excellent book of 1722, *Chirurge Oculist de St Côme* by M. de Saint Yves, written 'with approval and privilege of the King'.

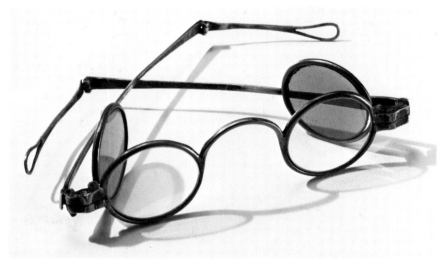

17. *Double glasses, as patented by J. Richardson in 1797. The second, tinted, pair could protect the eyes at the side against draughts or in the front against dazzle. Note the wide nose-piece.*
(Ramstein Collection, Basle)

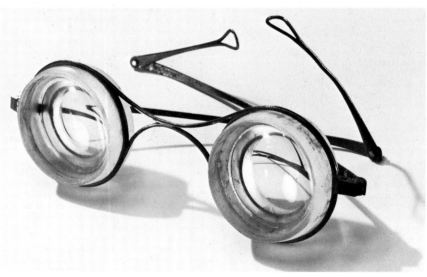

18. *Spectacles for the myopic; glass and steel frames, c. 1800.*
(Ramstein Collection, Basle)

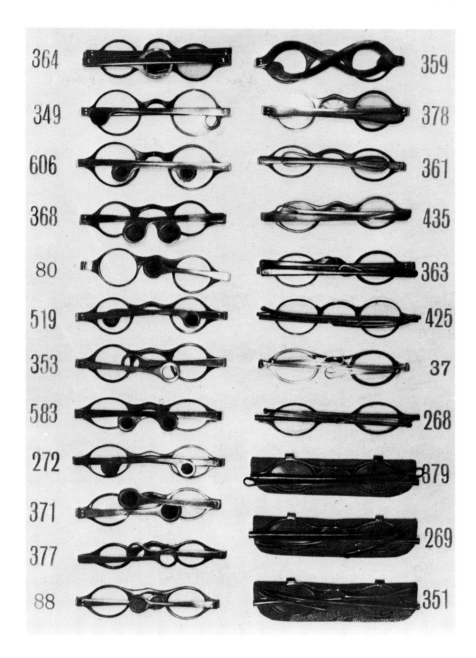

19.   Spectacles, c. 1700–1830 showing the
variety of side-piece, some ringed to take a
riband; the curving shape of the tortoise-shell
frames of No. 359, c. 1700, is of interest.
(British Optical Association Library)

The eighteenth century brought an ever increased use of the single eye-glass or quizzing glass by the fashionable, and these were now highly ornate and made of the richest materials. Richard Corson suggests that the true quizzing glass was a small looking glass made for the Beau Nash *monde* to see what was going on behind them (possibly the small mirrors referred to as dental mirrors in Chapter 9 (col. pl. V and pl. 21, p. 210), though this is not the opinion of the present writer.

However, spectacles were even more popular with those who merely wished to see more clearly. Tortoise-shell frames, a steel spring nose-piece, and a hinge folding one lens over the other were common; cases were usually of sharkskin or shagreen. In 1773 it was possible to buy a good pair for 1s but shoddy German spectacles with badly ground green glass and plated frames were 4d. At this time there was a higher standard in this country than elsewhere, and English spectacles were much prized. Men like Dollond and Ramsden, who were self-educated, rose through diligence to work with leading scientists and it was not considered bizarre that Dollond should become a Fellow of the Royal Society.

About 1728 Edward Scarlett at last invented spectacles with rigid side pieces; 'temple-spectacles' they were called. The side pieces ended in large rings which held them in place and the frames were of steel, silver, gold, horn, or brass. Later on, in 1752, sliding or hinged extensions were added. Lenses might be either clear or tinted blue or green. By the end of the century, Benjamin Franklin, tired of coping with two sets of spectacles, had made for himself the first pair of bifocals with a half lens from each pair inserted into one frame. A variation on this was double spectacles with one pair of lenses made to swing away when the other was required.

Monocles or magnifying glasses for reading became popular at the end of the century and were often encased in an ornate shell back which looked like a medallion when hanging round the neck. Popular among the dandies were scissor glasses, a kind of lorgnette with a handle for each glass coming together under the nose and looking as if it would cut it off. 'Prospect glasses' were a highly ornate type of telescope for the opera and other entertainments. In 1797 Dudley Adam introduced his patent spectacles (patent not applied for) designed to relieve the nose and temples from pressure. The lenses could be raised or lowered, rotated, or the separation varied to suit anyone. The Science Museum shows eye-glasses attached to the cap for hunting or shooting; ingenuity knew no bounds.

During the nineteenth century, there was greater acceptance of

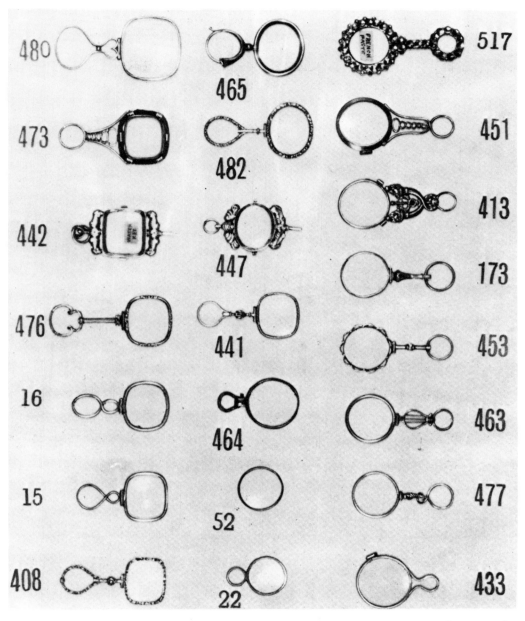

20. Quizzing glasses, c. 1800 to c. 1860. Numbers 442 and 447 are combined with a watch key. 6·5 cm. (British Optical Association Library)

spectacles, if only among men, and gradually pince-nez became the grudging compromise for both sexes. Early in the century someone thought of putting two telescopes together and the single one was superseded, making the first binoculars. Decoration was profuse, with mother-of-pearl, gold and seed-pearls for the fashionable opera goer. From these and the scissor glasses evolved the lorgnette

241

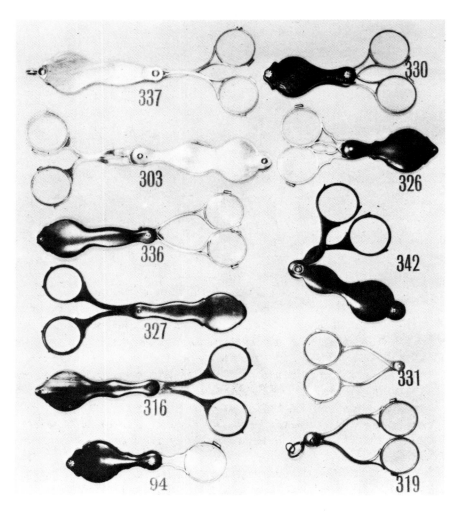

21. *Folding lorgnettes, c. 1800–1830.*
(British Optical Association Library)

as we know it—a pair of spectacles on a side-handle—which became popular for the woman of fashion.

In the early years of the century, probably about 1805, monocles were introduced. Sometimes two might be carried, one for long-sight and one for reading. They were of every conceivable shape—round, oval, square, rectangular, and octagonal—and the frames were of every material, gold, silver, horn, and shell, or were diamond-studded, or rimless, with a hole in the corner for the cord. They were severely ridiculed by Dickens in *Little Dorrit*. His character, Barnacle Junior, could not keep his monocle in. 'He had a superior eye-glass dangling round his neck, but unfortunately had such flat orbits to his eyes and such limp little eyelids that it wouldn't stick in when he put it up . . . that discomposed him very much.' Monocles

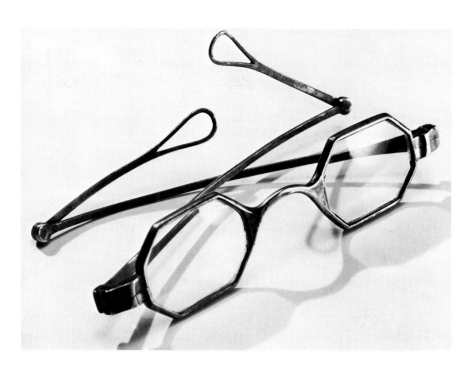

22. Octagonal framed spectacles with folding sidepieces, c. 1820. (Ramstein Collection Basle)

were very much frowned on by the medical profession as they were used indiscriminately as an adjunct of fashion whether they were needed or not, and obviously did much harm to the eyesight. Nevertheless, they remained in vogue, mainly with the English and Germans until the First World War, with a brief revival in the 1920s.

Spectacles in the nineteenth century were still chosen by the customer as and how he thought fit, or were ordered by post by the out-of-town, who merely stated their age. Silver was most commonly used for frames. By 1820 lenses were usually oval, octagonal, or rectangular as these were considered more elegant than round. Occasionally one finds glasses intended to correct a squint, with inner frames of wood or tortoise-shell, sometimes with only a tiny hole in the centre left to see through—such as the pair in the Science Museum described as 'diaphragm' spectacles. Double-jointed frames became popular although it was said that 'if a single-jointed frame is fastened round the head with a riband it may be kept on almost as steadily and comfortable as a double-jointed frame.'

The appalling conditions in the nineteenth century, particularly among needlewomen, lace-makers, and underpaid clerks working in ill-lit premises through long hours, resulted in a need for cheap spectacles, and they sold wholesale at the rate of 18s per dozen. Of not much help to these customers was the advice given in the *Cyclopaedia of Practical Medicine* in 1833—'The absolute necessity of purchasing glasses under the direction of a qualified person and of not going into a shop at random and just taking what the shopman gives you, has already been pointed out. In the mechanical arrangement of the lenses there are two or three points worthy of attention. The frames should be of metal and sufficiently strong to prevent twisting or loss of weight. Steel is probably the best though some people prefer gold.'

The nineteenth century saw every kind of nose piece introduced, X-shaped, K-shaped, followed by a W-type in mid-century. Half-glasses appeared for the first time; bifocals and even trifocals came in, terms first used and patented in 1827 by John Isaac Hawkins. This type of spectacle was much ridiculed by Edward Lear in *More Nonsense*, 1872—'The Perpendicular Purple Polly who read the Newspaper and Ate Parsnip Pie with his spectacles'. Astigmatism was understood for the first time and glasses were made to correct it by Fuller of Ipswich in 1827.

In 1861, J. Braham of Bristol patented auxiliary spectacles attached to the main pair by a spring, and there were special protective glasses for road and rail travel (col. pl. VIII). Smoked glass came in about 1820; coloured glass as a protective measure was now under censure and green glass was considered vulgar. *Good Society*, published in 1860, said, 'smoke-coloured glasses are best; green glass are detestable'! Other types of protection such as crêpe head shields were introduced and cocquilles or 'shell-specs' which covered the eyes as in a cup were an alternative. Among all this great variety of *aide-voir*, the nineteenth-century favourite was undoubtedly the pince-nez. This had first appeared as early as the sixteenth century but did not become really popular until now. Pince-nez were made with heavy rims, light rims, or no rims; with ribbons, chains, no anchorage; circular, oval, rectangular, or half-moon; and with every type of nose piece. They were the fashionable perquisite of that backbone of the nineteenth century, the middle and professional classes, and must have been considered becoming or they would have been removed before photography.

As early as 1845 Sir John Herschel suggested the idea of contact lenses, but it was not until the end of the century that it was put into practice.

Spectacles revolutionised man's attitude to the world; no longer was he entirely dependent on his physical limitations and such natural factors as the length of daylight.

Artificial limbs

Ambroise Paré (1509–90) was the first to tackle the problem of producing artificial limbs and the first to establish their feasibility. He became a military surgeon in 1536 and consequently was surrounded by the need for these aids. He was unique for his ingenuity in simulating natural functions with mechanical gadgetry. His inventions were mainly designed for wounded soldiers and he devised for them several arms and hands that were successful. One of his ideas was a reproduction of the human hand with a holder for a quill pen; another most complicated device was a hand with individually moving fingers on a system of cog wheels and levers. His work in this field was widely accepted when he became surgeon to Charles IX of France.

After Paré, Scultetus invented various artificial limbs, eyes, and noses in the seventeenth century. Little quite so advanced was attempted again until the nineteenth century when a variety of cumbersome limbs appeared in the catalogues. Few have survived and it is difficult to date so much as a crutch with certainty. Hugh Ryder in 1685, described a tin case he had devised for the leg of a patient with a compound fracture, in which there were little doors to open and shut 'for the opportunity of making applications to the wounded parts', but this hardly counts as an artificial limb (pls. 23–28).

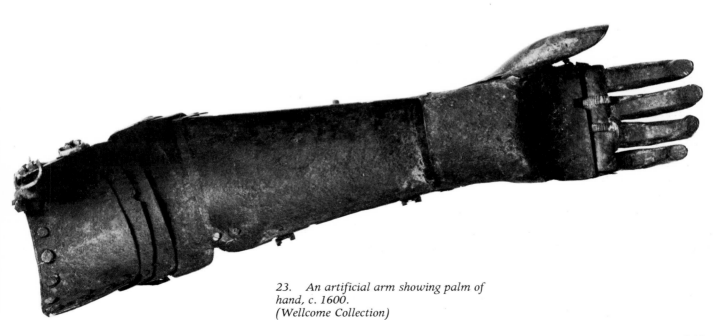

23.   An artificial arm showing palm of hand, c. 1600.
(Wellcome Collection)

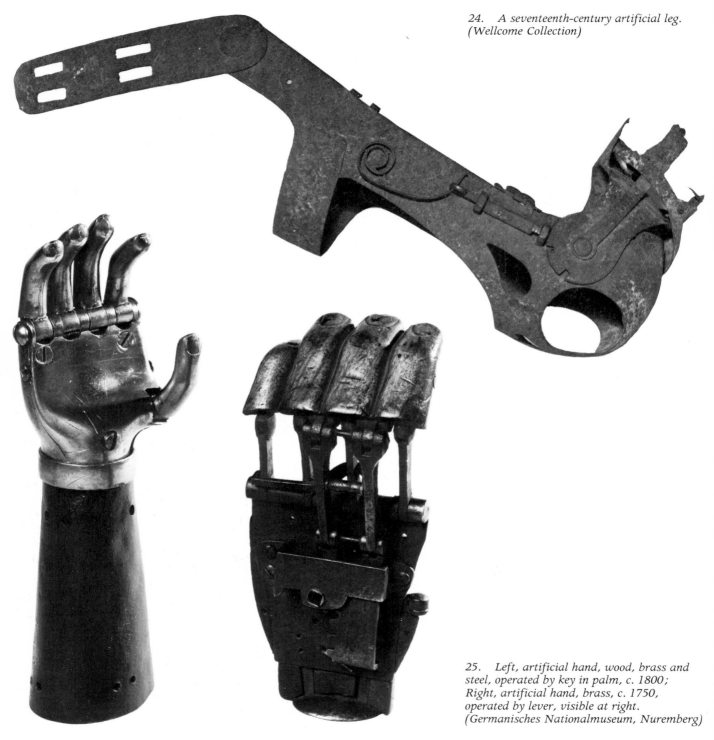

24.   *A seventeenth-century artificial leg.*
(Wellcome Collection)

25.   *Left, artificial hand, wood, brass and*
steel, operated by key in palm, c. 1800;
Right, artificial hand, brass, c. 1750,
operated by lever, visible at right.
(Germanisches Nationalmuseum, Nuremberg)

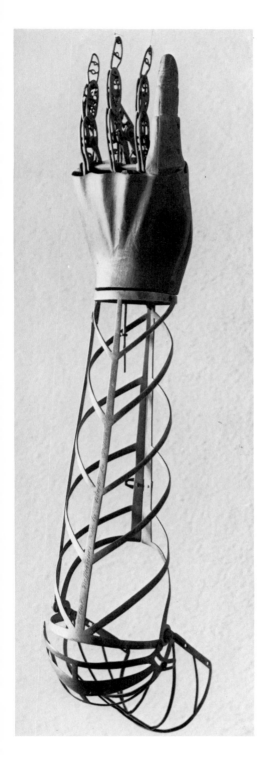

26. *Artificial arm, c. 1794, inscribed 'Aux deffenseurs de la liberté la patrie reconnaissance'.*
(Musée Crozatier, Puy)

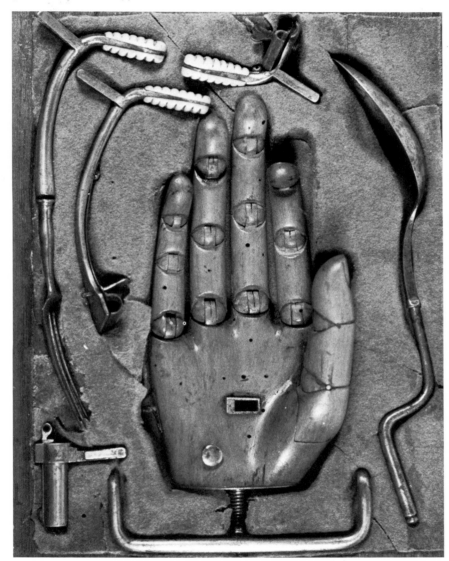

27. *Articulated artificial hand, wood, made to unscrew and alternate with spoon, fork, etc. Made in London, 1807, and presented to a Danish Naval Officer who lost his hand in a sea battle with the British.*
(Museum of Historical Medicine, Copenhagen)

247

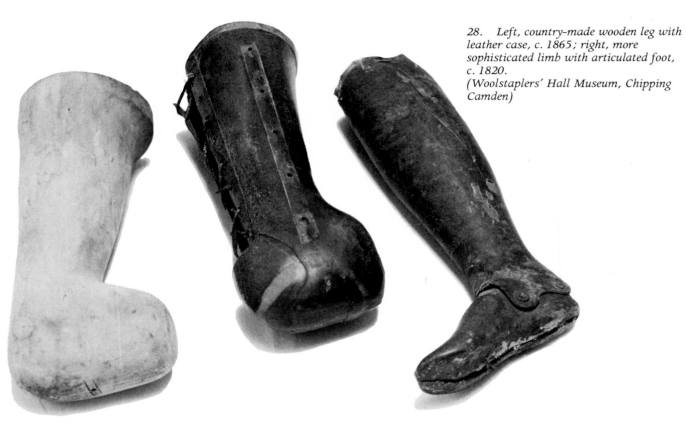

28. Left, country-made wooden leg with leather case, c. 1865; right, more sophisticated limb with articulated foot, c. 1820.
(Woolstaplers' Hall Museum, Chipping Camden)

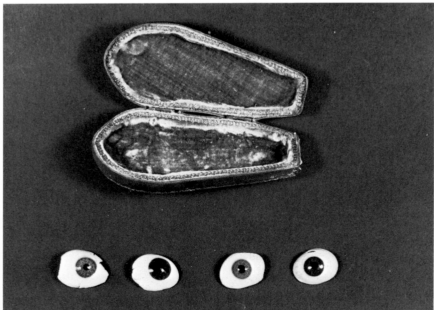

29. Set of glass artificial eyes, cased, c. 1810.
(Museum of Historical Medicine, Copenhagen)

248

Artificial teeth

It is unlikely that any but the most specialised collector would wish to form a collection of false teeth, but as countless numbers have long been dependent on their provision, it is worth mentioning something of their history. The Etruscans—the best dentists of the ancient world—made partial dentures with gold bridge work as early as 700 B.C. The teeth were carved from bone or ivory or were human teeth from other mouths. In England the very rich might have had dentures by the end of the seventeenth century. The mouth would have been measured with compasses and the false teeth tied onto the natural ones with silk. A full lower set would be hand carved, often from one piece of ivory, but upper sets, being more difficult to keep in place, presented more problems. Walrus ivory was favoured but rhinoceros was used too. Sometimes human teeth were set in tinted ivory gums (in desperate cases, animal teeth were used). For fashionable use at Court, teeth might be of silver or mother of pearl, and Lord Hervey astonished his friends in 1735 by appearing with teeth carved from Italian agate. In 1730, the London goldsmith, Pezé Pilleau Junior, referred to himself as 'Goldsmith and Maker of Artificial Teeth'—a diverse combination but one that suggested gold teeth were desirable too. All these teeth had to be removed for eating, though some women had their gums pierced with hooks to keep the teeth in place. The Parisian dentist Fauchard, in the early eighteenth century, fastened the upper and lower sets together with a steel spring, but constant pressure was needed to keep the mouth closed. The claim was made that it was perfectly possible to masticate with these dentures, but since a certain dentist undertook to make them without the necessity of seeing the patient, one is sceptical of the possibility.

There was great interest in the possibility of replanting sound teeth that had been accidentally knocked or pulled out of their sockets. Guy de Chauliac (1300–1367) found transplanted teeth from another mouth could last for years and Paré, writing about 1540, again found they could be successfully replanted. John Hunter, at the end of the eighteenth century, was a great supporter of this endeavour which is now becoming popular again today.

Teeth made of bone, ivory, or other organic substances were decayed by oral fluids so it was a great step forward when, just before the French Revolution, a Parisian dentist produced all porcelain teeth baked in one piece. From about 1845 individual porcelain teeth were available to be set in plates. Meanwhile 'Waterloo teeth' still sat in the jaws of ageing Regency bucks. Good prices were paid for teeth from plundered graves, and battlefields provided a rich source. Tooth-drawers collected copious numbers at Waterloo, and teeth from the dead in the American Civil War were sent to England by the barrel. However, from America came the introduction of a vulcanite setting so that by mid-century, devices such as the suction pad and spring coil became obsolete.

More attractive for the collector are the pottery and porcelain stands made in the nineteenth century to hold the dentures at the bedside during the night. Some of these can be seen in the Wellcome Collection (pl. 30).

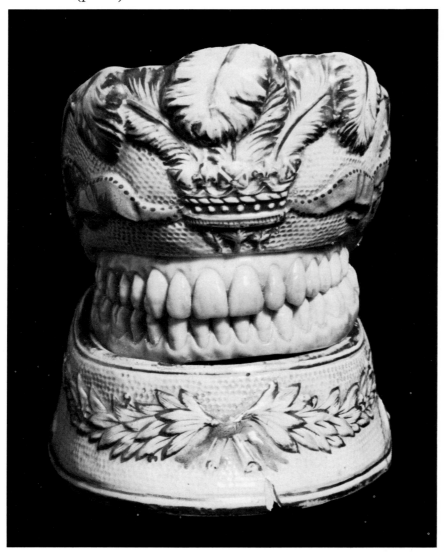

30. An early nineteenth-century pottery holder for dentures. (Wellcome Collection)

250

CHAPTER TWELVE

Medicine receptacles

Medicine spoons

One of the earliest examples of a medicine spoon must be that of *c.* 1698 in the Burrell collection at Pollock House, Glasgow, which has a covered bowl, but spoons of this time are rare as medicine was sold in single dose bottles. It was not until well into the eighteenth century that larger bottles made special spoons of an accurate size necessary (col. pl. VII). The earlier ones are mostly silver, similar to a normal dessert spoon, but with a short, often recurved, stem. By the end of the eighteenth century pewter spoons were being made, and those in silver were often partially or entirely gilt. Early Victorian spoons were double-ended for two sizes of dose (pl. 1) and spoons usually formed part of most toilet services (see Chapter 15).

1.   Medicine spoons. Left to right: pewter Gibson spoon inscribed 'Gibson, Inventor', c. 1835; double-ended silver-gilt spoon, 1860, T.J.; double-ended silver spoon, 1873, H.H.; silver Gibson spoon, 1829, William Knight. Gibson spoon 11·5 cm. (Simon Kaye Ltd, London)

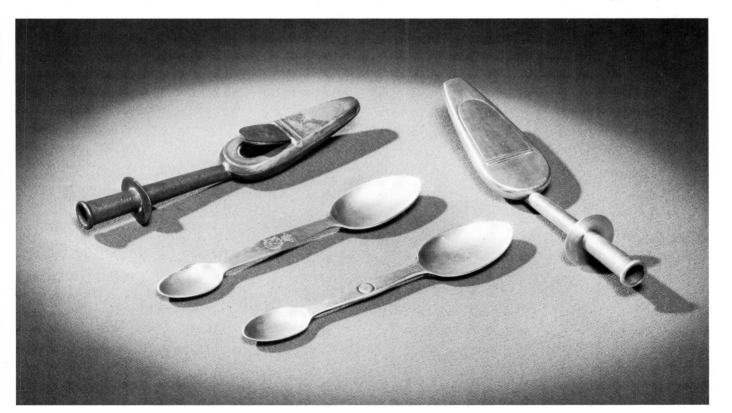

In 1827 Charles Gibson introduced a celebrated spoon that has become known as the castor oil spoon (pl. 1). Made in silver, pewter, Britannia metal, and pottery, it had a hinge cover to the bowl which opened for filling, and a small orifice for administering the medicine. There was a flange halfway down the hollow tubular stem, the end of which was covered by the thumb. When the thumb was removed, air was admitted and the liquid was forced down the patient's throat. The hollow stem was not, as has been repeatedly asserted, to blow through. The use of the Gibson spoon spread rapidly and it was soon listed in no less than three sizes by J. S. Maw, and Dixon of Sheffield. Types of medicine, such as castor oil, were apparently rendered tasteless by this spoon, and it was found helpful in feeding the insane as much as the invalid.

By the middle of the nineteenth century, porcelain spoons with recurved handles allowing them to stand firmly for filling, first appeared (pl. 2). White earthenware ones followed in profusion, and these sometimes had feet and were occasionally half covered. They were mostly plain white, but some had floral decoration or gilt borders. One type had dosage rings marked in the bowl, i.e. table, dessert, and tea.

2.   *A group of mid-nineteenth-century medicine spoons in creamware. (Pharmaceutical Society of Great Britain Museum)*

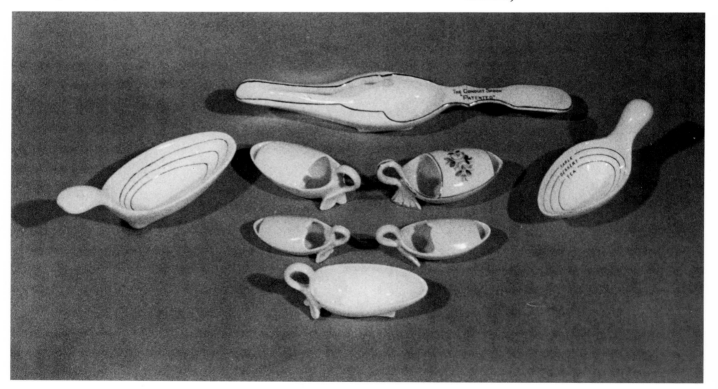

Medicine cups

Cups of silver and silver-gilt appeared in the middle of the eighteenth century and were usually of perfectly plain bucket-shape. Some had a short foot and are found described as eye-baths, but the medicine cup is soon seen to be unhipped and wider in the bowl than would fit into the eye socket. They often formed part of travelling toilet services and a fine one of 1814, formerly belonging to Queen Charlotte, is in col. pl. XV. A beautifully made small silver beaker type with folded rim has been found, made in Exeter in 1835. As glass became cheaper to produce in the nineteenth century, this became the favourite material and they appeared in many different shapes, both with feet and without, some with the doses engraved on them (pl. 3).

Another type of medicine cup was of hour-glass shape formed of two bowls of different sized doses. These were made in the eighteenth century of silver, pewter, pottery, and turned boxwood. Boxwood was used, both polished and unpolished, for the tiniest medicine cups, some even as small as 2·5 cm high.

3.   Timothy Lane minim measure, cased, c. 1810, 5 cm; glass eye bath, c. 1815; medical bougie-box, silver, c. 1750, Edward Medlycott; cased medicine glass, c. 1820. (Simon Kaye Ltd, London)

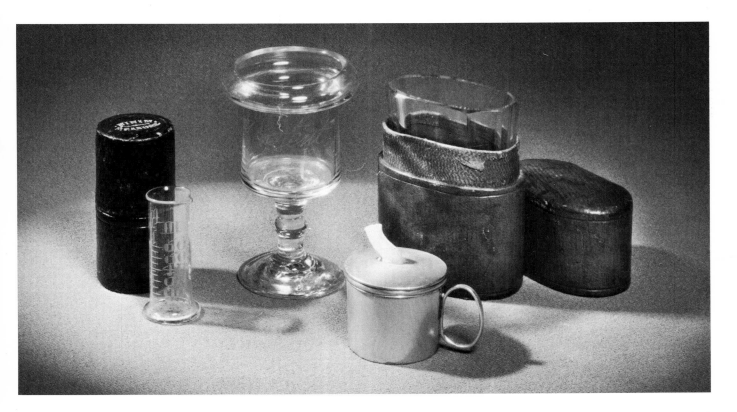

Medicine bottles

A very few small phials for single doses still survive from the seventeenth century. These are dark green, of slightly 'bubbly' glass, and are either hexagonal or bulbous in shape. By the eighteenth century, either the same dark green or a soft blue-green glass was used. The bottles were larger, bulbous or cylindrical, and had a high, pushed up kick and unpolished pontil mark. The pontil mark remained prominent until about 1850 when moulded glass began to appear, usually with the doses marked on the glass. A beautiful blue, Bristol glass bottle (*c.* 1820) is in col. pl. VII. The obligatory dark ridged glass poison bottle was introduced in 1850 from an earlier prototype by Savory and Moore, but many ways of drawing attention to poison had been tried before that. All of them were of designs that could be differentiated in the dark as well as by day. Some were made so that they could not stand up, some were boat-shaped, others had an extraordinary serpentine neck, and another type had a bell around the neck or attached to the stopper (pl. 4).

Some small nineteenth-century medicine bottles—evidently to hold the more expensive and precious preparations—fitted into turned boxwood cases with domed covers over the stoppers. Fine glass bottles with silver stoppers were often supplied to rich customers by Savory and Moore, and have probably come from a travelling medicine chest (col. pl. IX).

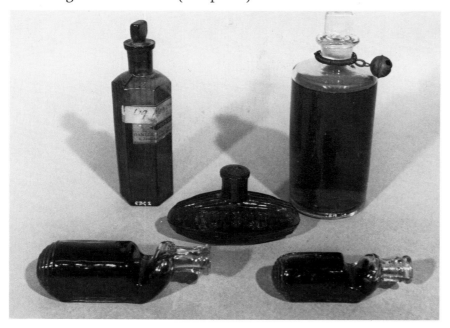

4. *A group of poison bottles showing the standard type introduced c. 1850 and the earlier alternatives.*
(Pharmaceutical Society of Great Britain Museum)

Drug jars

Sometimes described as gallipots as they were imported in galleys; they are found in every variety of decorated pottery, both labelled and otherwise. These more properly belong to the field of the apothecary and are well described in *Antiques of the Pharmacy* by Leslie G. Matthews, to which the reader should refer (pl. 5).

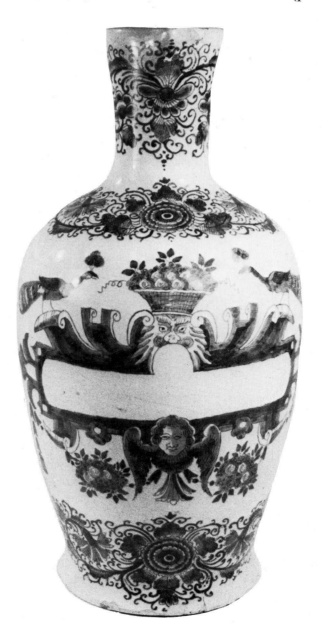

5.   *An early eighteenth-century Delft apothecaries' jar. (Stedelijk Museum, Amsterdam)*

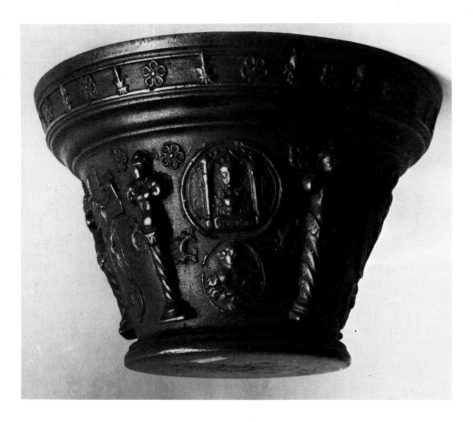

6.   *A seventeenth-century bronze apothecaries' mortar.*
(Musée Crozatier, Puy, France)

Inhalers

Various drugs have been inhaled as a form of medication since the Egyptians first used a reed over a fire to benefit from the soporific and anaesthetic qualities of their preparations. Herbs, particularly balsam, have been used in a form from which the vapour facilitated breathing, and even pure steam was inhaled by asthma patients and others. The use of inhalers in the anaesthetic field in the nineteenth century made medicinal progress. The first inhalation preparations for which official formulae were prescribed were set down in the *British Pharmacopoeia* of 1867 (the first to be published under the Medicines Act of 1858). The five preparations were: 'Inhalations of Hydrocyanic Acid, of Chlorine, of Conia [extract of Hemlock], of Creosote, and of Iodine.'

The general function of the inhaler was to facilitate entry of the agent to the nose, mouth, or both, either as a vapour or a fine spray. By the middle of the nineteenth century the anaesthetic properties of ether (Morton, 1846) and chloroform (Simpson, 1847) had stimulated the use of medicaments by inhalation. Most involved a

256

bag or bellows to induce a flow or air to vapourise the liquid used. Dr John Mudge invented a pewter inhaler which he is said to have patented in 1778. This took the form of a pint tankard into which warm water was poured, the height being controlled by air holes. A metal tube was soldered to the cover, and to this a mouthpiece could be attached. Air rushed in when suction by mouth was applied. Although this inhaler bears the incised wording 'Mudge: Patent', no patent is recorded in the Patent Office in London. These inhalers are a very rare find (pl. 7).

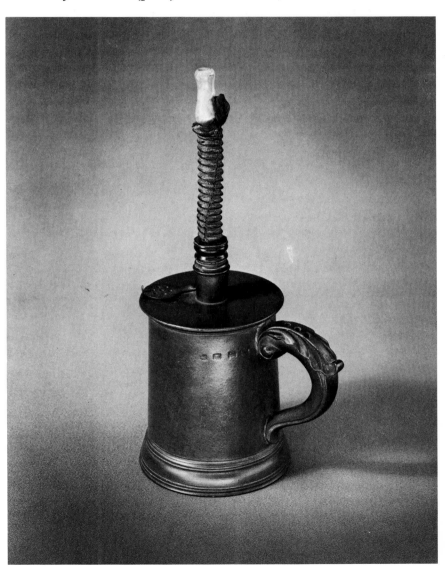

7. *Mudge's patent pewter inhaler of 1778, made by Pitt & Dudley, c. 1820. 17·8 cm. (Simon Kaye Ltd, London)*

257

Inhalers generally were made in pottery of many designs, mostly variations on 'Dr Nelson's Improved Inhaler'—a bulbous container in white or marbled glazed earthenware, about 17 cm high with an air inlet and a bulbous spout at an angle to which a mouthpiece could be attached (now invariably missing). Nelson's name and instructions for use are printed in black on the side. Other variations in the middle of the nineteenth century were introduced by S. Maw and Son, later S. Maw & Thompson, and others, by changing the shape or adding a valved mouthpiece. Some were made as high as 25·5 or 30·5 cm and had a flexible tube of silk-covered rubber attached to the top, ending in a shaped mouthpiece of pottery or glass.

Pill boxes and drug boxes

One of the rarest pill boxes known is made of silver, c. 1635, and must be one of the few for which the use is undoubted. Octagonal in shape, an inner lid is inscribed like a clock with a movable hand that can be set to indicate the time of the next dose. This covers the main compartment where the pills were kept. Such a box is unique and of all the proliferation of small silver and enamel boxes made between then and the mid-nineteenth century, it is not often possible to say with any accuracy which were intended to hold pills. Obviously many could and would have been put to a variety of uses. On the whole, pills were large, and globular in shape, covered in gelatine, varnish, or fine talc (pearl coating). They could be silvered or gilt for important patients. It is unlikely that they were often carried about on the person. For the purpose of coating the pills, spherical boxes on a circular foot were needed in which they might be rolled and tossed. They were made usually in yew, boxwood or fruitwood. A pill-silverer is in col. pl. XIV.

By the end of the eighteenth century, pharmacists began to produce their own boxes. These were either of pottery with the name transferred on the lid (this was usual with patent preparations such as ointments, toothpastes, etc.), or were circular wooden 'chip' boxes with a close fitting lid which were more usual for pills. They were hand-made from shavings of willow, and the walls, base, and lid were glued. James Goddard patented their manufacture in 1809 but when the patent expired makers rushed to provide the pharmacists with these cheap containers. Even a collection of the labels of these boxes makes an absorbing study, particularly those for patent remedies.

Medicine chests, usually of brass-bound mahogany, fitted with compartments, bottles and drawers (illustrated in col. pl. IX)

PLATE IX

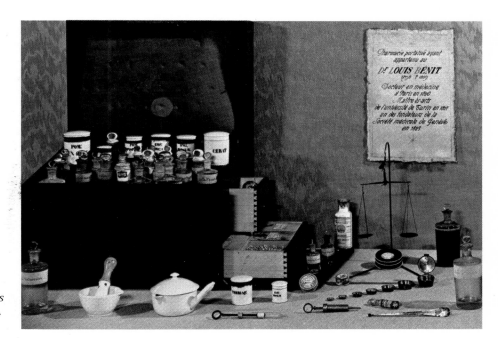

The chest and all the medicine receptacles of Dr Louis Bénit (1798–1869) of Lancy. (Musée d'Histoire des Sciences, Geneva)

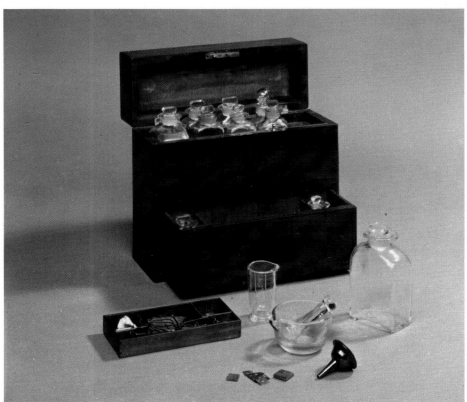

Medicine chest with mahogany case containing bottles, measures, scales, pestle and mortar and funnel, c. 1810. Height 23cm. (Simon Kaye Ltd, London)

PLATE X

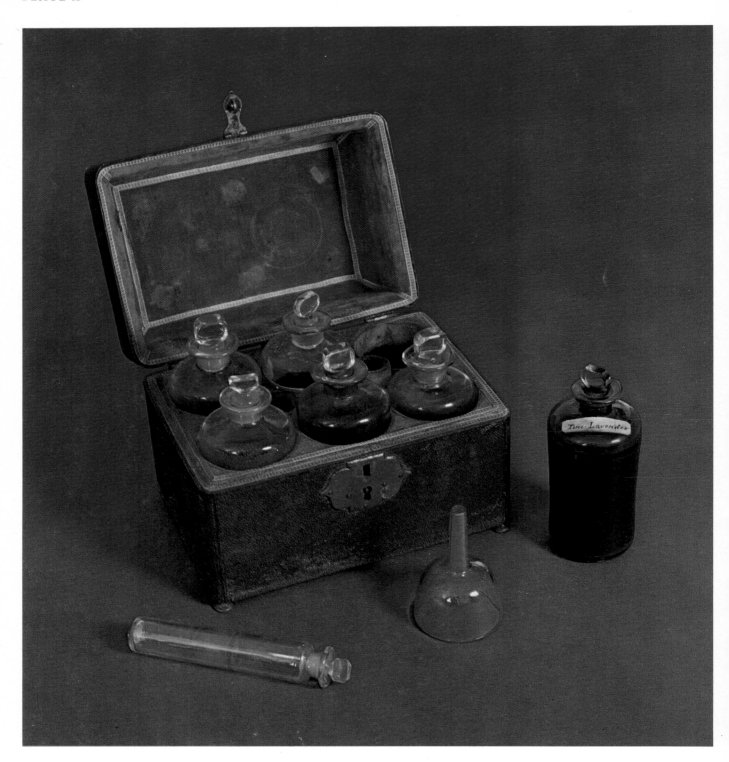

Colour plate
Fish-skin apothecaries case with velvet lining
containing six bottles, funnel and measure,
c. 1750. Height 15 cm.
(Simon Kaye Ltd, London)

were made from the eighteenth century for private households and travellers, and are hardly the province of this book. Occasionally, one finds the small drugs' box of the individual doctor; a japanned metal example was found recently. This oval box, with a most secure fastening, opens to reveal five compartments. The shape of these is repeated on the inside of the lid where the various potions are inscribed for each place.

Glass measures

Apart from the many medicine cups, spoons, and bottles with incorporated measures described previously, there was a growing tendency from the mid-eighteenth century towards more accurate measurement when mixing medicines. Apothecaries were, therefore, no longer prepared to use the time honoured brass, pewter, and wooden measures of the previous centuries, and demanded the precise measurements that only glass could give. Horn measures with a degree of translucency were practical where breakage was likely, and these were used both prior to the eighteenth century and afterwards on the battlefield. A set of such measures used at

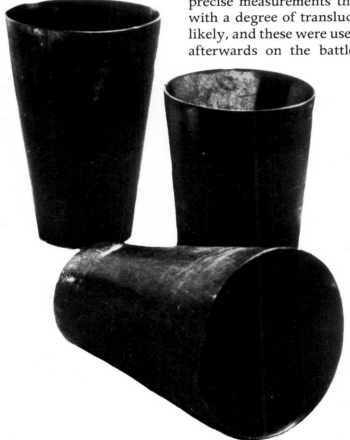

8. *Set of three horn measures, c. 1850.*
10 cm.
(Woolstaplers' Hall Museum, Chipping Camden)

259

Waterloo is in the R.A.M.C. Museum, and another at Woolstaplers' Hall, Chipping Camden (pl. 8). Savory and Moore provided them for the Crimea.

The earlier glass measures were conical, but cylindrical measures were in use by 1790. Timothy Lane patented in 1801 a graduated measure, usually referred to as a 'minim' measure, which was claimed to have a high degree of accuracy and is marked 'Lane' (pl. 3). In 1829 Beatson Clark and Co. were making plain measures with or without feet, the graduations to be specified by the client. Glass measures, either conical, bucket-shaped, or cylindrical, may be found, capable of containing quantities of up to a pint. They continued the same until the recent introduction of the metric system.

Medicine funnels

Usually part of a medicine chest, these small funnels are sometimes found on their own. They are identical to a wine funnel but are about half the size, and were made in silver and silver-gilt, in addition to glass (col. pl. IX).

CHAPTER THIRTEEN

Infant and invalid feeding utensils

Apart from the obvious circumstance of the death of the mother or her physical inability to feed her infant, fashion and other particular factors have necessitated the manufacture of babies' feeding bottles for many centuries. They were made in ancient Babylon *c.* 2000 B.C., the Greeks and Romans had them, and only the Jewish people appear to have managed without. A Roman pottery type was of breast-shaped pottery with a nipple-like mouthpiece. Arnold Haskell suggests that this could equally well have been a wine jar although one such find bears the inscription MAMO. There is a Roman example of glass in the Castle Museum, Colchester.

The earliest form, in use from the Middle Ages until the early eighteenth century, was an inverted cow's horn with an opening made in the tip. This was then wrapped in cloth to form a teat. Sixteenth and seventeenth-century part-glazed pottery feeders with a spout and handle are occasionally to be found in museums, but the nipple tip is usually missing. Elizabethan portraits show feeders of pressed leather (which were possibly from Italy) and a globular wooden feeder with tapering nipple. Teats were stitched in the shape of the finger of a glove and were filled with cotton waste, though calves' teats were frequently used. The india-rubber teat came in during the 1840s and was developed here by Maw, who also made ivory teats.

By the eighteenth century, feeders were usually of three types—pear-shaped, round with flattened sides (mostly of continental origin), or like a sugar-castor with a pewter or silver top. In 1777 Dr Hugh Smith introduced his pottery 'Bubby-pot' which he invented for use in his own family. He published a description in *Letters to Married Women on Nursing and the Management of Children* in 1772. 'The pot is somewhat in form like an urn; its handle and neck or spout are not unlike those of a coffee pot except that the neck of this arises from the very bottom of the pot and is very small . . . The end of the spout is a little raised and forms a roundish knob . . . This is perforated by three or four small holes . . .' Bubby-pots were made in creamware for the poor, or with transfer decoration for the more affluent. A variation on this idea was the tin can of Pennsylvania called a 'mammale', in use at the end of the eighteenth and the first half of the nineteenth centuries.

At about the same time, the flat boat-shaped feeding bottle made its first appearance. The bottles were filled from a central hole in the upper side, which was covered by the thumb in feeding to control the flow; some of the later ones had a screw plug of boxwood, seldom of cork, which could be adjusted for the same purpose. The spouts, to which teats would have been attached, were usually short and straight, but some are long and curve gracefully upwards. This type of bottle was made by most of the Staffordshire potteries, undecorated at first, though occasionally ribbed—Spode decorating them with Chinoiserie and pastoral scenes from about 1810. They

1. A group of pottery feeding bottles, two with blue and white decoration, c. 1820. 15 cm.
(Strangers' Hall Museum, Norwich)

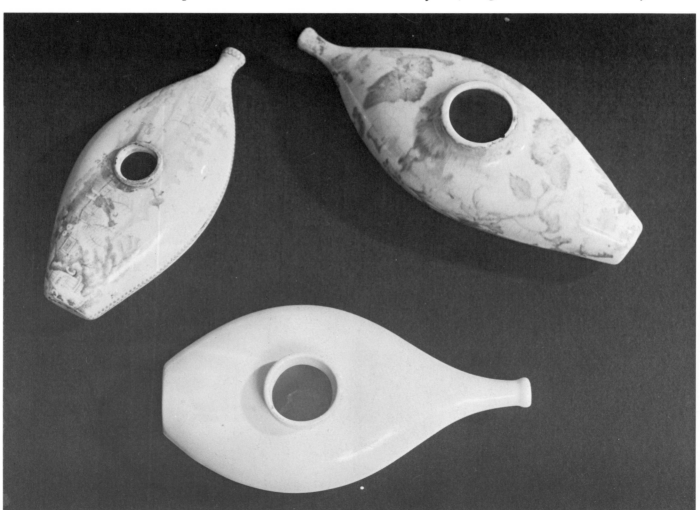

were also made in pewter and there are several silver examples in American museums dating from about 1840. Arnold Haskell considers many to be Indian Colonial; an unmarked example is in pl. 2. A brown stoneware feeding bottle appeared *c*. 1840 which took the form of a bust of Queen Victoria; a patriotic concept of the monarch nurturing the nation, quite unsuitable for a queen who described breast-feeding, with distaste, as 'making a cow of oneself'.

Glass feeders of similar design to those in porcelain were introduced in the first quarter of the nineteenth century and largely replaced porcelain (pl. 2); this material resulted in the blowing of other forms, notably conical and gourd-shapes. Some were fluted

2.   *Glass feeding bottle, c. 1840 and a silver feeding bottle, c. 1810. 15 cm. (Simon Kaye Ltd, London)*

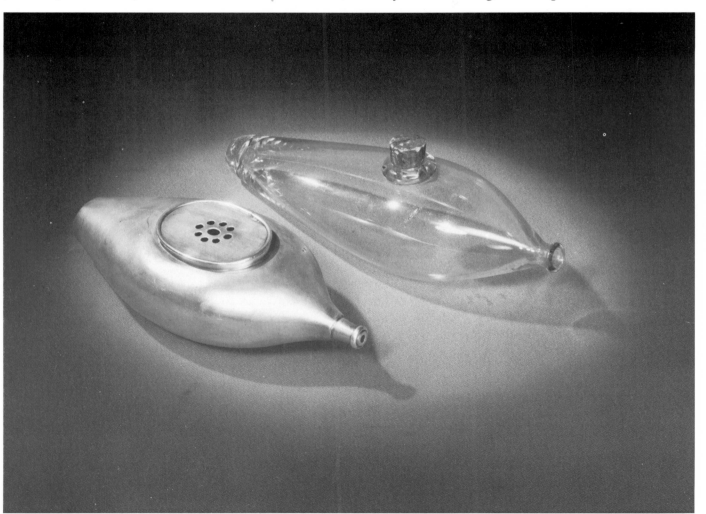

and some had the design obtained by pouring molten glass on to wire netting. A French bottle, the biberon, was on show at The Great Exhibition of 1851, a mass of tubes and ivory pins to regulate the flow. The *Lancet* reported it had 'never seen anything so beautiful'. Another ingenious invention included an artificial breast to be worn, filled with milk, 'by the female in the position of the breast, keeping the food warm all night and day'. Matthew Tomlinson, in 1863, advertised a coloured glass pear-shaped bottle called 'The Cottage'. Priced at 1s, he thought it 'so well adapted to the working man's household'.

In 1864 came the 'Siphonia' bottle, afterwards banned in many American States, and often referred to as a 'Murder bottle'. It was an upright glass bottle from which came a long india-rubber tube leading to the teat—'a bacterial paradise' has been a latter-day comment (pl. 3).

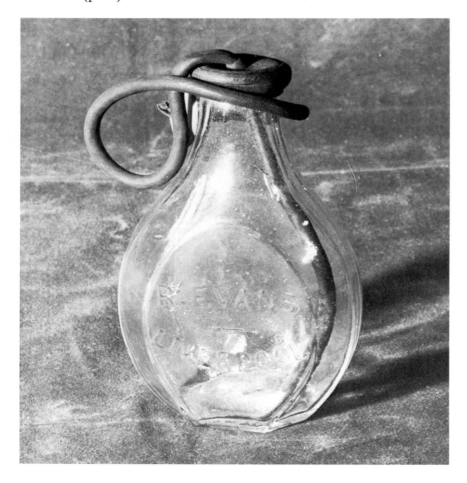

3.   *Siphonia feeding bottle, Evans, Liverpool, c. 1865. 12·7 cm.*
(Castle Museum, York)

The feeding bottle was sometimes considered better than a wet-nurse as there was thought to be no danger of the child inheriting the nurse's characteristics. However, in the nineteenth century it was still fatal to 7 out of 8 babies for whom it was used and it was considered a great achievement to have reared a child 'by hand' as Pip found in Dickens's *Great Expectations*.

Spout cups and feeding cups

The early spout cups are usually of straight-sided tankard shape with lidded or semi-lidded top, and a side spout of curving shape. The larger ones were certainly not for invalids but were probably loving cups or posset cups (gravy and coffee have even been suggested). The earliest of the small invalid variety is recorded in 1689, and the Wellcome Collection has one of 1698. They are usually silver but occasionally glass. A London Delftware example of the large type of *c.* 1680 is in the Manchester City Art Gallery (pl. 4). An interesting travelling feeding cup of silver, made about 1745,

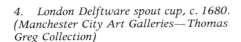

4. *London Delftware spout cup, c. 1680. (Manchester City Art Galleries—Thomas Greg Collection)*

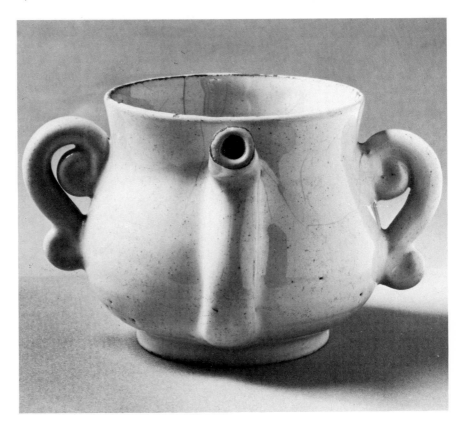

has a detachable handle and spout of beautifully carved horn; the ivory finial to the spout is detachable in itself (pl. 5). Spout cups of later design were made up to the end of the eighteenth century. A very familiar type, semi-spherical and with a half cover, has the handle and spout at right angles for easy use by a right-handed person (one has yet to be found for a left-handed person). This type is 7·5 to 10 cm high and was made, in the eighteenth and nineteenth centuries, in silver, pewter, and glass. Liverpool produced tin-glazed Chinoiserie versions in the latter half of the eighteenth century, and Lowestoft, about 1770, made them in blue floral porcelain; those in cream-ware came from Leeds. By the nineteenth century there was even more variety in the decoration; some decoration was inside the cup. Even Copeland Garret was making them. By the latter half of the nineteenth century, mass produced versions with transfer decoration were in many households. There were, in addition, pewter and silver cups like bachelor teapots, but without lids; these were later copied in glass, with long curving spouts (pl. 7).

5.   Silver travelling invalid's cup, detachable spout and handle of horn, c. 1745, 7·5 cm; inverted cone-type feeding cup, plaited twine cover, silver rim, glass body, 1829, John Driver; pewter spout cup, c. 1790. (Simon Kaye Ltd, London)

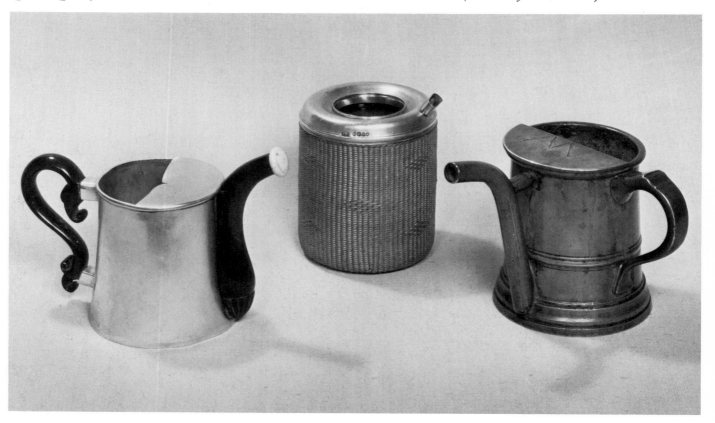

Another type, made in the early years of the nineteenth century and much more rarely found, was a cylinder of glass, usually silver-mounted, with an inverted glass cone cover. This allowed air to pass into the cup while the beverage was sucked from a side hole to which a tube was attached, making it impossible to spill the liquid. That in pl. 5 has the outer glass encased in finely woven twine and is dated 1829, maker's mark possibly of John Douglas. The suggestion that this vessel was intended for mixing drinks—an early cocktail shaker—is refuted by the present writer.

6. *Small-size Lowestoft black and white spout cup, c. 1780. 5 cm.*
(Castle Museum, Norwich)

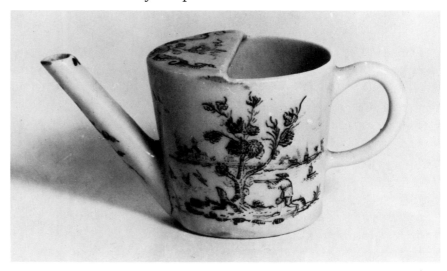

7. *Victorian glass spout cup, c. 1860,*
6·5 cm; Old Sheffield Plate spout cup,
c. 1765, Tudor and Leader.
(Simon Kaye Ltd, London)

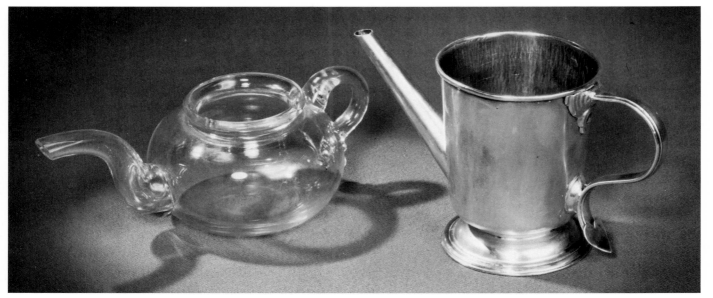

Sick syphon or cobbler tube

This is a scroll-shaped silver tube with a hook on one side to attach it to the cup of liquid in which it was inserted. The lower end is closed by a hinged and pierced cover to strain the food. Michael Clayton has found them to be usually of American origin, though this is not the experience of the author. A pottery version appeared in the Wedgwood pattern book of 1803 and the silver examples in pl. 8 are all of the first quarter of the century.

8. *A group of silver sick syphons, 1800–1830; early creamware baby-feeder c. 1780. Height 10 cm.*
(Simon Kaye Ltd, London)

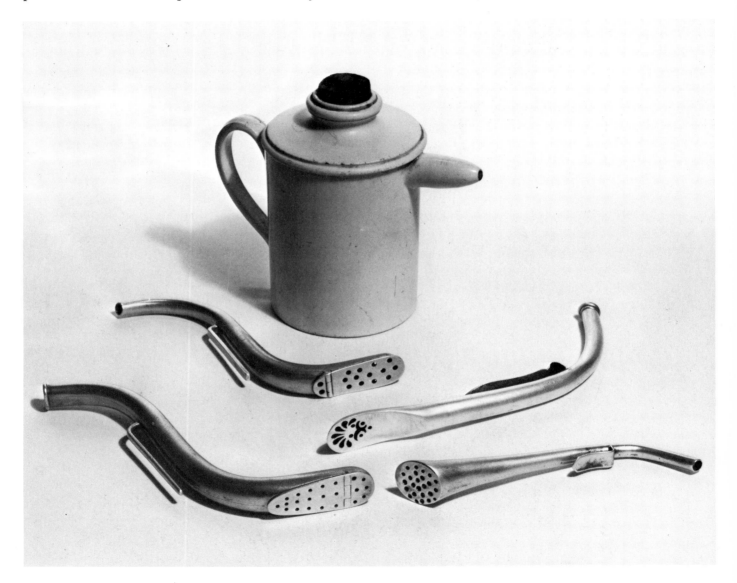

Pap boats

Pap boats probably date from about 1710, though Eric Delieb puts it a quarter of a century earlier; they were in use until the end of the nineteenth century. Open or half-covered boat-shaped vessels with a lip at one end, they were used to administer 'pap' to an infant or invalid. The preparation of the pap itself was from a piece of bread soaked in wine with meal and sugar added and was occasionally chewed smooth by the nurse, though obviously the boats were suitable for any semi-liquid food. Early pap boats were plain, later becoming highly decorated. They are known in porcelain, creamware, and glazed earthenware and have a great variety of decoration to delight the child; sometimes with a gilt rim and a coloured floral design in the bowl. Wedgwood made creamware boats with a scalloped edge. They were rarely made in glass but frequently in silver (col. pl. XI), Old Sheffield Plate and pewter; even gold ones are known. From plain rims they progressed to a reed edge and later to gadrooning; the most elaborate of the early

9.   From left: creamware half-covered pap boat, c. 1770, 14 cm; Lowestoft spout cup, c. 1775; pewter pap boat, c. 1810; glass posset cup, c. 1750 (the whey was poured off through the spout and the curds were eaten from the top with a spoon); blue and white earthenware pap boat, c. 1810. (Strangers' Hall Museum, Norwich)

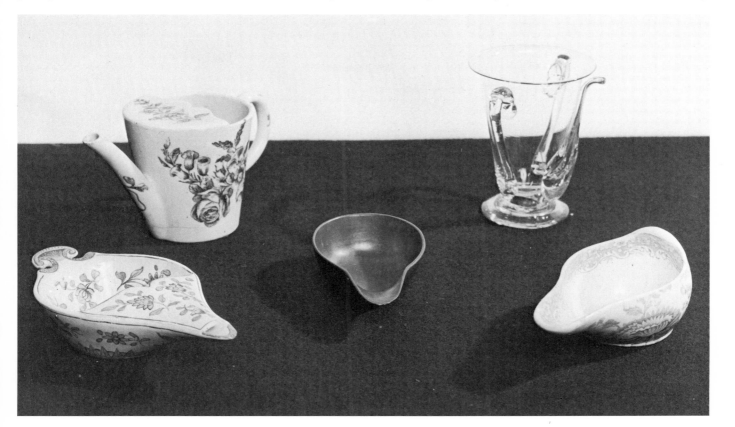

nineteenth century pap boats having gadroon and shell borders with acanthus leaf decoration, the bowls often gilded for cleanliness. One occasionally finds pewter examples made *c.* 1800 and stamped *FH*. These were apparently originally made to raise money for a Foundling Hospital. A very rare coquilla-nut pap boat is shown in col. pl. XII.

An interesting specimen in the Wellcome Museum and another in the possession of the Pharmaceutical Society have a spout at one end from which it is deduced that a mixture of liquids and solids was used in the feeding. It is occasionally asserted that the high infant mortality rate of this period is in some way attributable to the use of these uncovered pap boats which were no doubt left lying about waiting on the appetite of the child.

10. Dutch silver pap boat, c. 1800. (Stedelijk Museum, Amsterdam)

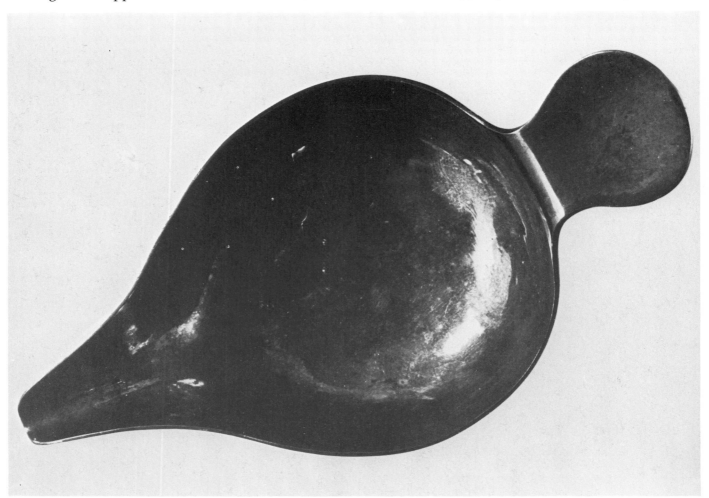

270

Nipple shields

Scultetus describes a nipple shield as follows, '. . . a silver cap and full of holes which is applied . . . to the breasts that nurses may suckle the infants without trouble' which, when children were breast-fed until long after their front teeth were cut, must have been very necessary. The more sophisticated type had a row of holes round the base for ventilation.

Nipple shields were known since the earliest days and were made in lead (obviously with dire results), pewter, horn, bone, ivory, wood, silver and glass, the latter sometimes of the most convoluted shapes. Unrecognised, they are often put to diverse uses and spoilt. The most frequently found examples are in silver from the turn of the eighteenth century, Phipps and Robinson having made many (pl. 11).

11. A group of nipple shields: silver, 1809, Phipps and Robinson; silver, 1801, Phipps and Robinson; glass, folded rim, c. 1840; rare treen version, c. 1800. Diameter 3·8 cm. (Simon Kaye Ltd, London)

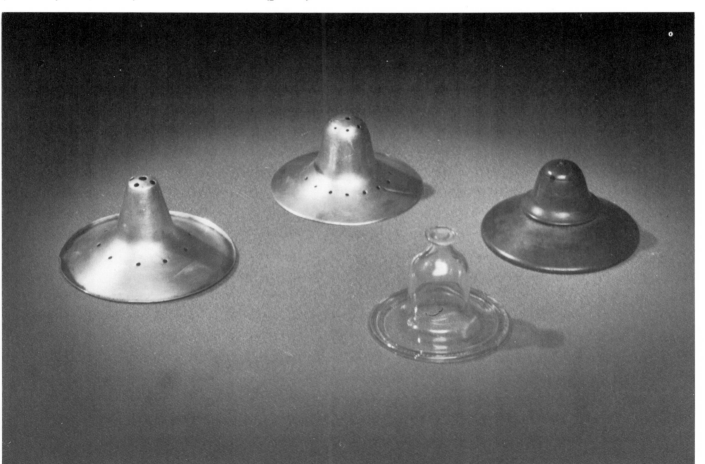

Food warmers

In the first half of the nineteenth century an apparatus for keeping food warm in the sick room appeared. It was a covered pottery vessel fitting into a second two-handled container of cylindrical shape. This had an aperture at the base to allow a short candle or taper to burn, thus heating the upper container (pl. 12).

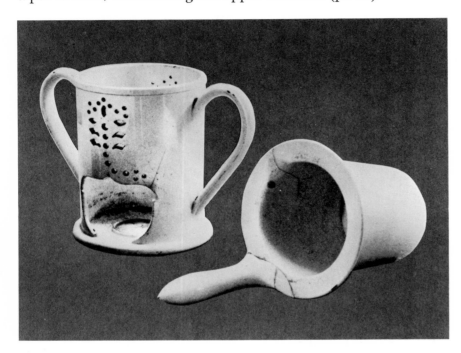

12. Creamware invalid food warmer, showing heating chamber and container, c. 1850. 25·5 cm.
(Woolstaplers' Hall Museum, Chipping Camden)

CHAPTER FOURTEEN

Articles of medical association

This covers a wide variety of most interesting pieces which though not specifically instruments, are so closely allied to the medical profession that they deserve a place in this book.

Instrument cases

Made specially to hold surgical instruments, these cases are still occasionally found, either with or without their former contents. Undoubtedly, prime among them, is the magnificent example belonging jointly to the Worshipful Company of Barbers and the Worshipful Company of Goldsmiths (pls. 1 and 2). It is unmarked but the official text ascribes it to about 1512—the late Commander G. E. P. How, however, allowed it to be a few years earlier. Apart from its interest as an instrument case, this piece must be one of the finest and earliest works of the silversmith's art to survive. Measuring 18·4 cm long and, at the top, 5·7 by 5 cm, it is made of parcel gilt with some coloured enamels. Each side and the top and bottom are heavily ornamented with arms, figures of saints, and engravings depicting scenes both religious and mythological. The cover fits closely over the wood and leather interior and is preserved from loss by a chain which passes from lion mask rings on the sides of the body through further rings on the sides of the cover. Inside is a slotted grille to take the instruments, none of which, unhappily, has survived. This must have been one of the most elaborate pieces of medical history of the profession, deserving pride of place in this book, but obviously it is doubtful if it was intended as anything more than a ceremonial presentation piece from King Henry VIII to the Barber–Surgeons.

A Hindu writer of *c*. 600 B.C. suggested a list of no less than 121 instruments suitable to accompany the King to the battlefield: for army surgeons in the time of the later Tudors, huge medicine chests to take both the instruments and medicines were made and a horse-drawn cart with a man to drive it were provided. An illustration of 1588 shows a wooden case, leather bound and studded, with three dozen bottles and drawers for instruments. George Solly, apothecary to Charles II, was appointed to make these

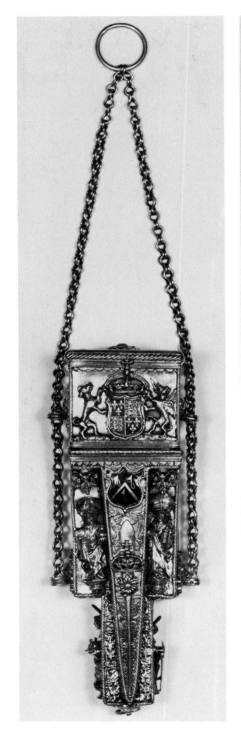
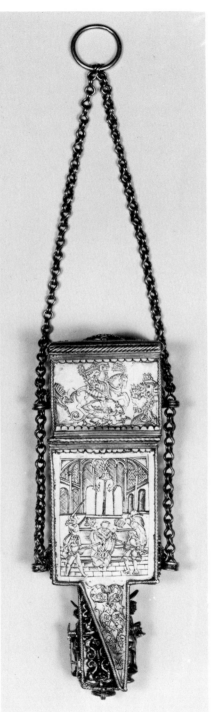

1.   Henry VIII instrument case, c. 1512, parcel-gilt and enamel. This side showing Royal Arms, the Arms of the Surgeons' Company and a spatula with crowned rose; flanking figures are SS Cosmas and Damien, the Patron Saints of the Barber–Surgeons. 18·4 cm.
(Worshipful Company of Barbers)

2.   Reverse side showing, curiously, the martyrdom of St Thomas à Becket and St George and the dragon.
(Worshipful Company of Barbers)

PLATE XI

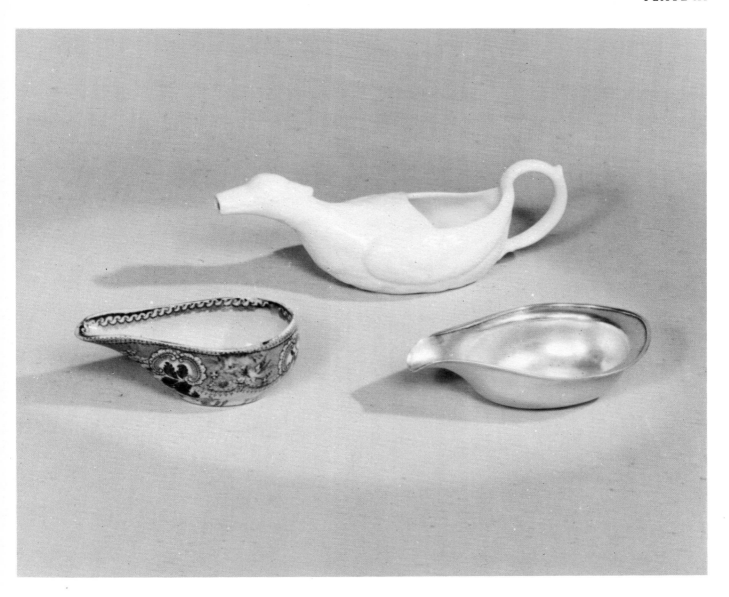

Porcelain pap boat (transitional spout cup)
c. 1860; Staffordshire pap boat, c. 1820;
silver pap boat, 1805, S. Hennell. Length of
left boat 14cm.
(Simon Kaye Ltd, London)

PLATE XII

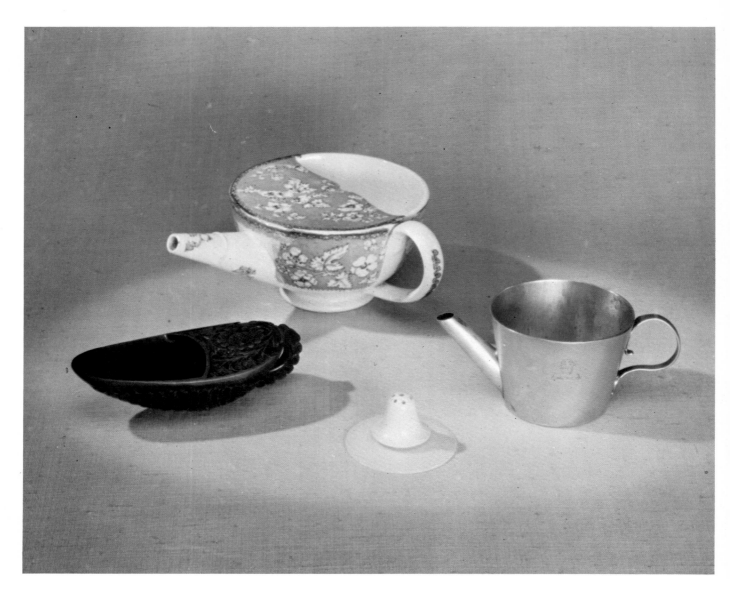

Rare Austrian coquilla-nut pap boat, c. 1800;
Staffordshire spout, cup, c. 1830; silver spout
cup, 1763, William Vere and J. Lutwych;
ivory nipple shield, c. 1810. Length of left
boat 10cm.
(Simon Kaye Ltd, London)

PLATE XIII

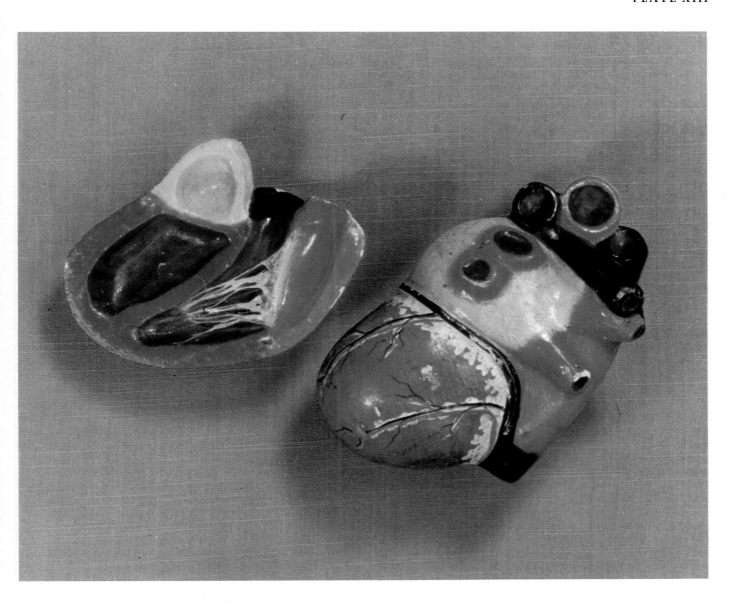

*Wood and plaster model of the heart, opening
to reveal interior. Diameter 10cm.
(Simon Kaye Ltd, London)*

PLATE XIV

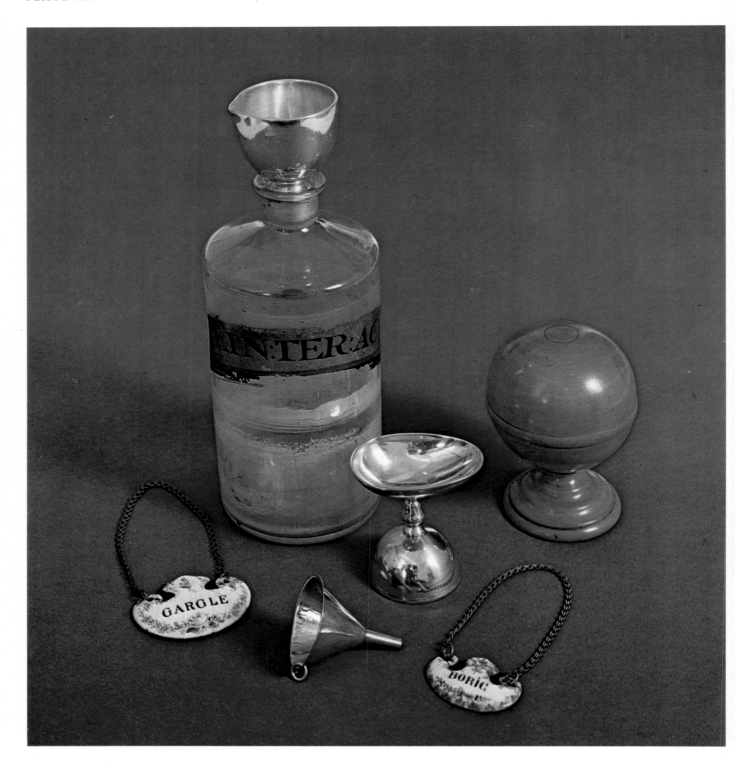

3. Carved wooden instrument case, dated
1528 and bearing the arms of Paumgärtner-
Dichtel, a medical family. This was made in
a Nuremberg monastery, post-Reformation.
20·3 cm.
(Germanisches Nationalmuseum, Nuremberg)

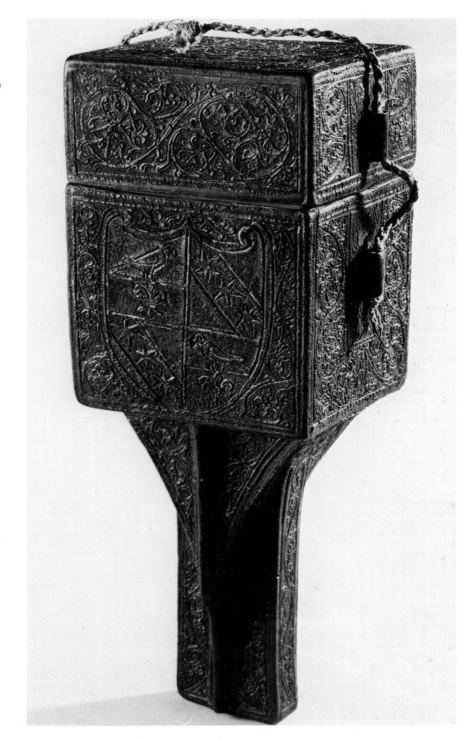

Colour plate
Medicine bottle with silver stopper/medicine
cup, 1839, Sebastian Crespell, London;
Boxwood pill-silverer, c. 1780; two Bilston
enamel labels, c. 1850; silver medicine
funnel, 1704, A. Hudson, London; double-
dose silver medicine cup, c. 1800. Unmarked.
Height of pill-silverer 10 cm.
(Simon Kaye Ltd, London)

cases for both naval and land warfare. He caused endless controversy as the Barber-Surgeons' Company claimed the surgeons' right to have them fitted where they wished. The seventeenth-century Prujean Collection, now in the Museum of London, includes a case with two trays of intricately-shaped compartments lined with marbled paper (pls. 4 and 5). Pocket cases opening flat in two halves were made in wood at the same period.

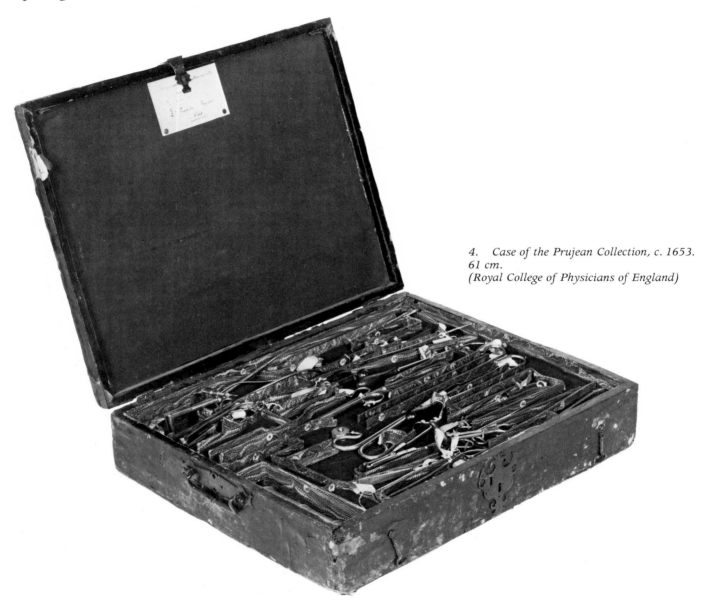

4.   *Case of the Prujean Collection, c. 1653. 61 cm. (Royal College of Physicians of England)*

There is a brass instrument case in the Victoria and Albert Museum, though shagreen seems to have been the most favoured material for these small cases throughout the seventeenth and eighteenth centuries, the boxes being about 12 to 15 cm long with rounded ends. Another particularly interesting example, apparently from 1672, is that shown with the instruments in pl. 13 (p. 62). This has a drawer in the base, presumably to hold the sharper instruments more safely. A similar one is in the possession of the Wellcome Collection. In col. pl. II are two others, of later date— without drawers but silver-mounted. From the mid-eighteenth

5. *Interior of the Prujean Collection case, showing divisions, c. 1653.*
(Royal College of Physicians of England)

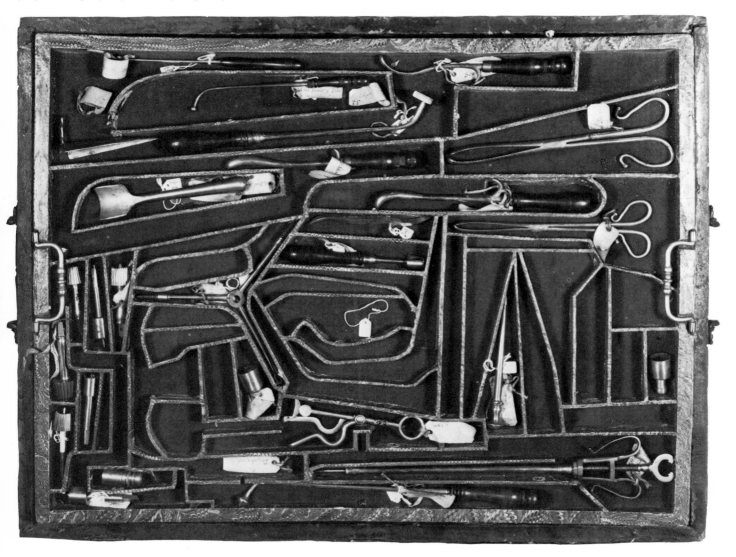

century and for most of the nineteenth century, instrument cases of leather, sharkskin, and brass-bound mahogany were standard, fitted inside with velvet-covered slots, larger ones having several trays and side-carrying handles. The sharkskin case for the dental instruments in col. pl. V and the beautifully made box for the trephine set in col. pl. I are typical.

Silver cases of the etui-type for lancets and, occasionally, other instruments, date from the early eighteenth century. They are of tapering design with the lid at the thicker end, often with intricate hinges and spring clasp; the interiors fitted with a slotted silver grille to hold the lancets. The one in pl. 6 is typical of the earlier, more robust design, while by 1780–90 they had become more delicate and attracted, very often, the prettiest and most intricate bright-cut designs (pls. 41 (p. 44) and 6). The suggestion that the small deep bruises often found on these cases were made by the patients having been given them to bite on during operations, can only be speculative! There is a beautifully made silver-mounted walking-stick in the possession of the Royal College of Surgeons of England, the handle of which opens to reveal a surgeon's etui still containing the original instruments (pl. 7). There, too, is a cylindrical silver case with flush cover of 1819. Cylindrical cases were popular for probes and forceps from the mid-eighteenth century.

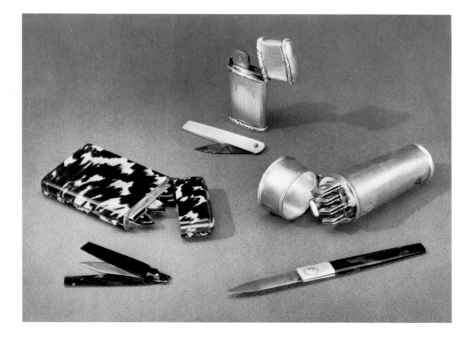

6. Tortoise-shell lancet case with 6 lancets, c. 1790 (identical to Sir John Hunter's own at Royal College of Surgeons), 6·5 cm; silver lancet case, 1819, Joseph Taylor; two lancets with mother-of-pearl guards; silver lancet case with 6 lancets, c. 1760. (Simon Kaye Ltd, London)

By the late eighteenth century less affluent doctors found it more convenient to carry small numbers of instruments, such as they would only need for routine visits and small operations, in folding leather pouches with fitted slots of the pencil case type. Many of these are found with the original instruments still in them at the Royal College of Surgeons. At the R.A.M.C. Museum, Aldershot, is a rare Sikh fighting knife, picked up during the Indian Mutiny, containing the following instruments concealed in the handle— finger saw, lancet, 2 forceps, probes, scoops, 2 knives, caustic holder, and spatula; it was the property of Surgeon-Major D. P. Berry.

7. *Buckston Browne's walking stick, showing instrument case in handle, c. 1872. (Royal College of Surgeons of England)*

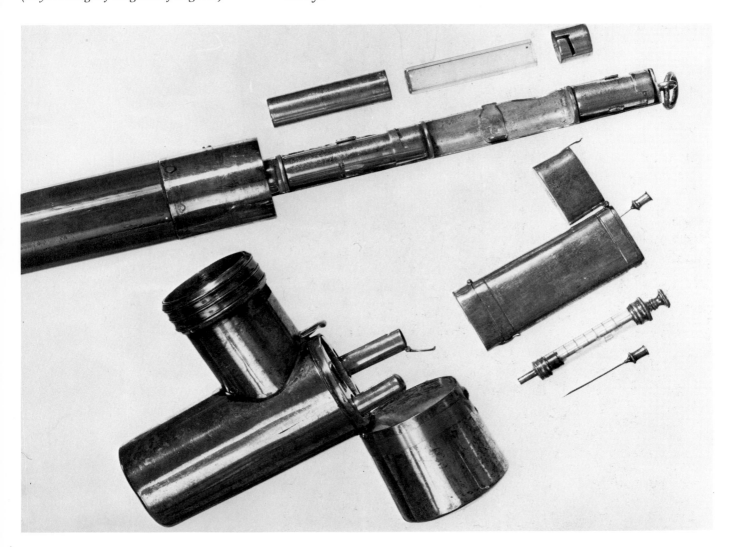

Stone and caul cases

To have survived an early operation for stone was obviously a drama that coloured one's whole life, and an occasion for special celebration. Samuel Pepys marked with thanksgiving and a good dinner each anniversary of his operation by Thomas Hollyer in 1658. In common with many people who had undergone a similar experience he retained the stone as a relic and later (in 1664) had a case made for it. 'Thence to my case maker for my stone case, and had it to my mind and cost me 24s which is very well done and pleases me.' He does not tell us, but it seems likely, that the case was of silver and probably inscribed.

A surgeon, writing about 1580, tells us 'In phlegmatic persons, stones are usually white, smooth, and grow rapidly (phosphates). In the melancholic they are black, rough, hard, and grow slowly (oxalates). In the choleric they are reddish and of rapid growth but sometimes soft (urates).' With such multi-coloured stones being removed, Pepys was not alone in marking his triumph of survival, and a case such as his must be a singular reward for the collector. One such box, half glass, half gold, and in its original shagreen case, is at St John's College, Oxford. It still contains the stone and has the inscription: 'This stone was taken from ye body of Doctor John King, Lord Bishop of London. Descended from ye Antient Kings of Devonshire who dyed ANNO 1621' (pls. 8 and 9).

Similarly rare are cases made to hold cauls, the membrane occasionally still covering the face of a baby at birth. Superstitions regarding the caul are very ancient and they were usually preserved, sometimes, we are told, for sale to sailors to prevent them from drowning. A heart-shaped silver case made in Exeter in 1830 is in the possession of the Birmingham Assay Office (pls. 10 and 11).

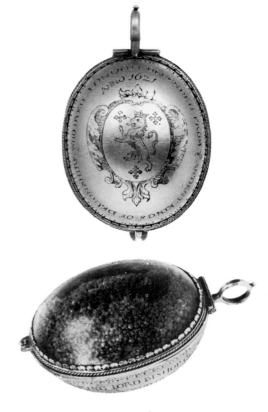

8 and 9.   *Gold and glass stone case, still containing stone. The inscription reads 'This stone was taken from ye body of Doctor John King, Lord Bishop of London. Descended from ye Antient Kings of Devonshire, who dyed ANNO 1621'.*
(St John's College, Oxford)

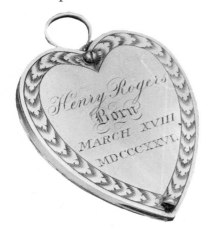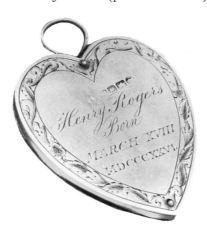

10 and 11.   *Silver caul case, Exeter, 1830, (prob.) Joseph Hicks.*
(Birmingham Assay Office)

Leech jars

Large pottery jars for storing leeches (some hundreds might be kept by a hospital) more properly belong to the province of the apothecary than the doctor. They may be found in glass and creamware of about 1780, made by Leeds Pottery, and in stoneware, often lavishly coloured in blues and puce with gilt embellishment, from the end of the eighteenth century. These can be very handsome as the collection of the Pharmaceutical Society shows (pl.

12. Eighteenth-century stoneware leech jar, puce and gilt decoration. 30·5 cm. (Pharmaceutical Society of Great Britain Museum)

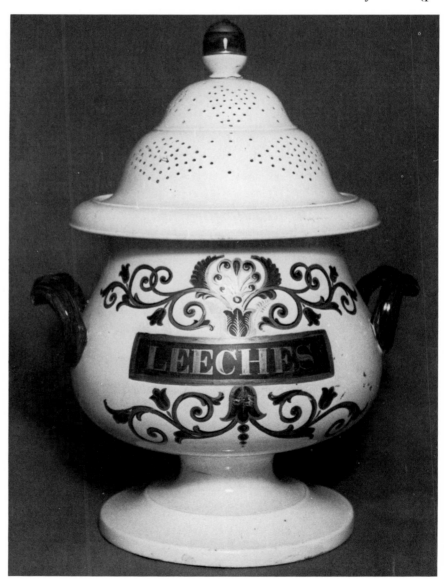

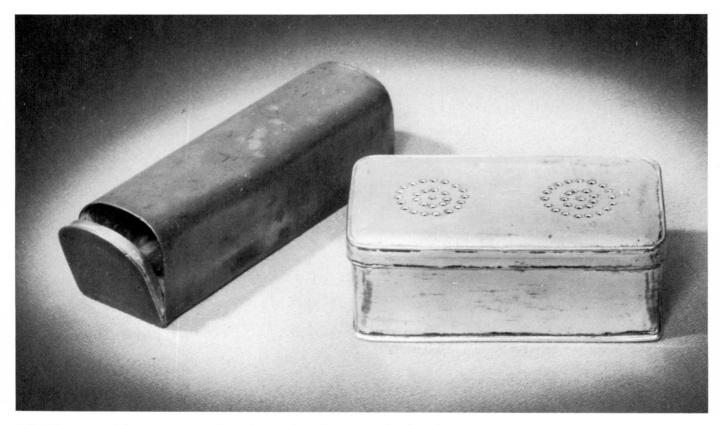

12). They are either urn-shaped with two handles, or cylindrical, about 25·5-30 cm high, all with perforated covers. J. & S. Maw listed a set of three Staffordshire glazed earthenware jars for leeches, honey, and tamarind (a fruit laxative) in 1839, and an innovation was a mid-nineteenth-century glass jar with perforated shelves so that the leeches could clean themselves by passing through the perforations. A stoneware 'Patent Leech Jar' is in the Wellcome Collection and has a band of holes two-thirds of the way up the cylindrical sides and a strong brass clip on the lid to prevent escape. Individual physicians and surgeons would have had smaller jars similar to the cupping glasses of about 1820 in pl. 41 (p. 44) or, for carrying to and from a patient, one of the rare travelling leech boxes such as those in pl. 13. The pewter version measures 12 cm in length and has a hinged and perforated lid to admit air—it could have held at least a dozen or so leeches. Considering the proliferation of complaints for which leeching was part of a cure, it is curious that more of these boxes have not survived. Leech tubes are mentioned in Chapter 4.

13. Pewter leech box, c. 1840; Old Sheffield Plate leech box, c. 1810. 10 cm, 5 cm by 8·9 cm.
(Simon Kaye Ltd, London)

14. Pair of Staffordshire vases, c. 1835, apparently used for leeches.
(Division of Medical Sciences, National Museum of History and Technology, Smithsonian Institution, Washington D.C.)

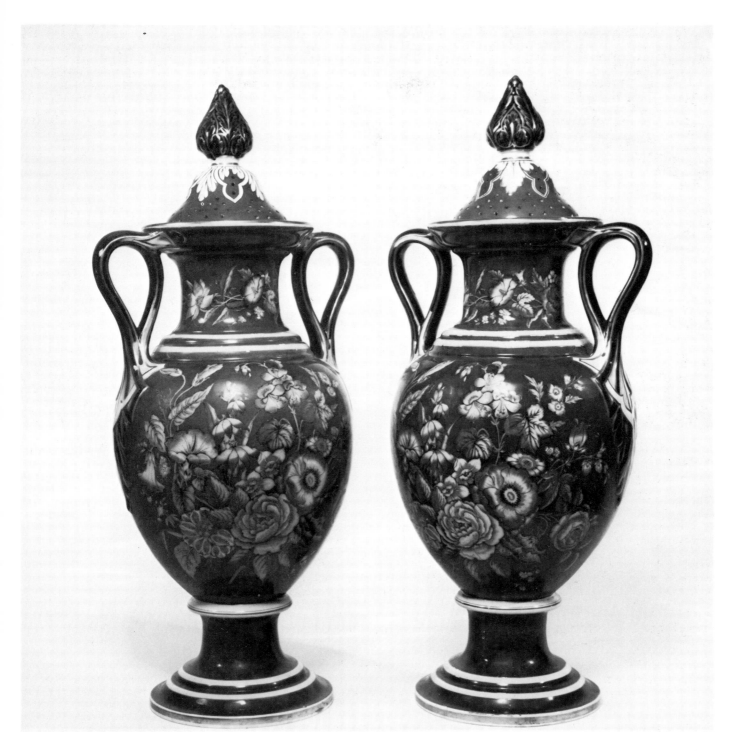

Taper boxes

Another helpful piece of equipment for the doctor, before the days of the electric torch, was some travelling source of light. Candles must, except in an exceptional case, have been readily available, but it seems obvious that, even in daylight, a small and concentrated light would have been needed for use with specula and for examining the mouth and throat. Very small wax taper boxes have occasionally been found, such as the silver one by Edward Medlycott of about 1750 in pl. 3; p. 253. This measures just under 3·8 cm in diameter and is quite large enough to hold a coiled taper that would burn for the relatively short period necessary. From 1807 reflected candlelight was used with a urethroscope and in 1853 a cystoscope was invented which used gaslight. Throughout the nineteenth century great strides were made in ingenious devices for use with a speculum but these are beyond the scope of this book.

Medicinal bottle labels

Some of the rarest finds for the collector are medicinal bottle labels to hang by a chain across the shoulders of a bottle, similar to wine labels though usually nearer the size of a sauce label. Eric Delieb found two silver ones of 1808 by Samuel Hennell for Arquebuzade (a lotion used on gunshot wounds) and Eau de Miel (evidently some similar preparation of a soothing nature) and he feels they were probably carried by an officer in the field. Two Bilston enamel labels from about 1850 for Gargle and Boric are illustrated in col. pl. XIV, and must have cheered any sickroom delightfully. Among the names on the bottle labels listed by N. M. Penzer the more medicinal include: 'Acid, Camphor drops, Camphor Julep, Eau Astringente, Eau Borique, Elixir Dentifrice, Huille des Anis, Mouth Wash, Poison, Poison Laudanum, and Tooth Mixture.'

Scales

Many physicians carried their own set of scales with them. These had many uses, from the pharmaceutical to the practice of weighing their fee before leaving the patient's side; very necessary when fraud abounded. John Bell (now John Bell & Croyden) who started business in 1798 says he was defrauded of half a guinea by a false coin on the first day of trade. There is a very early set of coin scales of about 1630 in the possession of the Pharmaceutical Society. There are ten weights, eight of which are stamped either with the head of James I, a thistle, or St Michael killing a serpent. Troy weight was not used, but the Roman system of the scruple, the drachm, and the grain. The larger scales were either of the equal arm or pillar variety, though doctors would also have carried small folding coin scales of the type in pl. 15, fitting into a case and either held in the hand for weighing, or hung from a metal stand. Scale making only became a specialist activity in the eighteenth century when T. Beach & Son (later becoming W. & T. Avery Ltd) and Young and Son (now Young, Son & Marlow Ltd) were established. Before that time it was the province of the silversmith, pewterer, clockmaker, or blacksmith. So many medicinal recipes of the eighteenth and nineteenth century called for accurate weighing that scales of this type are those most often found, the scale pans being silver, pewter, brass, copper, or glass, and either round or scoop-shaped. Some fit into cases as small as 11·4 by 6·4 cm. One sometimes finds scoops for

15. A set of silver scales, 1808, Thomas Meriton; a japanned metal case of scales, Old Sheffield plate pans, c. 1780. Diameter of scales 5 cm.
(Simon Kaye Ltd, London)

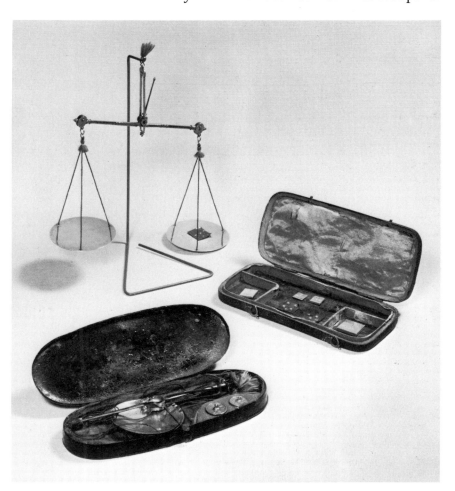

the various medicinal ingredients which could vary from powdered coral to peacock's dung; these were shaped like larger, flatter caddy-spoons. Tortoise-shell was favoured in the nineteenth century, while a silver scoop by Samuel Hennell which appeared on the market recently, seems without parallel.

16.   Late nineteenth-century suture case of Auguste Ruerdin; baby scales of Dr Robert Odier, c. 1870.
(Musée d'Histoire des Sciences, Geneva)

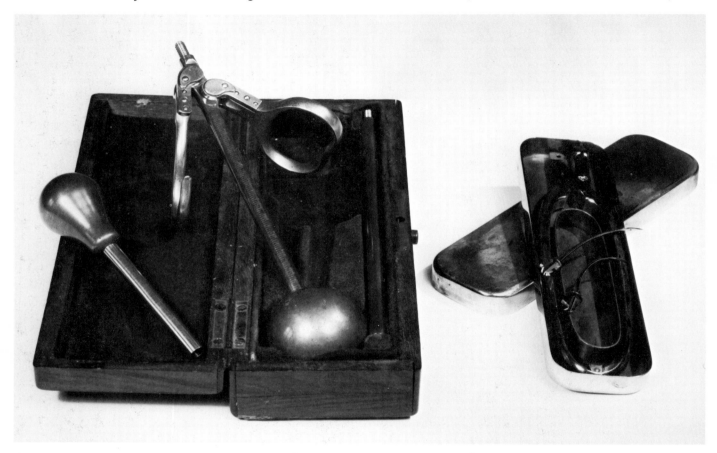

Demonstration models

A much rarer find is a demonstration model of part of the human body used in lecturing to students. The Italians seem to have been most adept at producing these and the Wellcome Museum has male figures of about 45·8 cm high made in wax showing the most precise anatomical details (pl. 17). Again from Italy is a stuffed leather and canvas semi-torso of a woman with foetus *in utero* and fully dilated cervix on which the various obstetrical forceps and hooks were

17. *Eighteenth-century Italian wax anatomical model of a man showing bones and muscles.*
(Wellcome Collection)

18. *Eighteenth-century ivory anatomical model of a pregnant woman.*
(Wellcome Collection)

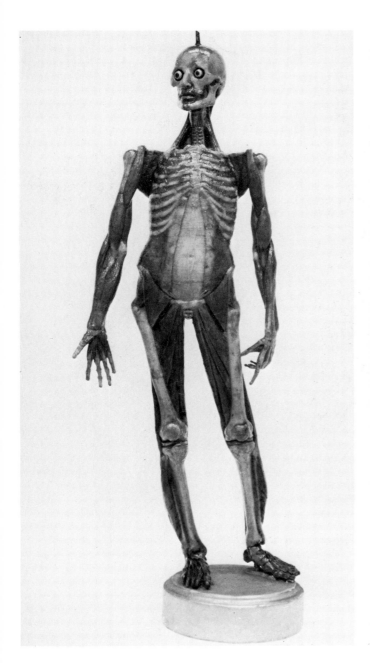

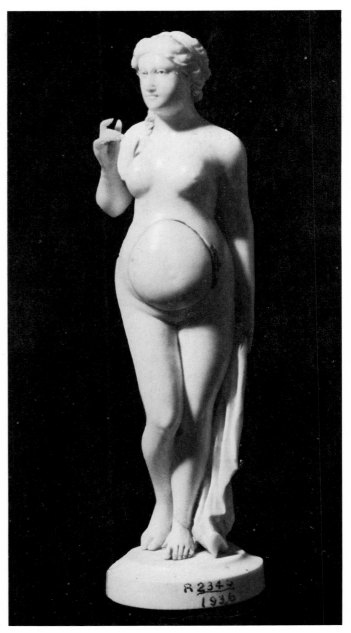

demonstrated and practised (see Chapter 6). However, English models of many types were made. One example is the life-sized wooden heart shown in col. pl. XII. It opens on pins to reveal the auricles and ventricles and all indications are that it is from about 1850.

The pseudo-science of phrenology, very popular from its introduction by J. F. Gall (1758–1828) until early this century, produced several models. Pottery busts showing the localisation of mental faculties are found from the mid-nineteenth century; Gall listed more than thirty faculties though there were variations on this. The Wellcome Museum has a phrenological bust by Fowler of Ludgate Circus in creamware with annotations in blue and black and a similar one is in pl. 20.

19. Ivory models of the ear, made to take apart and clip together by a series of pegs. Carved by the Zick family of Nuremberg, c. 1750.
(Germanisches Nationalmuseum, Nuremberg)

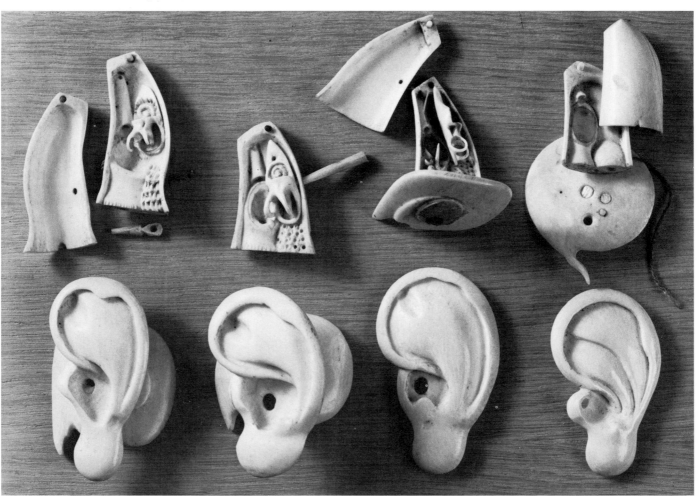

20.   Pottery phrenology bust, Fowler,
c. 1855. 30·5 cm.
(Castle Museum, York)

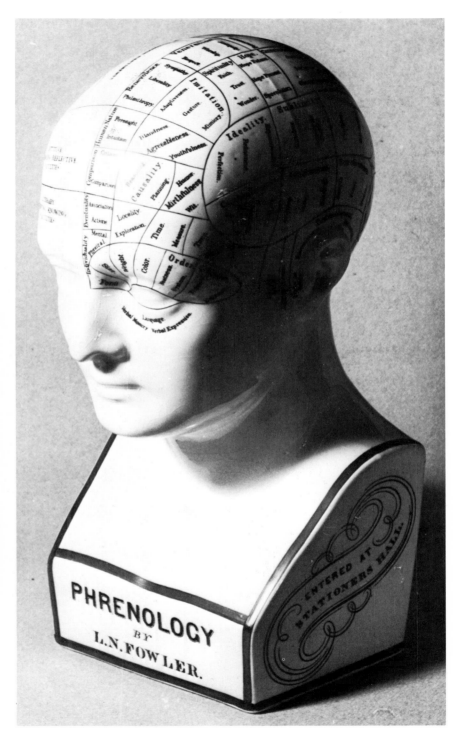

21.   Model of an eye on an ivory plinth,
c. 1810. 9 cm.
(Museum of Historical Medicine,
Copenhagen)

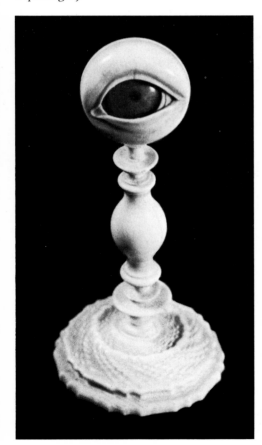

Pastille burners

Fumigating pastilles were burnt in the sickroom for combating odorous or poisonous air and vessels for the purpose were made between 1820 and 1850. One for a child, made like a house, is in the Wellcome Collection and pottery and porcelain examples with attractive decoration are often mistaken for pot-pourri containers.

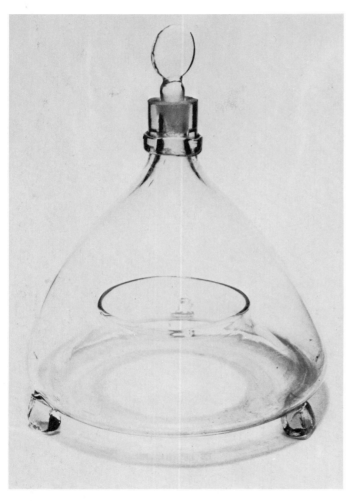

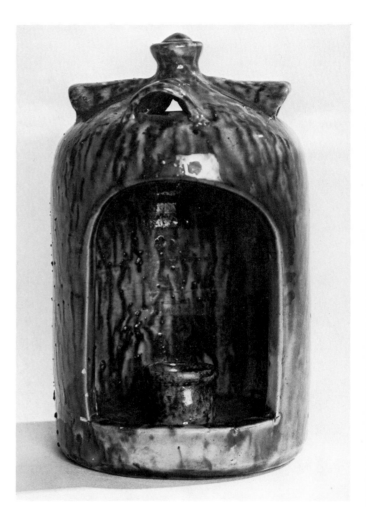

22.   Victorian glass fly catcher for the sick-room, c. 1840. Wine and water, or sugar and water were placed in the outer ring to attract the flies which flew in between the feet at the base and were then trapped. 18 cm. (Woolstaplers' Hall Museum, Chipping Camden)

23.   Green-glazed pottery invalid's candlestick, c. 1855. 18 cm. (Strangers' Hall Museum, Norwich)

PLATE XV

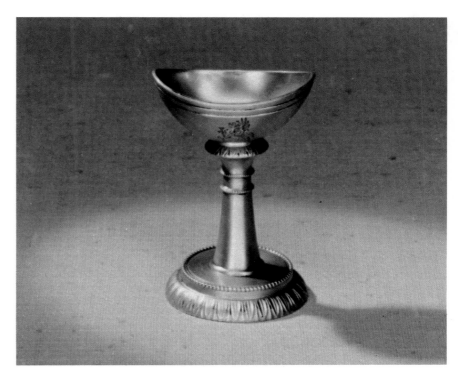

French silver-gilt eye-bath, c. 1815.
(Simon Kaye Ltd, London)

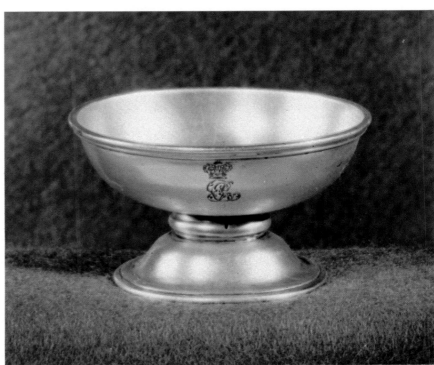

Silver-gilt medicine cup, 1814, Garrard.
Previously in the collection of Queen Charlotte
and the Princess Mary, and bearing their
ciphers. Height 6.5cm.
(Simon Kaye Ltd, London)

PLATE XVI

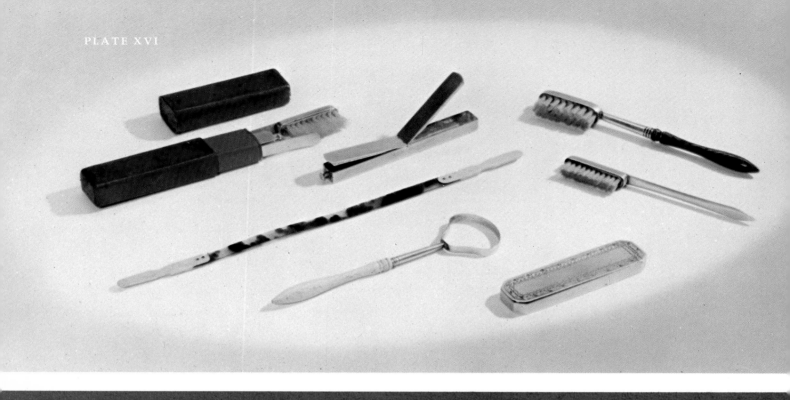

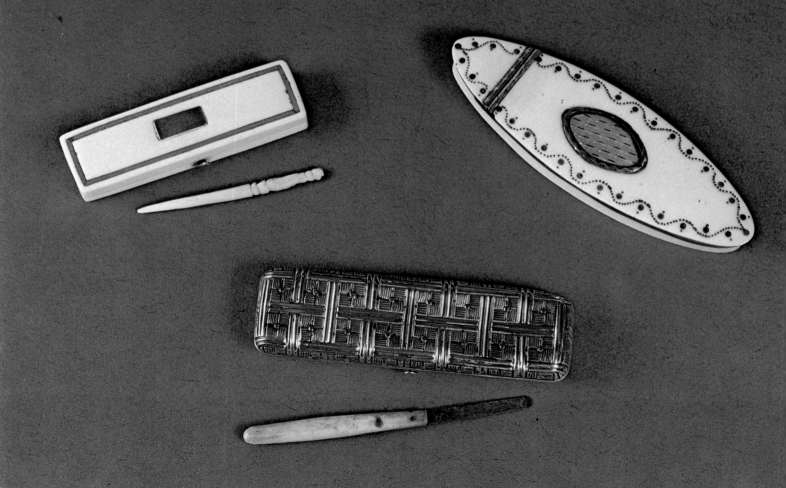

CHAPTER FIFTEEN

Toilet articles

There is sufficient overlap of pieces of sickroom equipment with everyday toilet articles found in most homes to deal briefly with some of them here.

Chamberpots, urinals and bordeloues

The earliest recorded chamberpot of silver appears in the household books of Queen Elizabeth I in 1575. By 1595 they were common enough to be satirised by John Marston and differed little in form from those of the present day. In 1672 a gold one is recorded as being pawned by a lady for £15. Pewter chamberpots were made early in the seventeenth century but with stoneware and porcelain examples being made on a large scale during the eighteenth century, metal chamberpots probably died out before their replacement by cheap enamel ones late in the nineteenth century. A tin-glazed pottery chamberpot, probably Lambeth, of the late seventeenth century is in the Wellcome Collection. It is worth recording that they were not merely part of the bedroom equipment but for the dining room as well, many a sideboard having a pot cupboard at the back (pl. 1). Pepys remembered that he 'surprised my Lady Sandwich upon her chamber pot'. Other, shallower types were made for travelling in fitted shagreen, leather, or wooden cases. The pottery and porcelain chamberpots of the nineteenth century are often so delightfully decorated that one feels it was done euphemistically—a thought taken a step further today, when one finds them in fashion on the other side of the Atlantic, filled with flowers.

Bedpans, specifically for the use of invalids, appeared in the seventeenth century. A pottery example in the Wellcome Collection is circular with a heavily inward-folding rim, both for comfort and to avoid spillage; it has a side spout for emptying. A similar one is in the Museum of London where it is dated as from the first half of the seventeenth century, though the writer feels this doubtful. Towards the end of the nineteenth century a metal bedpan was advertised shaped exactly like a Gibson spoon (see Chapter 12), but without a lid, for 5s 'much supplied to the Army'. Another, for use of male patients, has two holes, one for each function and is in pl. 3.

Colour plate
A group of toilet articles, c. 1810, showing toothbrushes, tongue scrapers, toothpowder box and toothpick box.

George III toothpick box, 1800, G. Hall, London, with ivory-handled toothpick; navette-shaped ivory and gold toothpick box, c. 1790; ivory and gold toothpick box, c. 1800, with toothpick. Length of box 9 cm. (Simon Kaye Ltd, London)

'When a man is sick with a fever,' said *The Family Physician* in the late nineteenth century, 'don't keep on talking to him under the impression that you are doing him good, for you are in all probability worrying him to death. When a man is really ill he doesn't want to be bothered with questions . . . you must remember that in ague there is often a good deal of irritation of the bladder, and that in certain cases your occasional absence from the room would be desirable.'

Male urinals of the upright flask type appeared around 1800 and were made in silver, pewter, pottery, porcelain, and later in glass. The Wellcome Museum has a blue and white Staffordshire one by E. Challinor.

Female urinals of slipper-shape were named after a French Jesuit priest, Louis Bordeloue (1632–1704), much famed for his mellifluous voice and eloquent oratory. However, so long were his sermons that his lady admirers had to have their maids send discreet urinals to the pew during the discourse. They were made in all possible materials until the end of the nineteenth century. The Wellcome Collection possesses a rare leather one of *c.* 1820 and another by Spode *c.* 1805. A pewter example *c.* 1780 is in pl. 10 and recently the silver bordeloue of Princess Augusta (granddaughter of Queen Victoria), fitted into a velvet-lined leather case, appeared on the market.

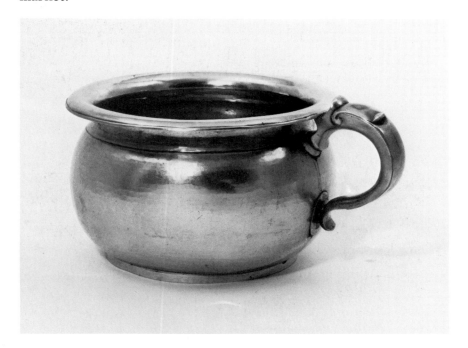

1. One of a pair of silver sideboard chamberpots, Anthony Nelme, 1730. (Sotheby Parke Bernet & Co. Ltd)

2.   *Two early eighteenth-century pewter bedpans.*
(Castle Museum, York)

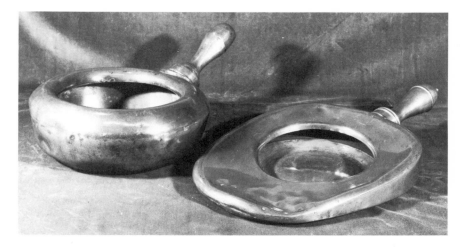

3.   *An unusual double-function bedpan for male use, in japanned metal, Aitken, York, c. 1870.*
(Castle Museum, York)

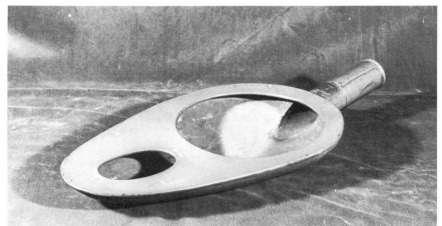

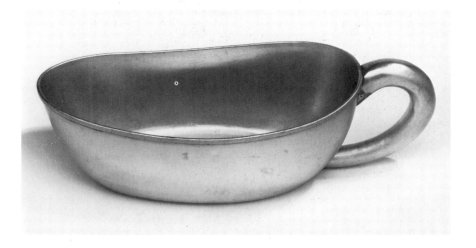

4.   *Old Sheffield Plate bordeloue, c. 1780. 22·9 cm.*
(Private Collection, United States)

Tongue scrapers

In days when a bottle of claret a day was both modest and commonplace, the use of a tongue scraper the next morning was desirable. 'A furred tongue', wrote a Victorian writer, 'is very common in the case of people who smoke much. When the fur is white, thickish, and tolerably uniform and moist, it usually indicates an open, active state of the fever, in which, though the symptoms may possibly be violent, there is little danger of any lurking mischief or of a malignant tendency. A yellowish hue of the fur is commonly indicative of disordered liver. A brown or black tongue is a bad sign, usually indicating a low state of the system and a general condition of depression.'

Tongue scrapers, it will be seen, were much needed and appeared either as part of a toilet service, or separately from the early eighteenth century onwards. They were made of silver, gold, silver-gilt, tortoise-shell, and ivory. They were formed from a strip of pliable silver or tortoise-shell either with a finial at each end and intended to be bent into a bow between the thumb and fingers, or they were already caught into a half-hoop with a handle. Other types included the 'wishbone' variety and a blade set at right angles to the handle as in an infant's 'pusher'. Silver tongue scrapers, if marked, exist from about 1800 onwards and often come in cases with a toothbrush and powder box (col. pl XVI). The dental profession in the United States is now, once again, advocating their use.

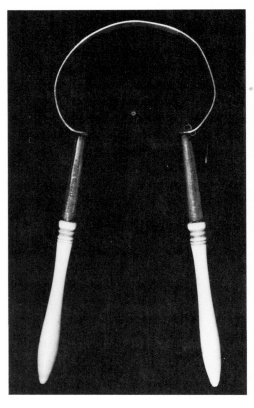

5. Tongue scraper with ivory handles, c. 1800.
(Royal College of Surgeons of Edinburgh)

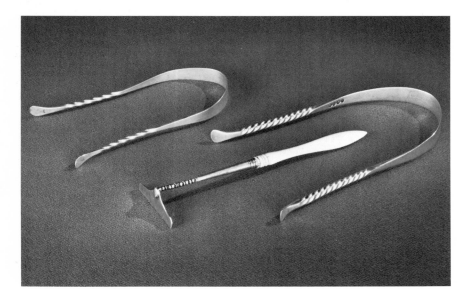

6. Silver 'wishbone' tongue scraper, c. 1800, John Death; silver and ivory tongue scraper, c. 1780, 10 cm; silver 'wishbone' tongue scraper, 1832, T.D.
(Simon Kaye Ltd, London)

Toothbrushes

Rudimentary toothbrushes formed of a bundle of animal bristles set in a tubular handle were developed in the second half of the seventeenth century, but one recognisable as such today did not appear until a hundred years later. Earlier than about 1780 they are very rare though we know Edward Finch ordered six from George Wickes in 1748. These early toothbrushes were invariably of silver, sometimes with an interchangeable pad of bristles. Later, delicately turned ivory handles appeared. They are sometimes found cased with a powder box (see below) (col. pl. XVI) and, occasionally, alone in a perforated silver case to keep them dry.

Toothpowder boxes

Rudimentary dentifrice presumably appeared at the same time as toothbrushes, and special containers were made for it. A recipe of 'Mr Ferens of the New Exchange appeared in 1660 and was so much approved at Court', though it makes horrific reading. Jacob Hemet took out a patent in 1773 for his Essence of Pearl and Pearl Dentifrice; his grandfather Peter Hemet had been 'Operator for the Teeth to King George II'. Clearly this early dentifrice was in powder form, mostly chalk, camphor, and borax, and the silver boxes found are long, narrow, and shallow, with a centrally hinged double lid

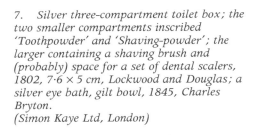

7. *Silver three-compartment toilet box; the two smaller compartments inscribed 'Toothpowder' and 'Shaving-powder'; the larger containing a shaving brush and (probably) space for a set of dental scalers, 1802, 7·6 × 5 cm, Lockwood and Douglas; a silver eye bath, gilt bowl, 1845, Charles Bryton.*
(Simon Kaye Ltd, London)

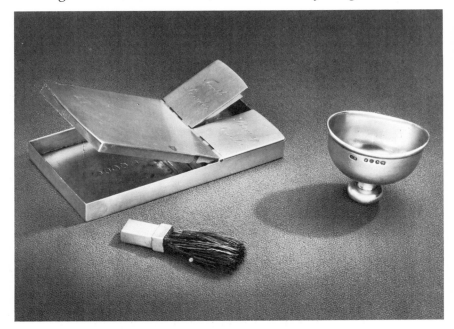

covering two compartments. Fine quality examples can be found with bright-cut decoration, and around 1800 they appeared as a set in a leather case with a toothbrush and scraper (col. pl. XVI). Toothpaste was later made in cake form and was sold in circular stoneware pots like those for pomatum with the maker's name transferred on the lid. A brand of about 1845 was made by John Coswell & Co. of London and patronised by the Queen. The pot lid describes it as 'Cherry Toothpaste (Extra Moist) for beautifying and preserving the teeth and gums'.

Toothpicks and toothpick boxes

Very thin silver and gold toothpicks were made from Elizabethan times onwards, often combined with an ear pick and sometimes folding on a hinge into a cover like a penknife. Later they were made of ivory, horn, or bone, with a prettily turned finial. As the material became less precious, toothpick boxes were made to contain a number of them. From the end of the eighteenth to the early nineteenth century these long thin boxes, usually with a mirror on the inside of the lid, were made in every type of highly decorative material from silver and silver-gilt with decoration in enamel and semi-precious stones to ivory, tortoise-shell, and finely inlaid wood (col. pl. XVI).

Eye-baths

Although silver eye-baths were mentioned in the sixteenth century, they were not in general use until the eighteenth century and then usually formed part of a toilet service (see p. 299). They were in much the same form as those of today, about 6 cm high on a stem with splayed foot (col. pl. XV). A silver one in a private collection is dated 1800 and a gold one of 1820 is recorded. Earthenware and porcelain eye-baths appeared in the second half of the eighteenth century, and Leeds creamware at about the same time. Lowestoft made them in fine porcelain, 1770–80, with floral spray decoration (pl. 8). Wedgwood, in the nineteenth century, made plain cream-coloured eye-baths and later made them in willow pattern. Victorian glass eye-baths have a wider oval bowl than pottery ones and look more like wine glasses on a short foot.

Eye-drop bottles of about 1840 often had the top of the bottle shaped for use as an eye-bath. These tiny globular bottles, 5–6·4 cm high, had a rubber-lined stopper with a hollow rod reaching to the bottom and appear efficient.

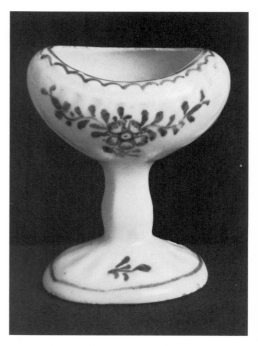

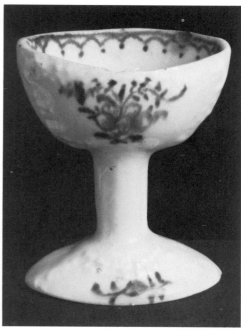

8. Two Lowestoft eye-baths c. 1770. 6·5 cm.
(Castle Museum, Norwich)

Shaving bowls and soap boxes

A shaving basin was mentioned in an inventory of 1521, but no surviving pieces are known earlier than Charles II. They are usually oval with a wide rim from which a semi-circle has been cut to take the neck of the man about to be shaved (pls. 9 and 10), while the (usually matching) jug is of flattened oval form. One basin, bearing the cipher of William III, was made the perquisite of his barber. A most interesting jug (1710, by Anthony Nelme) in the Ashmolean Museum is obviously a travelling set, as it comes apart to reveal a bowl and beaker (pl. 11). Other travelling sets are in fitted cases with soap boxes, shaving brushes, and heaters for the water. Later on all these items were made of porcelain and pottery, but the use of silver (pl. 12) or Old Sheffield Plate was retained for travelling well

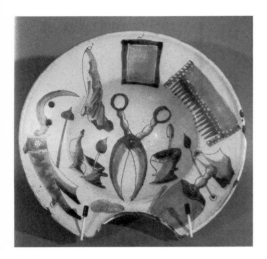

9. Blue and white London Delftware shaving bowl, c. 1720. 28 cm. (Pharmaceutical Society of Great Britain Museum)

10. Chinese export blue and white porcelain barber's bowl, c. 1750, 25·5 cm; pewter bordeloue, c. 1780; brass barber's bowl, c. 1780. (Simon Kaye Ltd, London)

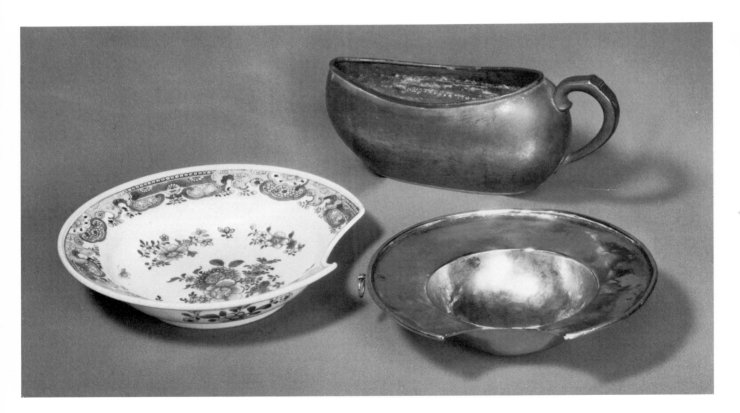

down the nineteenth century, and humbler sets are found in pewter, brass, and copper.

It is a long held contention that shaving bowls of the type described above were used by the Barber–Surgeons and were dual purpose. It is not proven either way, but attention here must be called to the collection of the Pharmaceutical Society in which there are several examples in English Delftware c. 1700, decorated in blue and white, with pieces of barbers equipment—combs, scissors, razors, and so on—but no surgical instruments (pl. 9).

Soap, being made in spherical form, had a spherical box on a rim foot to contain it. They are not found earlier than c. 1745 and were sometimes made to match similar boxes for sponges, the latter having a perforated top (pl. 13). Again, except for travelling, pottery and porcelain were used in the nineteenth century although silver and ivory remained the favourite material for the handles of shaving brushes. These are sometimes found with bristles that can be unscrewed and reversed into the handle, as in pl. 12, and often with a compartment for soap.

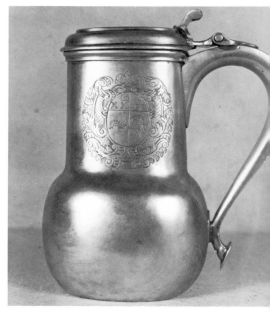

11.   Silver shaving jug, 1710, by Anthony Nelme, which takes apart to reveal a bowl and beaker.
(Ashmolean Museum, Oxford)

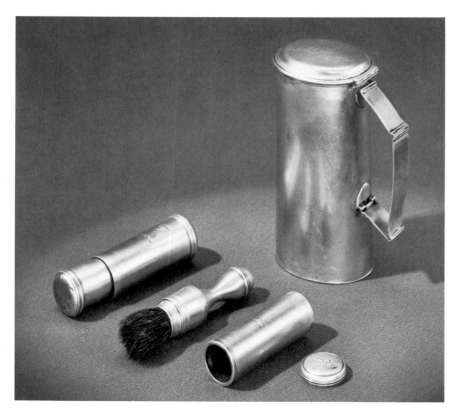

12.   Shaving-soap container of silver, 1798, J. Taylor, 7·5 cm; shaving brush in silver case, 1809, and a silver travelling hot-water can with collapsible handle, 1821.
(Simon Kaye Ltd, London)

13. Old Sheffield Plate sponge-box, c. 1790.
12·7 cm.
(Simon Kaye Ltd, London)

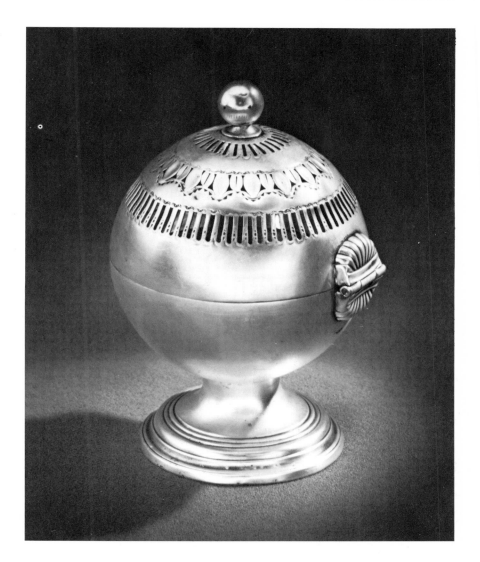

Toilet services

A travelling toilet service containing every conceivable personal item for a woman's toilet was introduced in the middle of the seventeenth century, and a hundred years later, similar cases for men including razors, pomatum boxes, etc. were made. One of the earliest of the former, of 1673, is at Knole, and Charles II presented a toilet service—very continental in style—to Catharine of Braganza in the same year. A very fine one in the Ashmolean Museum—the Treby Service—of 1724, is by Paul de Lamerie (pl. 15).

A good toilet service, in gold, silver-gilt, or silver, and fitting into a velvet-lined, layered case of leather or brass-bound wood, might contain all or some of the following:

Mirror
1 or 2 comb boxes
Many other assorted boxes for jewellery, patches, pomatum, powder, etc.
Ewer and basin
Candlesticks
Dressing weight (for tightening stay-laces)
Tongue scraper
Medicine spoon
Toilet water bottles
Hair brushes
Pin cushion
Toothpick
Tray
Whisk
Medicine cup
Eye bath
Corkscrew (probably for toilet water, not brandy)
Clothes hook
Bodkin, etc.
Pens, pencil and ivory-leaved *aide-memoire*
Scissors.

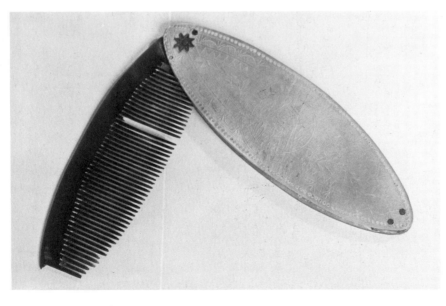

14.   Tortoise-shell comb folding into navette-shaped mother-of-pearl case engraved with chinoiserie design, c. 1790. 9 cm.
(Strangers' Hall Museum, Norwich)

15.   The silver-gilt Treby toilet service, 1724, Paul de Lamerie.
(Ashmolean Museum, Oxford)

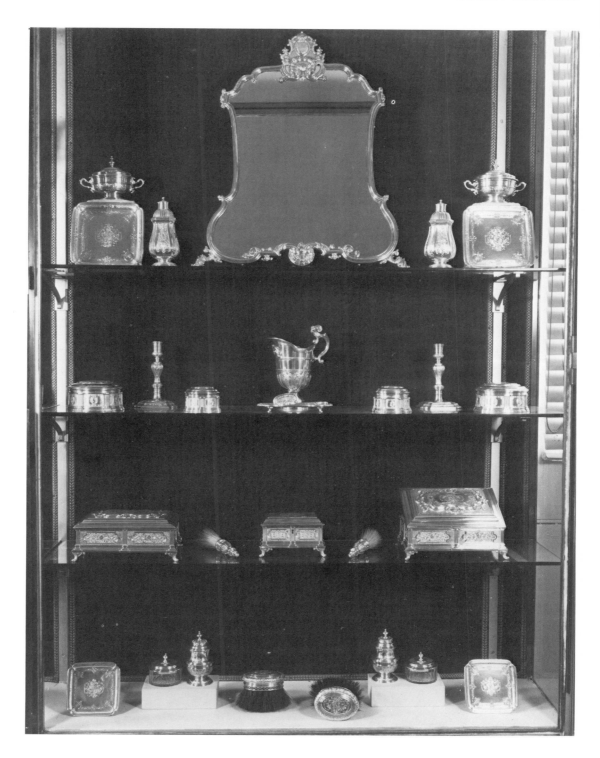

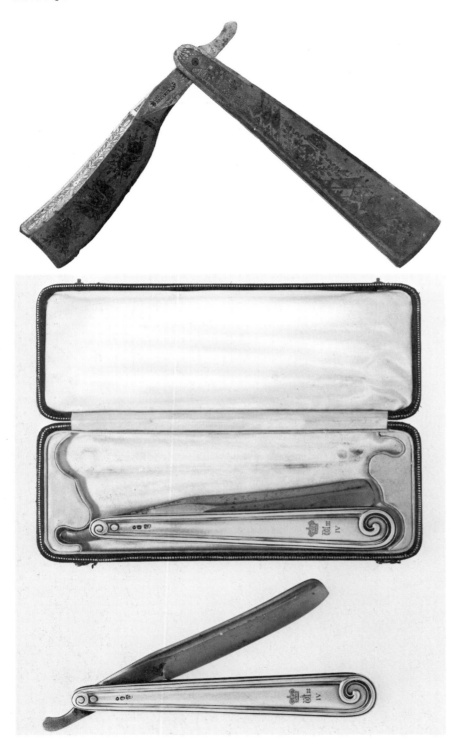

16.   *French razor, embellished with floral arms and trophies, c. 1680.*
(Musée le Secq des Tournelles, Rouen)

17.   *The silver razors of William IV, bearing his cipher, 1830, Paul Storr. 10 cm.*
(Simon Kaye Ltd, London)

Epitaph

The apparatus below was introduced by Joseph Lister in 1871 and marks the end of an era. From that time the recovery rate from surgical operations soared, but never again could medical instruments display the decorative craftsmanship which this book has tried to illustrate. The earlier surgeons had limited facilities, but any study of their lives and work shows most of them to have been men of humility. They did their best according to their own time and understanding. On their best, the surgeons of today have based theirs.

Lister carbolic spray. 20·5 cm.
(College of Physicians of Philadelphia)

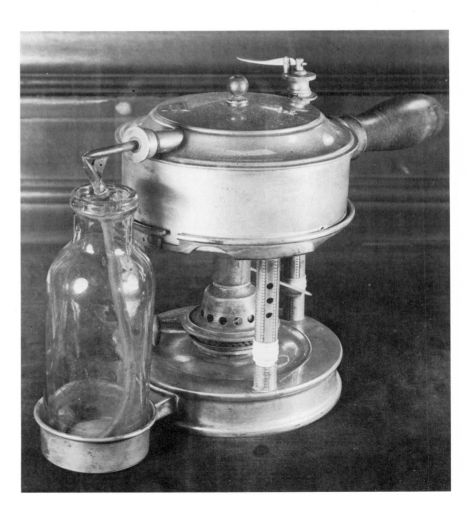

Directory of surgical instrument makers

From the middle of the eighteenth century onwards, instruments and their cases appeared stamped with the maker's name. It is therefore important, for purposes of accurate dating, to have as much information as possible about these makers. The makers listed below are known to have made instruments prior to 1870, though not all are known to have described themselves as surgical instrument makers as such. It has been decided to omit the majority of those firms established after 1870, although it is conceded that it might have been useful to list them separately as being too late for the context of this book. In many cases, long-founded makers still in existence have shown little interest in their origins, and the information forthcoming has not been conducive to accuracy; the British Surgical Trades Association was unable to help. However, thanks are due to Mr Wynne Davies whose own list, in the beginning, showed me the possibility of this type of directory; to the Library of the Royal College of Surgeons of England for permission to consult the Russell papers; and to those County Librarians across the country whose records have contributed towards the compiling of this list. Silversmiths who have made medical pieces are not included, and for these the reader should refer to: *English Goldsmiths and their Marks*, Sir Charles Jackson, London, 1921; and *London Goldsmiths 1697–1837*, Arthur G. Grimwade, London, 1976.

Abbreviations used are as follows:

C.	Cutler
CH.	Chemist
D.	Druggist
D.I.M.	Dental instrument maker
M.I.M.	Mathematical instrument maker
OC.	Oculist
OP.	Optician
S.I.M.	Surgical instrument maker
T.M.	Truss maker
V.I.M.	Veterinary instrument maker

United Kingdom instrument makers

Aitken

1820	Established. Henry A. Aitken
1858	Known to have made percussion hammer introduced by Henry Vernon of the Great Northern Hospital
1861–76	Henry Aitken, 16 Railway Street, York
1886	Henry Aitken & Co.
1910	Henry Aitken & Co., 13 Micklegate (later renumbered 29), York

Allcard & Edgill

1845–9	Allcard & Edgill, 6 Union Lane, Sheffield
1852	Allcard & Co., 6 Union Lane, Sheffield

Allen & Hanbury

1715	Established London, E.2 as Bevan
1774	Samuel Mildred
1795	Mildred & Allen, 2 Plough Court
1797	Surgical instruments first mentioned in catalogue
1856	Allen & Hanbury
c. 1870	Moved to Wigmore Street
1878–9	Manufacture of instruments at Bethnal Green factory
c. 1972	Taken over by Escham Bros. & Walsh

Amesbury

1843	Joseph Amesbury, 8 Berners Street, London

Archer & Co

(known 1817)	Strand, London

Armitage

1843	John Armitage, 2 Hampton Street, Walworth Road, London

Arnold

(Post Office Directory 1883: 'by appointment to St Bartholomew's Hospital. Manufacturers of surgical instruments and general cutlery, trusses, elastic stockings, belts, bandages and bougies, catheters, artificial legs, arms, hands, eyes, etc. Veterinary instrument maker by appointment to the Royal Veterinary College, St Pancras').

1819	J. & S. Arnold (CH. and D.), 59 Barbican, London
1829	James Arnold, (S.I.M.)
1837	James & John Arnold, (S.I.M.)
1845	James Arnold, (S.I.M.) } 35 West Smithfield, London
1857	James Arnold & Son, (S.I.M.)
1866	Arnold & Sons, (S.I.M.)
1928	Incorporated into John Bell & Croyden, 50–52 Wigmore Street, London

Ash

1814	Ash & Son, Silversmith and Jeweller, 64 St James's Street, London
1835	C. Ash, 9 Broad Street, Golden Square, London
1840	C. Ash, 9 Broad Street, Golden Square. Manufacturers of mineral teeth.
1844	C. Ash & Sons, 9 Broad Street, Golden Square. Manufacturers of mineral teeth.
1846	C. Ash & Sons, 8 & 9 Broad Street, Golden Square. Manufacturers of mineral teeth.
1859	Claudius Ash & Sons, 6, 7, 8 & 9 Broad Street, Golden Square. Manufacturers of mineral teeth and dental material.
1875	C. Ash, (D.I.M.), Factory in Kentish Town, London Now Amalgamated Dental Co. Ltd, 26 Broadwick Street, London W.1

Atlee

| 1847 | T. Atlee & Co. (ether inhaler in Wellcome Museum) |

Auchinleck

| 1776 | Gilbert Auchinleck, (C.), Nether-bow, Edinburgh |

Bailey

1833	Established, (T.M.)
1843	William Huntley Bailey, (T.M.), 418 Oxford Street, London
1873	William Huntley Bailey, (T.M.), 16 Oxford Street, London
1894	W. H. Bailey & Son, (T.M.), 38 Oxford Street, London

Baker

| 1765 | Established |
| 1894 | Baker, 243 High Holborn, London |

Ballard

| 1843 | Henry Ballard, 42 St John's Square, London |

Barker

1797	Geo. Barker, (c.), Fargate, Sheffield
1817	Geo. Barker, (c.), Hawley Croft, Sheffield

Bartrop

1843	Henry Bartrop, 33 Crawford Street, London

Battensby

1821	John Battensby, (c. and s.i.m.), Groat Market, Newcastle
1827	John Battensby, (c., s.i.m. and t.m.), 15 Groat Market, Newcastle
1829	John Battensby, (c., s.i.m. and t.m.), Middle Street, Newcastle
	No trace by 1833

Bayne

1823	Charles Bayne, (c.), High Street, Oxford
1846	Bayne & Chadwell, (c.), 2 Grove Street, Oxford
1854	Bayne & Chadwell (c.), 112 High Street, Oxford
1867	Mrs Chadwell, (c.), 112 High Street, Oxford
1872	Mrs Chadwell, (c.), $30\frac{1}{2}$ Cornmarket, Oxford
1880	Chadwell, & Long, (c. and s.i.m.), $30\frac{1}{2}$ Cornmarket Oxford
1884	Wemborn (late Chadwell), (c. and s.i.m.), $30\frac{1}{2}$ Cornmarket, Oxford
	In business until 1912

Beach

Mid-18th century	Established as T. Beach & Son, Scale Makers Now W. & T. Avery Ltd., London

Beatson Clark

18th century	Established as makers of glass measures as Beatson Clark & Co., London

Beauchamp

	Instruments at Royal College of Surgeons, London

Bell (1)

1798	Established, (ch. and d.) Now John Bell & Croyden. See Arnold

Bell (2)

1839	Thos. Bell, (c.), 15 Cornmarket, Belfast
1850	Thos. Bell, (c. and s.i.m.), 15 Cornmarket, Belfast Last mentioned 1880

Bernadoue

c. 1736   James Bernardoue, Russell Court, Drury Lane, London
No trace by 1744

Best

c. 1690   John Best

1750   John Best, Lombard Street, London. (Made Smellie's forceps, *c.* 1750. Trade card known to date from 1690–1760). No trace by 1843

Bickerstaff

1678–*c.* 1700   Thos. Bickerstaff, (C.), Princes Street, Drury Lane, London

Bigg

1751   Established. Henry Bigg

1832–4   Sheldrake & Bigg, 29 Leicester Square, London

1842   Henry Bigg, 9 St Thomas's Street, Borough, London

1852   Bigg, St Thomas's Street, Southwark, London

1858   Heather Bigg, 29 Leicester Square, London

1858–9   Bigg & Millikin, 8 St Thomas's Street, London. (Apparently took over the Laundy business)

Blackwell

1817   J. Blackwell

1826   Charles Blackwell, 3 Bedford Court, London

1843   William Blackwell, 3 Bedford Court, Covent Garden, London

Blair

c. 1735   Thomas Blair, (C.), Edinburgh

Louis Blaise & Co

See Savigny

Blyde

1841   Established. John Blyde Ltd, London.
See Down

Bodker

1765   Henry Bodker, (S.I.M.), Poultry, London

1768   Richard James Bodker, (S.I.M.), Poultry London

1770   Jane & Richard Bodker, (S.I.M.), Poultry, London

1774   Richard Bodker, (S.I.M.), Poultry, London

1777   Richard Bodker, (S.I.M.), 2 Colman Street, London

308

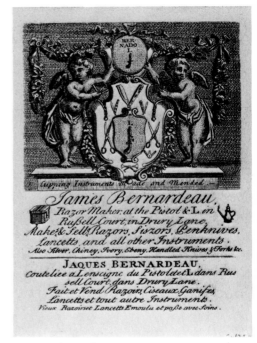

1. Trade card.
(Sir Ambrose Heal Collection, British Museum)

2. Trade card.
(Sir Ambrose Heal Collection, British Museum)

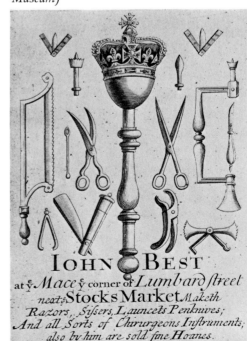

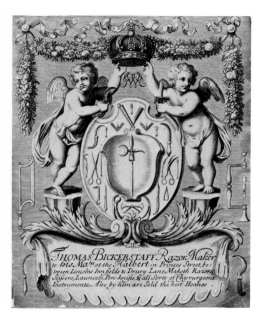

3. Trade card.
(Sir Ambrose Heal Collection, British Museum)

Bond

Arthur Bond, Euston Road, London.
Instrument at Royal College of Surgeons, London

Boog

1748	Robert Boog
1779	Andrew Boog, College Street, Edinburgh
1784	Alexander Boog
1800	Andrew & Alexander Boog, Netherbow, Edinburgh
1820–6	Andrew & Alexander Boog, 13 High Street, Edinburgh
1830	Thomas Boog, (C. and S.I.M.), 105 High Street, Edinburgh

No trace after 1859

Borthwick

Early 19th century   B. Borthwick, College Street, Edinburgh

Borwick

1791	Roger Borwick, (C.), Sheffield
1817	Roger Borwick, (C.), Bailey Lane, Sheffield
1825	Samuel Borwick, (C.), Bailey Lane, Sheffield

No trace after 1860

Botschan

19th century   Joseph Botschan, 35 Worship Street, Finsbury, London

Bourne & Taylor

Mid-19th century   Bourne & Taylor

Boyce

1751–60   Samuel Boyce, Maiden Lane, London

Bradford

Mid-19th century   136 Minories, London

Brady

1855	Established as Henry Bowman Brady, (CH.)
1857	Henry Bowman Brady, (CH.), 40 Mosley Street, Newcastle
1869	Henry Bowman Brady, (CH.), 29 Mosley Street, Newcastle
1879	Brady & Martin, 29 Mosley Street, Newcastle
1883	Brady & Martin, (CH. and S.I.M.), 29 Mosley Street, Newcastle

ANTIQUE MEDICAL INSTRUMENTS

Brailsford

Early 18th
century   John Brailsford, St Martin's Court, London

Brand

Early 19th
century   Brand

Brennand

1843   Pearson Brennand, 217 High Holborn, London

Brookwick Ward

19th century   Brookwick Ward & Co., (V.I.M.), 8 Shepherds Bush
                 Road, London

Brown

1822   John Brown, Wire worker, 2 Whitechapel Road,
                 London
1852   John Brown, (C.), 2 Townsend Road, London
1858   John Brown, (C.), 17 Connaught Terrace, London
                 No trace after 1861

Bruce

1832–3   Henry Bruce, (C. and S.I.M.), 66 Southbridge, Edinburgh

Bullen

1858   Established. C. S. Bullen, (S.I.M.), 89 Mount Pleasant,
                 Liverpool

Butler

c. 1681   Established. George Butler, Sheffield
c. 1810   George and James Butler, (C.), 4 Trinity Street, Sheffield
1865   George and James Butler, (C.), 105 Eyre Street, Sheffield

Capron

19th century   Capron. Hernia bistoury found

Cargill

1739   John Cargill, Lombard Street, London
1773   Peter Cargill, Lombard Street, London
1789   Peter Cargill, (C.), Lombard Street, London

Carr

                 Edward Carr, Newcastle

Carsberg

1798 — Established. Carsberg, 38 Great Windmill Street, London

Cartwright

c. 1760–80 — Paston Cartwright, Lombard Street, London

Casella

19th century — L. Casella, Hatton Garden, London (Made Aitken's clinical thermometer)

Chadwell — see Bayne

Chandler

Late 18th century — Chandler

Charlwood

1770 — Yeeling Charlwood, (C.), Russell Court, London. 'Successor to the late Mr Gordon, c. 1760' see Underwood

Chasson

c.1770 — J. Chasson, (C. and S.I.M.), Newgate Street, London
1789 — Mary Chasson, (C.), 68 Newgate Street, London

Clark

1818 — G. Clark, (C.), 5 York Buildings, Bath
1828 — G. Clark, (C.), 16 Vineyards, Bath
1832 — G. Clark, (C.), 3 Bond Street Buildings, Bath No trace after 1832

Clarke (1)

c. 1832 — Invented electromagnetic machine

Clarke (2)

c. 1861 — J. Clarke, 225 Piccadilly, London

Cluley

1813 — Francis Cluley, (S.I.M.), Westbar Green, Sheffield
1825 — Francis Cluley, (S.I.M.), 4 Surrey Street, Sheffield No trace after 1837

Cole

c. 1760 — Henry Cole, Strand, London

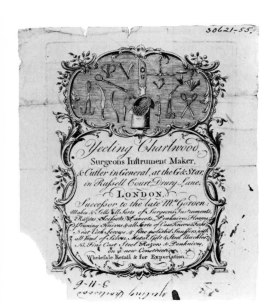

4.   *Trade card.*
(Sir Ambrose Heal Collection, British Museum)

Collings

1817	James Collings (registered mark London Assay Office)
1822	James Collings, Spectacle Maker, Bowling Green Lane, London
1835	James Collings, (OP.), 5 Skinner Street, London
	No trace after 1839

Cooke

1670	John Cooke
c. 1686	George Cooke
1698	George Cooke, Old Lombard Street, London

Coombes

before 1730	John Coombes, Cross Inn, Oxford

Corcoran

Late 19th century	Corcoran, Dublin?

Corneck

1768	James Corneck, (C.), Cheapside, London

Courtney

c. 1710	Richard Courtney, Hatton Gardens, London

Cox

	See Savigny and Krohne & Seseman

Coxeter

1836	Established
1843	J. Coxeter & Co., 23 Grafton Street, London
1863	J. Coxeter
1870	J. Coxeter & Son
1894	James Coxeter & Son, 4 & 6 Grafton Street, London
1923	Coxeter Ltd, London

Craddock

1843	Geo. Craddock, 35 Leicester Square, London

Crawford

1817	W. Crawford, 68 Charles Street, London

Crookes

1826	John Crookes, (C.), Fetter Lane, London

312

Crooks

1787	John Crooks, Razor Maker, Great Turnpike, Holborn, London
1826	John Crooks, 1 Back Church Lane, Whitechapel

Cruickshank

1765	Cruickshank, London (made Pott's fistula knife)

Curry & Paxton

c. 1878	Curry & Paxton, (OP.)

Cuzner

1825	Henry Cuzner, Engraver, 36 Lower Arcade, Bristol
1832	Henry Cuzner, truss manufacturer and surgical mechanic, 36 Lower Arcade, Bristol
1849	Cuzner & Pearce, truss manufacturer and surgical mechanic, 36 Lower Arcade, Bristol
1850	Pearce & Co., truss manufacturers and surgical mechanic

Dalton

1852	Dalton, 85 Quadrant, London

Davies

Late 18th century	Davies, (S.I.M.)

Day

1840	Established. Day & Sons, Crewe, Cheshire
?	Day Son & Hewitt, (V.I.M.), 22 Dorset Street, London

Delolme

c. 1885	Delolme, Stethometer

Dick

1865	James Dick, (C. and bandage maker), 28 St Enoch Wynd, Glasgow
1866	James Dick, (C. and bandage maker), 92 Glassford Street, Glasgow
1871	James Dick, (C. and bandage maker), 45 Renfield Street Glasgow
1872	James Dick, (C., bandage and artificial limbs maker), 45 Renfield Street, Glasgow
1874	James Dick, (S.I.M.), 45 Renfield Street, Glasgow
1896	James Dick, (S.I.M.), 107 West George Street, Glasgow
1921	Went out of business

Dixon

1843   William Dixon, 2 Tonbridge Street, New Road, London

Dong

Mid-19th   Dong, (v.i.m.), to H.M. Queen Victoria
century

Donnell

Mid-19th   J. E. Donnell, 384 Strand, London
century

Down

1874   Down Bros. Ltd
1879   Millikin & Down, St Thomas Street, Borough, London
1894   Down Bros. 5–7 St Thomas Street, Borough, London
              Now Down Surgical Ltd, Mitcham, Surrey,
              incorporating Mayer & Phelps, Blyde & Gray.

Druce

Early 19th   H. Druce
century

Dungworth

1861   John Dungworth, 146 Broomhall Street, Sheffield

Dunsford

c. 1780–1800   Dunsford

Durroch

1788   Wm. F. Durroch established
1847   Wm. F. Durroch, (s.i.m.), 2 New Street, London
1860   Wm. F. Durroch, (s.i.m.), 28 St Thomas's Street, London
1862   Wm. F. Durroch, (s.i.m.), 3 St Thomas's Street, London
              No trace after 1869. See Smith

Dyer

1823   Wm. Dyer, (c.), Old Town Street, Plymouth
1830   Wm. Dyer, (c. and s.i.m.), 5 Old Town Street,
              Plymouth
1844   Daniel Dyer, (c. and s.i.m.), 5 Old Town Street,
              Plymouth
1857   Daniel Dyer, (c. and s.i.m.), 59 Old Town Street,
              Plymouth
1864   Alfred Dyer, (c. and s.i.m.), 59 Old Town Street
              Plymouth
1873   Alfred Dyer, (c. and s.i.m.), 99 Old Town Street,
              Plymouth

1890   Daniel Dyer, 8 Whimpole Street, Plymouth and 13
                Marlborough Street, Devonport
                In business until 1923

Eagland
1826   Charles Eagland, 10 Poland Street, London

Einsle
1843   Edward Einsle, 46 St Martin's Lane, London

Elam
1843   Alfred Elam & Bros, 403 Oxford Street, London

Elliott
1824   John Elliott, (C. and S.I.M.), Spring Gardens, Clitheroe
1848   John Elliott, (C. and S.I.M.), Church Brow, Clitheroe
1851   Robt. Elliott, (S.I.M.), Church Brow, Clitheroe
1855   Robt. Elliott, (S.I.M.), Waddington Lane, Clitheroe
                No trace after 1858

Ellis
1843   Wm. Ellis, 3 Thanet Place, London

Ernst
1863   Gustav Ernst, 19 Calthorpe Street, London
1869   Gustav Ernst, 80 Charlotte Street, London

Evans (1)
1676   John Evans, Blacksmith
1783   David Evans, (S.I.M.), 10 Old Change, London
1803   David Evans & Co., (S.I.M.), 10 Old Change, London
1811   John Evans & Co., (S.I.M.), 10 Old Change, London
1854   John Evans & Co., (S.I.M.), 10 Old Change and 12 Old
                Fish Street, London
1855   John Evans & Co, (S.I.M.), 12 Old Fish Street, London
1867   Evans & Stevens, (S.I.M.), 6 Dowgate Hill and
                31 Stanford Street, London
1874   Evans & Wormall, (S.I.M.), 31 Stanford Street, London
                'By Appt. to Army, Navy, and Indian Government'.
                Principal suppliers to the Navy. *c.* 1812—instruments
                marked with crown

Evans (2)
Late 18th   Evans, Oswestry
century

Everill   See Savigny

Evrard

1808	Jean Evrard, 32 Charles Street, London
1837	Jean Evrard, 35 Charles Street, Middlesex Hospital, London
1865	Jean Evrard, (principally D.I.M.), 34 Berners Street, London

Ewing

Mid-19th century	Ewing, Liverpool

Fannin

1829	Established. Fannin, 41 Grafton Street, Dublin Still in business

Ferguson

1822	Daniel Ferguson, (S.I.M.), 14 Castle Street, London
1826	Daniel Ferguson, (S.I.M.), 44 West Smithfield Street, London
1828	Daniel Ferguson, (S.I.M.), 21 Giltspur Street, London
1851	Ferguson & Son, 21 Giltspur Street, London
1858	John Ferguson & Co., 21 Giltspur Street, London No trace after 1869

Ferris

c. 1770	Established
1775	Till Adams
1783	Till Adams, (M.D.), Union Street, Bristol
1787	Till Adams, Ann, Apothecaries, Union Street, Bristol
1812	Fry & Gibbs, (D.), 3 Union Street, Bristol
1820	Fry Gibbs & Ferris, (D.), 4 Union Street, Bristol
1826	Fry Gibbs & Ferris, (D. and CH.), 4 Union Street, Bristol
1834	Ferris Brown & Capper, (D. and CH.), 25 Union Street, Bristol, and 1 Mall, Clifton
1837	Ferris Brown & Score, (D. and CH.), 25 Union Street, Bristol, and 1 Mall, Clifton
1842	Ferris & Score, (D. and CH.), 4–5 Union Street, Bristol
1856	Ferris, Townsend, Lamotte & Bourne, (D. and CH.), 4–5 Union Street, Bristol
1865	Ferris, Townsend, Bourne & Townsend (D. and CH.), 4–5 Union Street, Bristol
1869	Ferris, Bourne & Townsend, (D. and CH.), 4–5 Union Street, Bristol
1893	Ferris & Co. Still in business

Figgett

1843   J. L. Figgett, 29 Trafalgar Street, Walworth

Fisher

1805   John Fisher, 34 Wapping Street, London

1843   James Fisher, 7 Cannon Street Road, London

Ford

1846–85   John Ford, Flint Glass manufacturer, Canongate and North Bridge, Edinburgh

Fraser

c. 1830   Fraser. (Not listed by the Post Office between 1840 and 1860)

Froggatt

Mid-19th century   Froggatt

Fuller (1)

1832   John Fuller, Whitechapel Road, London

1843   John Fuller, 239 Whitechapel Road, London
No trace after 1860

Fuller (2)

1827   Fuller. Made spectacles, Ipswich, but not recorded in Post Office Directory of 1839

Fuller Spongs

c. 1860   Fuller Spongs, Thermometer

Gardner

Mid-19th century   J. Gardner & Son, 32 Forrest Road, Edinburgh

Gay

1817   John Gay, (C.), 68 Kirkgate, Leeds

1822   John Gay, (C. and S.I.M.), 68 Kirkgate, Leeds

1826   John Gay, (C. and S.I.M.), 5 Kirkgate, Leeds

1839   John Gay, (C. and S.I.M.), 10 Kirkgate, Leeds

1842   John Gay, (C. and S.I.M.), 10 Kirkgate, Leeds, Bradford

1845   John Gay, (C. and S.I.M.), 132 Briggate, Leeds

1849   John Gay & Son, (C. and S.I.M.), 132 Briggate, Leeds

1851   John R. Gay, (C. and S.I.M.), 132 Briggate, Leeds

1878   Lavini & Gay, (C. and S.I.M.), 132 Briggate, Leeds

1882   J. R. Gay, (C. and S.I.M.), 132 Briggate, Leeds
No trace after 1886

Gibbs

c. 1740   Established. Gibbs
1756   Joseph Gibbs, 137 Bond Street, London
1772   James Gibbs, 137 Bond Street, London
1800   Gibbs & Lewis, 137 Bond Street, London

Gilkerson & McAll

1822   Gilkerson & McAll. Spectacles found

Gill (1)

1825   John Gill, (S.I.M.), 45 Salisbury Square, London

Gill (2)

c. 1810   Thomas Gill, (C.), 83 St James's Street, London

Gillett

c. 1800   Gillett. At 'The Case of Knives' in St James's Market, London

Goodall

1805   John Goodall, St Saviour's Churchyard, London

Gordon

c. 1740   Established
c. 1770   Jacob Gordon, Russell Court, Drury Lane, London
c. 1825   Succeeded by H. Underwood

Graham

c. 1800   Graham

Grant

c. 1745   Established. Grant
1791   Richard Grant, (C.), St Anne's, Soho, London

Gray (1)

1849   Established. Joseph Gray, 154 Fitzwilliam Street, Sheffield
1864   Gray & Lawson, 51 New George Street, Sheffield

Gray (2)

1841   Wm. Gray, (C., S.I.M. and T.M.), 28 Market Street, Newcastle
          No trace after 1847

Greer

c. 1790   C. Greer, 10 Charing Cross, London

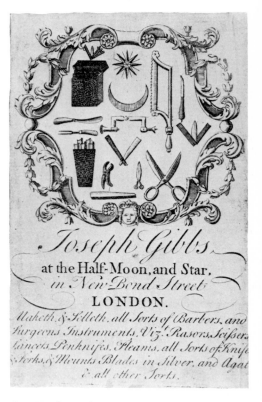

5.   Trade card.
(Sir Ambrose Heal Collection, British Museum)

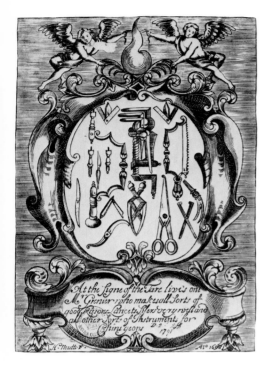

6. *Trade card.*
(Sir Ambrose Heal Collection, British Museum)

Grenier
1698   Isaac Grenier

Grice
c. 1800   Established. John Grice
1817   John Grice, 239 Whitechapel Road, London
1832   Grice & Fuller, Whitechapel, London

Grick
Mid-19th   Grick
century

Grover
c. 1680   Samuel Grover, London Bridge, London

Grumbridge
1843   J. Grumbridge, 42 Poland Street, London. (Stethoscopes)

Guest
Late 18th   Guest. Pieces in Wellcome Museum, London
century

Hales
1817   Henry Hales, 4 Manor Row, Tower Hill, London

Hall
1817   Thomas Hall, 8 Charles Street, London

Hammock
1826   Charles Hammock, 53 Chiswell Street, London

Harvey (& Reynolds)
1839   Thos. Harvey, (CH. and D.), 5 Commercial Street, Leeds
1841   Thos. Harvey, (CH. and D.), 13 Briggate, Leeds
1856   Harvey & Reynolds, (CH. and D.), 13 Briggate, Leeds
1861   Harvey, Reynolds & Fowler, (CH. and D.), 10 Briggate, Leeds
1864   Haw & Reynolds, (CH. and D.), Briggate, Leeds
1867   Haw, Reynolds, & Co., (CH. and D.), Briggate, Leeds
1872   Haw, Reynolds & Co., (CH.), 14 Commercial Street, and Briggate, Leeds
1886   Reynolds & Branson
                   Still in business today. (Makers of the first short clinical thermometer)

319

Hawkesley

1865	Thomas Hawkesley, 357 Oxford Street, London
1925	Hawkesley & Son Ltd. Now Gelman Hawkesley, Shoreham, Sussex

Hemmings

1843	Aug. F. Hemmings, 45 Chiswell Street, Finsbury, London

Hentsch

1826	Fred. C. Hentsch, 18 Dukes Court, London
1843	Fred. C. Hentsch, 25 Bartlett Buildings, London
1894	Fred. Hentsch, 49 Greek Street, London

Higden

Early 19th century	Higden, Edinburgh

Higham

1843	Mrs Priscilla Higham, 48 Jermyn Street, London

Hilliard (1)

1834	Established. W. B. Hilliard & Sons, Buchanan Street, Glasgow
1856–7	W. B. Hilliard & Sons, 65 Renfield Street, Glasgow
1909	W. B. Hilliard & Sons, 157 Hope Street, Glasgow
1920	W. B. Hilliard & Sons, 123 Douglas Street, Glasgow. (Made many instruments for Lister)

Hilliard (2)

1834	H. & J. E. Hilliard, 57 Arcade, Glasgow
1837	Harry Hilliard, 28 Argyll Street, Glasgow
1842	Hilliard & Chapman, 28 Argyll Street, Glasgow
1848	Harry Hilliard, 28 Argyll Street, Glasgow
1851–64	Hilliard & Chapman, 28 Argyll Street, Glasgow

Hilliard (3)

1832	Established. Hilliard
1850–51	H. & H. Hilliard, (s.i.m.), 7 Nicolson Street, Edinburgh Now trading as Ross & Hilliard

Hills

c. 1825	Monson Hills
1853	Henry J. Hills, 46 King Street, Borough, London

Hobbs, Robert & Swayne

1628	Hobbs, Robert & Swayne, Makers of Prujean Collection

7. *Trade card.*
(Sir Ambrose Heal Collection, British Museum)

Hockin

19th century   Hockin

Hodge

Early 19th   J. Hodge
century

Holborn Surgical Instrument Co. Ltd

c. 1870   (V.I.M.), 15 Charterhouse Street, London

Holmes & Laurin

c. 1760   Holmes & Laurin, (T.M.)

Hooper-Halse

1844–6   W. M. Hooper-Halse, 5 Pelham Crescent, London.
               (Medical Galvanist)
1850–4   W. M. Hooper-Halse, 22 Brunswick Square, London.
               (Medical Galvanist)
1857–66   W. M. Hooper-Halse, Addison Terrace, London
               (Medical Galvanist)
1866–c. 1885   W. M. Hooper-Halse, 40 Addison Road, London.
               (Medical Galvanist)

Hughes

1843   Francis Hughes & Co., 247 High Holborn, London

Huish

c. 1870   C. H. Huish & Co., (V.I.M.), 12 Red Lion Square, London

Hunter

1843   Hunter Mason & Co., 44 Webberrow, Blackfriars,
               London

Hutchinson

1825*   Wm. Hutchinson & Son, Razor Makers,
               10 Pinstone Street, Sheffield
1833   Wm. Hutchinson & Son, Razor Makers, (S.I.M. and
               V.I.M.), 10 Pinstone Street, Sheffield
1841   Wm. & Henry Hutchinson, (S.I.M. and V.I.M.), 76
               Norfolk Street, Sheffield
1859   Wm. Hutchinson & Co., (S.I.M. and V.I.M.), 78 Norfolk
               Street, Sheffield
1871   Wm. & Henry Hutchinson & Co., (S.I.M. and V.I.M.),
               36 Duke Street, Sheffield
1879   Wm. & Henry Hutchinson & Co., (S.I.M. and V.I.M.),
               36 Matilda Street, Sheffield
               Now see Skidmore (1922)
               *Said to be 'founded 30 Years before Simpson was born'

(1811) presumably, therefore, 1781. During the American Civil War a ship bound for the US was wrecked and found later to have large numbers of surgical instruments marked 'W. H. Hutchinson'.

Jackson

1821–2   James Jackson, (C.), 30 Bell Yard, Lincoln's Inn, London

Jamieson

Early 19th   Jamieson
century

Jarvis

Early 19th   Jarvis
century

Jessop

1774   Established. Wm. Jessop & Sons, Sheffield
1818   Wm. Jessop & Sons, Spring Street, Sheffield

Johnson

1818   Geo. Johnson & Son, Furnivall Street, Sheffield
1856   Geo. Johnson & Son, 13 Porter Street, Sheffield

Johnstone

c. 1860   Johnstone, Near Long Acre, London

Kettlebutter

1636   Registered. Richard Kettlebutter
1694   Mentioned

Kidston

1850   W. Kidston & Co., 18 Bishopsgate Street, London

Krohne & Seseman

c. 1860   Established. Krohne & Seseman by Mr Grice
1878   First Catalogue. 8 Duke Street, Manchester Square, London, and 241 Whitechapel Road, London
1926   Bought by Alfred Cox (Surgical) Ltd. Now trading in that name. See Savigny

Lane

c. 1730   James Lane, Fleet Street, London

Laundy

1783   Sam. Laundy, (S.I.M.), 12 St Thomas's Street, Borough, London

c. 1790	S. Laundy, (S.I.M.), 12 St Thomas's Street, Borough, London
1802	J. Laundy, (S.I.M.), 12 St Thomas's Street, Borough, London
1802	Laundy & Son, (S.I.M.), 12 St Thomas's Street, Borough, London
1803	J. Laundy & Son, (S.I.M.), 12 St Thomas's Street, Borough, London
1811	Joseph Laundy, (S.I.M.), 12 St Thomas's Street, Borough, London
1814	Laundy & Son, (S.I.M.), 12 St Thomas's Street, Borough, London. (No trace at this address after 1820)
1805	S. Laundy & Son, (S.I.M.), 9 St Thomas's Street, Borough, London
1813	Joseph Laundy, (S.I.M.), 9 St Thomas's Street, Borough, London
1816	Joseph Laundy & Son, (S.I.M.), 9 St Thomas's Street, Borough, London
1819	Joseph Laundy, (S.I.M.), 9 St Thomas's Street, Borough, London
	Business ceased in this name *c.* 1843. Afterwards, 1844, H. Bigg, 9 St Thomas's Street, Borough, London. See Bigg

Laurie

1826	John Laurie, 2 St Bartholomew's Close, London

Lawley

1866	Wm. Lawley, 78 Farringdon Street, London See Milliken

Leavers

1817	T. Leavers, 28 Charles Street, Hatton Garden, London

Lindsey

Mid-19th century	Lindsey

Lings

Mid-19th century	Lings

Logan

Early 19th century	Logan

Long

1817	Richard Long, (v.i.m.), 46 High Holborn, London
1826	Richard Long, 217 High Holborn, London
c. 1840	H. Long, 158 High Holborn, London. ((v.i.m.) to the Prince Regent)

Mackenzie

1835	Donald Mackenzie, (c.), 48 Nicholson Street, Edinburgh
1839	Donald Mackenzie, (c. and s.i.m.), 48 Nicholson Street, Edinburgh
1850	Donald Mackenzie, (c. and s.i.m.), 48 Nicholson Street, Edinburgh, and 58 South Bridge Street, Edinburgh
	No trace after 1876

MacLeod

1813	John MacLeod, (c. and s.i.m.), 17 College Street, Edinburgh
1818	John MacLeod, (c. and s.i.m.), 2 College Street, Edinburgh
1836	John MacLeod, (c. and s.i.m.), 3 College Street, Edinburgh
	No trace afer 1837 in this name, but then:
1838	James Simpson, 3 College Street, Edinburgh
1844	James Simpson, 80 South Bridge, Edinburgh

McLellan

1805	Wm. McLellan, St Martin-le-Grand, London
1852	Wm. McLellan, 3 Twiner Street, London

McQueen

1847	Robt. McQueen, (c. and s.i.m.), 52 Grainger Street, Newcastle
1873	Robt. McQueen, (c., s.i.m. and oc.), 52 Grainger Street, Newcastle

Machin

c. 1820	Machin & Co.

Mann

1741	Established. Mann, Jeweller, (op.), The Cross, Gloucester

Mappin

1818	J. Mappin, 3 Whitecroft, Sheffield
c. 1850	J. Mappin, Bull Street, Birmingham
	Later J. Mappin, (s.i.m.), 17 Motcomb Street, London
	Now Mappin & Webb Ltd

Marr

1878	David Marr, 27 Little Queen Street, London. (Made many of Lister's instruments)

Mather

1848	Wm. Mather, (CH. and D.), 105 Chester Road, Manchester
1858	Wm. Mather, (CH. and D.), 109–111 Chester Road, Manchester
1868	Wm. Mather, (D. and S.I.M.), 14 Bath Street, London, and 109 Chester Road, Manchester
1877–8	Wm. Mather, (D. and S.I.M.), Dyer Street, Manchester

Mathews

1846	Wm. Mathews, 10 Portugal Street, London
1851	Wm. Mathews, 8 Portugal Street, London
1865	W. Mathews & Co., 8 Portugal Street, London
1878	Mathews, London
1894	Mathews Bros, 10 New Oxford Street, London

Maw

1807	Established as Hornby & Maw, Fenchurch Street, London
1814	Hornby & Maw, Plaster Factory, Whitecross Street, London
1826	Geo. Maw & Son, Aldermanbury, London
1828	J.& S. Maw, 11 Aldersgate Street, London
1830	First Catalogue (illustrated by Cox, J. F. Lewis and Turner)
1860	S. Maw & Son
1868	Second Catalogue
1870	S. Maw, Son & Thompson
1901	S. Maw, Son & Sons

Mayer

1864	Jos. Mayer, (S.I.M.), 51 Great Portland Street, London
1869	Mayer-Meltzer, (S.I.M.), 59 Great Portland Street, London
1874	Mayer-Meltzer, (S.I.M.), 71 Great Portland Street, London
	(Factory at 83a Dean Street, London)
	After, see Down

Mayer-Meltzer

See Mayer

Mayer & Phelps

1863	Established. See Down

Meesham
1855	T. Meesham, (C.), Market Place, Salisbury
1865	Meesham & Son, (C.), Oatmeal Row, Market Place, Salisbury
1875	Henry Meesham & Co., (C.), 19 Market Place, Salisbury

Migden
Late 18th century	Migden. Instrument in Wellcome Museum, London

Millikin
1822	J. Millikin, (S.I.M.), 301 Strand, London
1826	Millikin & Wright, (C. and S.I.M.), 301 Strand, London
1846	John Millikin, 161 Strand, London
1860	Millikin & Lawley, 161 Strand, London
1860–61	Millikin (late Bigg & Millikin), 9 St Thomas's Street, London
1863	Millikin (late Bigg & Millikin), 33 St Thomas's Street, London
1865	John Millikin (late Bigg & Millikin), 12 Southwark Street, London
1875	John Millikin, 3 St Thomas's Street, London (see Bigg)

Montague
	J. H. Montague, see Savigny

Mountaine
c. 1750	Established. Richard Mountaine, (C.), High Street, Portsmouth
1798	William Mountaine, (C.), High Street, Portsmouth

Moyes
c. 1825	Moyes

Mundy
19th century	Mundy

Norie (or Norrie)
1801	W. A. Norie, (C.), 77 Hutcheson Street, Glasgow
1813	W. A. Norie, (C.), 618 Argyll Street, Glasgow
1821	W. A. Norie, (C. and S.I.M.), 5 Argyll Street, Glasgow
1824	W. A. Norie, (C. and S.I.M.), 94 Glassford Street, Glasgow
1826	W. A. Norie, (C. and S.I.M.), 12 Glassford Street, Glasgow

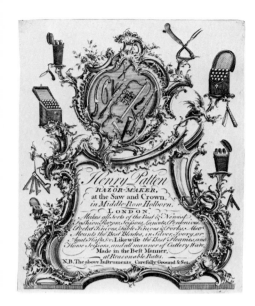

8. Trade card.
(Sir Ambrose Heal Collection, British Museum)

1833	Mrs W. A. Norie, (C. and S.I.M.), 12 Glassford Street, Glasgow
1839	L. Norie, (C. and S.I.M.), 12 Glassford Street, Glasgow
1840	Mrs Norie, (C. and S.I.M.), 12 Glassford Street, Glasgow
1841	W. A. Norie, (C. and S.I.M.), 12 Glassford Street Glasgow
	No later trace

Nowill

1700	Thomas Nowill, (C.), Sheffield
1788	Nowill & Kippax, (C.), 27 High Street, Sheffield
c. 1800	Hague & Nowill, (C.), 7 Meadow Street, Sheffield
1861	John Nowill & Sons, (C.), 115 Scotland Street, Sheffield

Oliver & Ogle

| 1818 | Oliver & Ogle, Sycamore Street, Sheffield |

Orok

| 1774 | John Orok, (C.), Head of Barrenger's Close, Edinburgh |
| | No trace after 1778 |

Page

| Late 18th century | Page (V.I.M.) |

Paget

| 1822 | Established. Richard Paget |
| 1826 | Richard Paget, 184 Piccadilly, London |

Palmer

| Mid-19th century | Palmer |

Patten

| c. 1750–80 | Henry Patten, Middle Row, Holborn, London |

Payne

| Mid-19th century | Payne, (V.I.M.) |

Peacock

1867	Aaron Peacock, (M.I.M.), 10 Clarence Street, Newcastle
1929	Peacock, (S.I.M.), Newcastle
	Still in business

Pearce

| | See Cuzner |

Pepys

John Pepys, (c.), St Helen's, Bishopsgate, London.
(d. 1760)
Wm. Hasledine Pepys (nephew), (c. and s.i.m.),
Poultry, London. (b. 1748, d. 1805)
Wm. Hasledine Pepys f.r.s. (son), (c., s.i.m. and ch.),
Poultry, London. (b. 1775, d. 1856)
Robt. Edmond Pepys (son), (s.i.m.), Poultry London.
(b. 1819, d. 1883)
Continued in business until 1863 when Poultry was
pulled down

Perkins
1826   Jonathan Perkins, 15 Portland Street, London

Philp, Whicker & Blaise
See Savigny

Plum (1)

Plum. In business for himself before entering
Weiss, c. 1830

Plum (2)
1822   R. Plum, (c.), 4 Dolphin Street, Bristol
1826   R. Plum, (c. and s.i.m.), 4 Dolphin Street, Bristol
1841   G. Plum, (c. and s.i.m.), 3 Dolphin Street, Bristol, and
                262 Strand, London
1851   G. Plum, (c. and s.i.m.), 3 Dolphin Street, Bristol, and
                448 Oxford Street, London
1880   G. Plum, (c. and s.i.m.), 6 Dolphin Street, Bristol
                Went out of business 1932

Plum (3)
1854–1939   Robt. Plum, (c. and s.i.m.), 3 St Augustine's Parade,
                Bristol

Pratt
1852   J. F. Pratt, (s.i.m. and d.i.m.), 10 Chase Street,
                Middlesex Hospital, London
1855   J. F. Pratt, (s.i.m. and d.i.m.), 420 Oxford Street,
                London

Price
Mid-19th   Price
century

Prockter
1826   Henry James Prockter, 12 Barton Street, London

Pryor

1826	Thomas Pryor, 67 Minories, London
	Now Pryor & Howard Ltd, London

Quiney

19th century	Quiney

Quixall

c. 1800	Quixall

Raeburn

1805	George Raeburn, 22 Little Queen Street, London

Rauschke

19th century	Rauschke, Leeds. (Late Mayer & Meltzer)

Read (1)

1826	John Read, (V.I.M.), Bridge Street, Newington Causeway, London. (Inventor of the stomach pump)
1829	John Read, (S.I.M.), 35 Regent Circus, London
1848	Richard Read, (S.I.M.), 35 Regent Circus, London

Read (2)

1670	James Read, Sword Cutler, Blind Quay, Dublin
1718	James Read, Granted freedom of Dublin
1735	James Read, Warden of Cutlers Guild (d. 1744)
1745	John Read, (C.)
1746	John Read, (C.), Crane Lane, Dublin. Also 4 Parliament Street (font door), Crane Lane (back door)
1776	Thomas Read, (C.), Crane Lane, Dublin. Also 4 Parliament Street (front door), Crane Lane (back door)
1800–1900	(S.I.M.)

Reay & Robinson

1829	Thomas Reay
1837	Reay & Robinson, 87 Church Street, Liverpool
1851	Partnership ended, thereafter Thos. Reay

Rein

1851–64	F. Charles Rein, Aurist and Acoustic Instrument Maker, 108 Strand, London
1865–6	Rein & Son, 108 Strand, London
1867–1917	Frederick C. Rein, 108 Strand, London

Remm

Early 19th century	Remm

329

Reynolds

c. 1840   Reynolds, Liverpool

Rhodes

1818   Rhodes & Son, Wicker, Sheffield
1868   W. C. & J. Rhodes, Castle Hill, Sheffield

Richardson (1)

1832   John Richardson, (C. and S.I.M.), 92 South Bridge,
             Edinburgh

Richardson (2)

c. 1750   John Richardson, Prescot Street, London

Richardson (3)

1800   Thos. Richardson, (C.), 31 Maguire Street, Liverpool
1805   Thos. Richardson, (C.), 121 Dale Street, Liverpool
1807   Thos. Richardson, (C.), Post Office Place, Liverpool
1810   Thos. Richardson, (C. and S.I.M.), Post Office Place,
             Liverpool
1825   Wm. & Thos. Richardson, (C.), 74 Church Street,
             Liverpool
1827   Thos. Richardson, (C. and S.I.M.), Post Office Place,
             Liverpool
1829   Thos. Richardson Jun., (C.), 72 Church Street, Liverpool
1832   Richardson Sen., (C. and S.I.M.), 72 Lord Street,
             Liverpool
1832   Richardson Jun., (C.), 70 Church Street, Liverpool
1841   Thos. Richardson Jun., (C. and S.I.M.), 70 Church
             Street, Liverpool
1862   Thos Richardson, Jun., (C. and S.I.M.), 18 South Street,
             Waterloo, Liverpool
             No trace after 1862

Risley

1826   Wm. Risley, 18 Roy Street, London

Roberts (1)

1844   Benjamin Roberts, Surgeon–Dentist, 15 North Parade,
             Bradford
1844   Benjamin Roberts, (C. and T.M.), 6 Darley Street,
             Bradford
1849   Benjamin Roberts, (C. and T.M.), 5 Darley Street,
             Bradford
1849   Benjamin Roberts, Dentist, 42 Darley street, Bradford
1861   Benjamin Roberts, Surgeon–Dentist, 8 Little Horton
             Lane, Bradford

Roberts (2)

c. 1800 Moses Roberts, New Street, Covent Garden, London

Robinson

1826 John Robinson, 19 Kingsland Road, London

Rodgers

c. 1820 J. Rodgers & Sons, London

Rooke

c. 1800 Rooke

Rudford

c. 1850 Rudford, Manchester

Ryley

1826 J. W. Ryley, 4 Duke Street, London

Salt

1773 Wm. Salt, (c.), Cock Street, Wolverhampton

1781 Wm. Salt, (c. and Toy Dealer), Cock Street, Wolverhampton

1822 Richard Salt, (c.), 4 Dale End, Wolverhampton

1828 Sarah Salt, (c.), 4 Dale End, Wolverhampton

1830 Sarah Salt & Son, 4 Dale End, Wolverhampton
Thomas P. Salt
Salt & Son
Edward W. Salt
Salt & Son Ltd, Orthopaedic Appliances

Saunders

19th century Saunders

Savigny

c. 1720 Paul Savigny, succeeded to business of late Widow How, (c.), Halbert and Crown, St Martin's Churchyard, London

1726 John Tessier Savigny, (s.i.m. and Razor Maker), Acorn and Crown, Gerrard Street, London

1784 John Henry Savigny, (s.i.m.), 129 Pall Mall, London

1794 John Henry Savigny, (s.i.m.), 28 King Street, London

1798 First Catalogue issued

1810 Savigny, Everill & Mason, (s.i.m.), 67 St James's Street, ('removed from Pall Mall and King Street') London

c. 1850 Everill, Philp & Whicker (late Savigny & Co.)

1855 Philp, Whicker & Blaise, 67 St James's Street, London

1856 Whicker & Blaise, (s.i.m.), 67 St James's Street, London

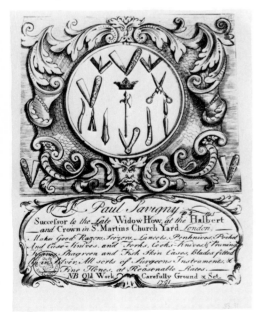

9.   Trade card.
(Sir Ambrose Heal Collection, British Museum)

ANTIQUE MEDICAL INSTRUMENTS

1868	Louis Blaise & Co. (late Savigny & Co.)
1872	Louis Blaise & Co., 67 St James's Street, and 276 Westminster Bridge, London
1885	C. Wright & Co. (from Louis Blaise & Co. late Savigny & Co.), 108 New Bond Street, London
1896	Alfred Cox (late partner of C. Wright & Co. from Louis Blaise, late Savigny & Co.), 108 New Bond Street, London
1896	J. H. Montague (late partner of C. Wright, etc.), 101 New Bond Street, London

Savory & Moore

1794	Thos. Paytherus, (CH. and D.), 136 New Bond Street, London
1806	Paytherus, Savory & Moore, (CH. and D.), 136 New Bond Street, London
1811	Savory, Moore & Dennys, (CH. and D.), 136 New Bond Street, London
1814	Savory, Moore & Co., (CH. and D.), 136 New Bond Street, London
1818	Savory Moore & Davidson, (CH. and D.), 136 New Bond Street, London
1826	Savory Moore & Co., (CH. and D.), 136 New Bond Street, London
c. 1840	Savory Moore & Co., (CH. and D.), 143 New Bond Street, London
1845	Savory & Moore, (CH. and D.), 143 New Bond Street, London
1854	John Savory & Sons, (CH. and D.), 143 New Bond Street, London
1861	Savory & Moore, (CH. and D.), 143 New Bond Street, London
1902	Savory & Moore Ltd, (CH. and D.), 143 New Bond Street, London
	Now amalgamated with McCarthy's and John Bell & Croyden, but still under name of Savory & Moore Ltd

Sawyer

19th century	Sawyer

Schmalcalder

1808–44	Schmalcalder, (OP., Philosophical and M.I.M.), 80 Strand, London

Schmidt & Robinson

19th century	Schmidt & Robinson, 267 Strand, London

332

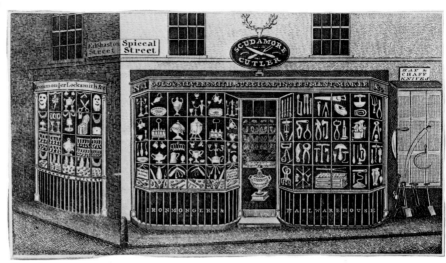

10.   Trade card.
(Sir Ambrose Heal Collection, British Museum)

Scudamore

c. 1700   Scudamore, Spiceal Street, London

Settle

19th century   Settle

Sharp

1851   James Sharp, (S.I.M.), 26 Market Street, Newcastle
              No trace after 1866

Sheldrake

1790   Timothy Sheldrake, (T.M.), 483 Strand, London
1796   Timothy Sheldrake, 50 Strand, London
1805 {   Timothy Sheldrake, 50 Strand, London
              William Sheldrake, 483 Strand, London
1820 {   Timothy Sheldrake, 10 Adams Street, London
              William Sheldrake, 483 Strand, London
1823   William Sheldrake, 483 Strand, London
              See Bigg

Shrimpton & Fletcher

1810   Established. Shrimpton & Fletcher. Premier Works,
              Redditch. Manufacturers of suture needles. Later made
              needles for Lister

Simpson (1)

1788   Robt. Simpson, (C.), 9 Clerkenwell Green, London
1803   Simpson & Smith, (C.), 16 Strand, London
1822   Simpson & Smith, (C.), 55 Strand, London
1863   Henry Simpson, 55 Strand, London

333

Simpson (2)

See MacLeod

Skidmore

1851   Wm. Skidmore, (S.I.M.), Awarded prize at Great Exhibition, 1851

1898   Wm. Skidmore & Co. Ltd, Sheffield

See Hutchinson

Smale

19th century   Smale

Smith (1)

1826   Benjamin Smith, 68 Cromer Street, London

Smith (2)

1803   Wm. Smith, 4 St Saviour's Churchyard, London

1831   Wm. Smith, (S.I.M.), New Street, London

1847   See Durroch

Snidall

1818   James Snidall, 52 Pond Street, Sheffield

Spurr

1818   Peter Spurr, Arundel Street, Sheffield

Staniforth

1864   G. H. Staniforth, (C.), 10 Church Street, Cardiff

1885   G. H. Staniforth, (C.), 5 Church Street, Cardiff

1889   G. H. Staniforth, (C.), 6 Church Street, Cardiff

Still in business at Staling Road, Penarth

Stanton

1738   Edward Stanton, Lombard Street, London

No trace after 1744

Stevens

c. 1830   J. Stevens, (S.I.M.), 159 Gower Street, London

Later Stevens & Pratt

Stevenson

1822   John Stevenson, (C.)

Still (1)

1799   Alexander Still, (C. and S.I.M.), Infirmary Street, Edinburgh

1835   Alexander Still, (C. and S.I.M.), 3 Infirmary Street, Edinburgh

Still (2)

1817   Charles Still, (T.M.), 9 Leicester Street, London

Stirling (1)

1828   Robt. Stirling (C.), 19 New Vennal, Glasgow
1834   Robt. Stirling, (C. and S.I.M.), 19 New Vennal, Glasgow
1836   Robt. Stirling, (C. and S.I.M.), 12 London Street, Glasgow
1837   Mrs Robt. Stirling, (C. and S.I.M.), 12 London Street, Glasgow
1839   Robt. Stirling & Co., (C. and S.I.M.), 12 London Street, Glasgow
1854   Robt. Stirling & Co., (C. and S.I.M.), 3 Saltmarket, Glasgow
              No trace after 1858

Stirling (2)

1851   James Stirling (C. and S.I.M.), 88 Gallowgate, Glasgow
              No trace after 1860

Stirling (3)

1856   Wm. Stirling, (C. and S.I.M.), 44 Trougate, Glasgow
1858   Wm. Stirling, (C.), 44 Trougate, Glasgow
              No trace after 1892

Stodart

1787   J. Stodart, (C. and S.I.M.), 401 Strand, London
1791   James Stodart, (C.), 401 Strand, London
1805   J. Stodart, (C.), 401 Strand, London
1826   David & Samuel Stodart, 401 Strand, London
1839   David Stodart, 401 Strand, London

Strange

1815   Wm Strange, (S.I.M.), 17 Cloisters Street, St Bartholomew's Hospital, London
1820   Wm Strange, (S.I.M.), 44 West Smithfield, London
1826   Taken over by Ferguson

Stubbs

c. 1860   Stubbs, (D.I.M.), Birmingham

Swain

c. 1735   Thomas Swain, Bedford Street, London. (Made Chapman's obstetrical forceps)

Tax

1705   Thomas Tax, (S.I.M.), Lombard Street, London

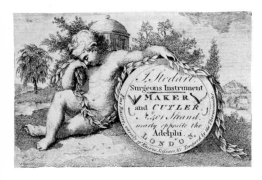

11.   Trade card.
(Sir Ambrose Heal Collection, British Museum)

335

Tempest

19th century   Tempest, (V.I.M.)

Thistlewaite

c. 1850   S. Thistlewaite & Co.

Thompson

1817   James Thompson, 42 Great Windmill Street, London

1826   James Thompson, 38 Great Windmill Street, London

1843   J. Thompson, 38 Great Windmill Street, London
        See Maw

Thompson & O'Neill

1833   S. Thompson, 6 Henry Street, Dublin

c. 1860   Thompson and O'Neill

Tully

1806   Geo. Tully (C.), 24 Maryport Street, Bristol

1808   Philip Tully, (C.), Somerset Street, Bristol

1813   George Tully, (C.), 24 Maryport Street, Bristol

1813   Philip Tully, (C.), Gay Street, Bristol

1816   George Tully, (C.), 4 Dolphin Street, Bristol

1818   Philip Tully, (C.), 17 St James Place, Bristol
        No trace of George Tully after 1821
        No trace of Philip Tully after 1828

Tymperon

c. 1735–70   Edward Tymperon, Russell Court, Drury Lane, London

Underwood

c. 1820   H. Underwood (late Charlwood), 56 Haymarket and
        Russell Court, Drury Lane, London
        See Yeeling Charlwood

Wade, Wingfield & Rowbotham

19th century   Wade, Wingfield & Rowbotham, (V.I.M.)

Walker

Early 19th   F. Walker, 16 Moorgate Street, London
century

Walsh

1839   Jonathan Walsh, 12 St Bartholomew's Street, London

Warren

1826   James Warren, 20 & 21 Chenies Mews, Bedford Square,
        London

1887   Warren & Rudgley

Weale

c. 1740   Richard Weale, Cannon Street, London

Weedon

1789   Thomas Weedon, (C.), 18 Little Eastcheap, London

c. 1830   Weedon, (C.), 41 Hart Street, Bloomsbury, London
(Pieces known until c. 1856)

Weiss

1787   Established. John Weiss, (C.), 42 Strand, London

1811   John Weiss, (C.), 33 Strand, London

1823   John Weiss, (C.), 62 Strand, London

1830   John Weiss & Son, 62 Strand, London

1831   First Catalogue

1843   Second Catalogue, 62 Strand and King William Street,
London

1863   Third Catalogue

1883   John Weiss & Sons, 62 Strand & 287 Oxford Street,
London

1889   J. Weiss & Sons, 287 Oxford Street, London

1894   J. Weiss & Sons, 287 Oxford Street (formerly 62 Strand)
Now 17 Wigmore Street, London

Well

c. 1800   B. B. Well, 431 Strand, London

Wenborn

19th century   Wenborn, (C. and S.I.M.), 30a Cornmarket, Oxford
See Bayne

Westbrook

1817   H. & J. Westbrook, (S.I.M.), 92 Broad Street, London

Westbury

1852   Established. Robt. Westbury, (S.I.M. and T.M.), 15 Old
Millgate, Manchester

1861   Robt. Westbury, (T.M.), 26 Old Millgate, Manchester

1865   Robt. Westbury, (S.I.M. and T.M.), 26 Old Millgate,
Manchester
In business until 1920

Whitford

1798   John Whitford, (C.), 2 Little Cloisters, Smithfield,
London

1814   John Whitford, (S.I.M.), 47 West Smithfield, London

ANTIQUE MEDICAL INSTRUMENTS

| 1822 | Elizabeth Whitford, (s.i.m.), 47 West Smithfield, London |
| 1823 | Whitford & Co., (c.), 2 Porter Street, London
No trace thereafter |

Whyte

| Mid-19th century | John Whyte, 58 Upper Sackville Street, Dublin |

Wight

| c. 1790 | Wight |

Wood (1)

1799	Joseph Wood, Spurriergate, York
1831	Joseph Wood & Son
1845	Joseph Wood
1850	Invented York razor
1871	Joseph Wood & Co.
1935	Closed business

Wood (2)

1833	J. & W. Wood, (c. and s.i.m.), 109 Piccadilly, Manchester
1836	J. & W. Wood, (c. and s.i.m.), 72 King Street House, and Grove Street, Manchester
1840	J. & W. Wood, (c. and s.i.m.), 72 King Street House and 4 Ardwick Place, Manchester
1845	J. & W. Wood, (c. and s.i.m.), 74 King Street, and 79 Market Street, Manchester
1850	J. & W. Wood, (c. and s.i.m.), 74 King Street, Manchester
1861	J. & W. Wood, (c., s.i.m. and t.m.), 74 King Street, Manchester
1881	William Wood & Son In business until 1929

Wood (3)

| 1868 | Wm. Wood, (s.i.m.), 95 Lord Street, Liverpool
No trace after 1875 |

Wood (4)

1864	John Wood, (s.i.m.), 81 Church Street, Liverpool
1878	John Wood, (s.i.m., op. and t.m.), 81 Church Street, Liverpool
1885	John Wood, (c. and s.i.m.), 81 Church Street, Liverpool No trace after 1916

Woolhouse
1818   John Woolhouse, 27 Smith Street, Sheffield
    Sam. Woolhouse, Orchard Street, Sheffield

Wotherspoon
1816   Geo. Wotherspoon, (C.), 17 New Vennal, Glasgow
1824   Geo. Wotherspoon, (C.), 7 Blackfriars Street, Glasgow
1825   Geo. Wotherspoon, (C.), 17 New Vennal, Glasgow
    No trace after 1828

Wright (1)
    See Savigny

Wright (2)
1794   John Wright, (C.), 7 Ships Alley, London
1809   Wm. Wright, (C. and T.M.), 7 Ships Alley, London
1825   Henry Wright, (S.I.M.), 13 London Road, Southwark, London
1832   Henry Wright, (S.I.M.), 32 London Road, London
1843   Henry Wright, (S.I.M.), 18 London Road, London
    No trace after 1867

Wright (3)
1782   William Wright, (C.), Morrison's Close, Edinburgh
1784   Wm. Wright, (C.), Blackfriars Wynd, Edinburgh
1795   Wm. Wright, (C.), Blairs Street, Edinburgh
1809   Wright & Son, (C.), Horse Wynd, Edinburgh
1815   Wright & Son, (C.), 31 West College Street, Edinburgh
1820   William Wright, (C.), 26 Potterrow, Edinburgh
1827   William Wright, (C.), 18 Middletons Entry, Edinburgh

European instrument makers

Anton   *Germany*

Becker   *Holland*
Beligne   *France*
Benois   *France*
Bernard   *France*
Birck   *Germany*
Blanc   *France*
Böhme   *Germany*
Boze   *Russia*

Canali   *Italy*
Carter   *France*
Chardin   *France*
Charrière   *France*
Clasen   *Belgium*
Collin   *France*
Conrad   *Strasbourg*
Creuzand   *France*

Delamotte   *France*
Denis   *Belgium*
Detert   *Germany*
Dewitt & Herg   *Germany*

Elser   *France*
Eppendorf   *Germany*
Esterlus   *Germany*

Faure   *Holland*
Fischer   *Hungary*

Galante   *France*
Gasselin   *France*
Gauet   *France*
Gauvin   *France*
Gentile   *France*
Gerber   *Russia*

Germain   *France*
Gilbert   *France*
Glitschka   *Belgium*
Goldschmidt   *Germany*
Graiff   *France*
Grangeret   *France*
Gribel   *Germany*
Grotewahl   *Germany*
Gueride   *France*
Guérin   *France*
Gugenbutter   *Germany*

Hajek   *Eastern European*
Hammer & Vorsak   *Germany*
Hansen   *Denmark*
Haran   *France*
Haufland   *Germany*
Hébert   *France*
Henry   *France*
Hersan   *France*
Hertel   *Germany*
Herzhause   *Germany*
Heynemann   *Germany*
Hunzinger   *Germany*

Jetter & Scheering   *Germany*
Jolivet   *France*
Joyant   *France*
Jung   *Germany*

Kraus   *Germany*

Lassère   *France*
Laurent   *France*
Lautenslager & Lautenslager   *Germany*
Leiter   *Austria*
Lemaître   *France*
Lépine   *France*

Leplanquais *France*
Lesueur *France*
Lichtenberger *Strasbourg*
Lipowsky-Fischer *Germany*
Loewenstein *Germany*
Lollini *Italy*
Lollins Frat *Italy*
Lowe *Germany*
Luer *France*
Lutter *Germany*

Magnet *Germany*
Malliard *Austria*
Mariand *France*
Mathieu *France*
Maug *Germany*
Menier *France*
Mette *Sweden*
Meyer-Ketsting *Germany*
Michault *France*
Moeke *Germany*
Molinari *Spain*
Morette *France*
Mossinger *Holland*
Müller *Germany*

Nachet *France*
Neupart *Germany*
Nyrop *Denmark*

Odelga *Germany*
Odoux *France*

Perret *France*
Personne *France*
Pohl *Holland*

Raillot *France*
Ratery *France*
Reiner *Austria*
Rizzoli *Italy*
Robert & Collin *France*
Rohrbeck *Germany*

Romelin *France*

Sabaj, Neck *Austria*
Samson *France*
Schaedel *Germany*
Schaffer *Switzerland*
Schaube *Russia*
Schmid-Luniger *Germany*
Schmidt *Germany*
Schutz, A. *Germany*
Serendal *France*
Simal *France*
Sirhenry *France*
Siries *Italy*
Songy *France*
Soubrillard *France*
Sousa-Ferreira, de *Portugal*
Soyez *France*
Stille *Sweden*
Suderie *France*

Varnout & Galante *France*
Verdin *France*

Walter-Biondetti *Switzerland*
Weber *France*
Windler *Germany*
Wulfing-Luer *France*
Wunsche *Germany*

341

North American instrument makers

Aloe *St Louis*

Boehun *Rochester*
Boekal *Philadelphia*
(Bonnerave *Argentina*)

Caswell Hasard & Co. *New York*
Chevalier *New York*
Codman-Shurtleff *Boston*
Crocker *Cincinnati*

Davis & Lawrence *New York and Montreal*

Ford *New York*
Frye *Portland*

Gardiner *Minneapolis*
de Garmo *New York*
Gemeric *Philadelphia*

Haenstein *New York*
Hernstein *New York*

Knauth Bros *New York*
Kolbe *Philadelphia*
Krug Sheerer Corp. *New York*
Kurmerle, J. F. *Philadelphia*
Kurn *Philadelphia*

Lane *New York*
Leach & Green *Boston*
Lentz *Philadelphia*
Leslie *St Louis*
Lufkin Rule Co. *? Michigan*

Otto *New York*
Otto & Reynders *New York*

Penfield *Philadelphia*
Pratt *Boston*

Queen *Philadelphia*

Reynders *New York*
Rochester Surgical
Appliances Co. *Rochester*

Sharp & Smith *Chicago*
Shepard & Dudley *New York*
Sherrard-Duffy *New York*
Snow *Syracuse*
Snowden *Philadelphia*

Taylor *New York*
Tiemann *New York*
Traux Greene & Co. *Chicago*

White *Philadelphia*

Yarnall *Philadelphia*

Bibliography

Henry d'Allemagne
  Decorative Antique Ironwork, Dover Publications, London, 1968
Theodore Beck
  The Cutting Edge, Lund Humphries, London, 1974
W. J. Bishop
  Early History of Surgery, Oldbourne, London, 1960
Howard L. Blackmore
  Hunting Weapons, Barrie & Jenkins, London, 1971
Edward de Bono
  Eureka, a History of Inventions, Thames & Hudson, London, 1974
Harold Burrows & Ronald Raven
  Surgical Instruments and Appliances, Faber, London, 1932
Ritchie Calder
  Medicine and Man, Geo. Allen & Unwin, London, 1958
Peggy Chambers
  Great Company, Bodley Head, London, 1954
Michael Clayton
  Collector's Dictionary of Silver and Gold, Country Life, London, 1971
Sir Frank Colyer
  Old Instruments Used for Extracting Teeth, Staples Press, London, 1952
Richard Corson
  Fashions in Eye-Glasses, Peter Owen, London, 1967
Very Rev. Rowland Davies
  Journal 1688–1690, Camden Society, London, 1857
Eric Delieb
  Silver Boxes, Herbert Jenkins, London, 1968
Eric Delieb
  'Medical Silver', article in *Apollo*, June 1961, London
Harvey Graham
  Surgeons All, Rich and Cowan, London, 1939
Arnold Haskell
  Infantilia, Dennis Dobson, London, 1971
R. W. Johnstone
  William Smellie, E. & S. Livingstone, Edinburgh, 1952
Christopher Lloyd and Jack Coulter
  Medicine and the Navy, 1200–1900, E. & S. Livingstone, Edinburgh, 1963

Ralph H. Major
   A History of Medicine, Blackwell, London, 1954
Leslie G. Matthews
   Antiques of the Pharmacy, G. Bell & Sons, London, 1971
Francis Mitchell-Heggs
   The Instruments of Surgery, Heinemann, London, 1963
Samuel Mihles
   Elements of Surgery, 1764
Vilhelm Moller-Christensen
   History of the Forceps, Oxford University Press, London, 1958
Phyllis Mortimer
   Only When it Hurts, Wolfe Publishing, London, 1974
Leonard J. T. Murphy
   The History of Urology, Charles C. Thomas, Springfield, Ill., 1972
Betty MacQuitty
   Battle for Oblivion, Harrap, London, 1969
A. M. Newth
   Britain and the World 1789–1901, Penguin, London, 1968
A. J. Patrick
   The Making of a Nation, 1603–1789, Penguin, London, 1967
N. M. Penzer
   The Book of the Wine Label, White Lion, London, 1947
Samuel Pepys
   Diary, 1659–1669
E. D. Phillips
   Greek Medicine, Thames & Hudson, London, 1973
Peter Quennell (Ed.)
   Four volumes of *The Memoirs of William Hickey*, Hutchinson, London, 1960
Walter Radcliffe
   The Secret Instrument, Heinemann, London, 1947
Sarah R. Riedman
   Masters of the Scalpel, Bailey Bros & Swinfen, Folkestone, 1973
John Scarborough
   Roman Medicine, Thames & Hudson, London, 1973
Maurice Smith
   A Short History of Dentistry, Allan Wingate, London, 1958
C. J. S. Thompson
   History and Evolution of Surgical Instruments, Schumann, New York, 1942
E. Ashworth Underwood
   Boerhaave's Men at Leyden, Edinburgh University Press, Edinburgh, 1977

E. T. Withington
  Medical History From Earliest Times, Holland Press, London, 1894
Bennet Woodcroft
  Index of Patentees of Inventions 1617–1852, Evelyn, Adams & Mackay, London, 1969

Further Reading*

John of Gaddesden   *Rosa Medicinae, c.* 1350
John of Arderne   *de Arte Medicinae, c.* 1370
John of Mirfield   *Breviarium Bartomolomaei* (Ms.)
John Scultetus of Ulm   *The Chirurgeon's Store-House*, translated English 1674
Benjamin Bell   *System of Surgery*, 1782
John Moyle   *The Sea-Chirurgeon*, 1693
Guy de Chauliac   *Chirurgia Magna*, 1478
Lorenz Heister   *General System of Surgery*, 1753
John Woodall   *The Surgeon's Mate*, 1617
John Markham   *Masterpiece*, 1668
Thomas Moresteyde   *Fair Book of Surgery, c.* 1440
William Northcote   *Marine Practise of Surgery*, 1770
Robert Liston   *Practical Surgery*, 1846
Samuel Sharp   *A Treatise on the Operations of Surgery*, 1739
Walter Ryff   *Major Surgery*, 1545

*These books are owned by some museum libraries for inspection.

345

Simple glossary of terms

Auriscope   Instrument for viewing the ear

Aneurysm   Abnormal dilation of the artery

Cautery, cauterising iron   Instrument used to burn tissue to arrest bleeding

Craniotomy   The act of breaking down the head of the foetus

Cannula   Tube or pipe

Caul   Membrane covering the head of some infants at birth

Cystoscope   Instrument used to examine cysts of the bladder

Clyster   An enema

Curette   Small-bladed knife used to remove growths and extraneous tissue

Calculus   A stone-like concretion which forms in the bladder and other parts of the body

Epistaxis   Bleeding from the nose

Epilation   Removal of hair

Fleam   Single-bladed instrument for venesection

Fenestration   A window-like opening

Gutta-percha   A rubber-like substance, but harder and not extensible

Hydrocephalus   An accumulation of serous fluid within the cranial cavity; dropsy of the brain

Hydrocele   Dropsy of the scrotum. Often suffered by climbing chimney-sweep boys in later life

Laryngotomy   The operation of cutting into the larynx

Laryngoscope   A mirror for examining the larynx

Metacarpal   Bones of the hand between wrist and fingers

Metatarsal   Bones of the foot between ankle and toes

Optometer   Instrument for testing and measuring sight

Ophthalmoscope   Instrument for examining the interior of the eye

Odontology   Science of the teeth

Phleam or Phleme   see Fleam

Polyp   A general term for a tumour arising from a mucous or serous surface

Pontil or Punty-Mark   Mark made by withdrawal of the rod used in holding and manipulating glassware during manufacture

Phrenology   A would-be science of mental faculties supposed to be located in various parts of the skull, and investigable by feeling the bumps on the outside of the head

Pleximeter   A small plate to receive the tap in examination by percussion

Scarificator   An instrument to make a number of lacerations on the surface of the skin

Schnappers   see Fleam

Styptic   An astringent for checking bleeding

Speculum   An instrument for viewing cavities of the body through its orifices

Stricture   The narrowing of a bodily passage

Trepan   To remove a piece of skull from the cranium

Tracheotomy   The surgical formation of an opening into the trachea

Urethroscope   Instrument for viewing the urethra

Venesection   Cutting into a vein for purposes of bleeding

Chronological chart

International contemporaries among the principal
surgeons mentioned in this book

Ancient World

2100 B.C. Hammurabi
1100 B.C. Archimathaeus
460 B.C. Hippocrates
25 B.C. Aulus Cornelius Celsus
130 A.D. Claude Galen

The countries listed are intended to include the geographical areas of those countries at the present time

Date of Birth	Gt. Britain	France	Germany	Italy	Spain	Switzerland	Austria	Holland	Belgium	Strasbourg	United States
570					Isadore of Seville						
936					Albucasis						
1114				Gerard of Cremona							
1170				Roger of Salerno							
1280	John of Gaddesden			Lanfranc c. 1280							
1298		Guy de Chauliac									
1307	John of Arderne										
1350	John Wryghtson										
1393	John of Mirfield										
1401	Thos. Morsteyde										
1477			Hans von Gersdorff	Bartolomeo Senarega c. 1477							
1500				Andrea della Croce		Jacob Rueff				Walter Ryff	
1507	Thos. Gale										
1509		Ambroise Paré									
1515				Alphonso Ferri							
1540	William Clowes				Francisco Martinez c. 1540						
1550		Jacques Guillemeau									
1556	John Woodall										
1560						Fabricius					
1572	Peter Chamberlen	Turquet de									

Date of Birth	Gt. Britain	France	Germany	Italy	Spain	Switzerland	Austria	Holland	Belgium	Strasbourg	United States
1799	Ferguson James Syme										
circa 1801	Thomas Machell	Armand Trousseau									
1808	William Ferguson										
1810		Louis Desmarres				G. G. Valentin					
1811	James Simpson										
1812	J. H. Bennett										
1813											J. Marion Sims
1816	Richard Quinn										
1819	Richard Butcher	A. Barde lieu									
1821			H. Helmholtz								
1827	Joseph Lister										
1830		Jules Pean									
1832											H. J. Knapp
1834			Herman Snellen								
1836	Clifford Allbutt John Brunton										
1838		Columbat	Karl Hueter								
1840											
1845	Robert Lowson Tait	Vidal de Cassis									G. P. Caniman c. 1845
circa 1854		Gely									
1857	Victor Horsley										

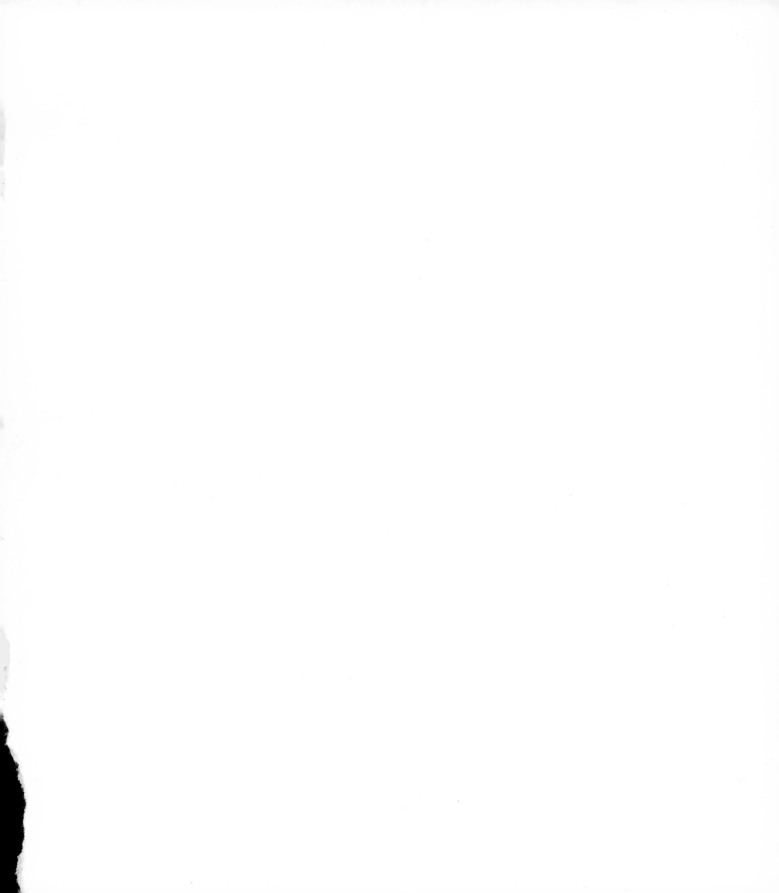

1595 — John Scultetus

1614 — James Cooke — François Moriceau

1622 — Richard Wiseman

1625 — Jean-Baptiste Denys

1641 — Covillard — Cornelius Solingen

1646 — James Yonge — François Tolet

1648 — Jules Clement

1650 — John Palfyn

1651 — Frère Jacques

1660 — John Moyle

1664 — Hugh Chamberlen

1668 — Herman Boerhaave

1669 — William Cockburn

1674 — Jean-Louis Petit

1679 — Dominique Anel

1683 — Lorenz Heister

1685 — John Atkins

1688 — William Cheselden — John Freke — Rene-Jacques Garengeot

1697 — William Smellie

1700 — Samuel Sharp — Claude-Nicholas le Cat

1702 — George Martine

1703 — Andrée Levret — Frere Côme

1710 — John Burton

1712 — Johann Schmucker

1715 — Percivall Pott — Samuel Mihles — Arnold van der Laar *c.* 1715

1718 — William Hunter — William Northcote — John Hunter — Baron de Wenzel — Juan Alexand Brambilla

Date of Birth	Gt. Britain	France	Germany	Italy	Spain	Switzerland	Austria	Holland	Belgium	Strasbourg	United States
1736	William Hey										
1744		P. J. Desault									
1749	Benjamin Bell / Edward Jenner										
1750		Charles Vial de St. Bel									
1756	James Currie	Antoine Dubois									
1759				Paolo Assalini							
1760	John Read										
1763							Franz Rudtorffer			Charles Laforgue	
1766	William Wollaston	Dominique Larrey									John Greenwood
1768	Astley Cooper										
1771		Pierre Bretonneau									
1772			Karl Himly								
1776			C. M. J. Langenbecke								
1781		René Laennec	Franz Reisniger								
1783	Henry Southey										
1787			Carl von Graefe								
1788	Thomas Smith / Neil Arnott										
1790			Johann Fricke								
1792			J. F. Dieff- enbach								
1794	William Dick										
1795	Thomas Wakley										
1796		Jean Amussat									
1797	Robert Liston										
		Leroy									

Index